# Cancer Etiology, Diagnosis and Treatments

nova
Medicine & Health
New York

# Cancer Etiology, Diagnosis and Treatments

**Burkitt Lymphoma: Diagnosis, Risk Factors and Treatment**
Douglas V. Berthelot (Editor)
ISBN: 978-1-68507-071-7 (Hardcover)
ISBN: 978-1-68507-083-0 (eBook)

**Bridging the Gap: In This Era of Cancer Immunotherapy**
Shiu Y. Tsao (Editor)
ISBN: 978-1-53619-900-0 (Hardcover)
ISBN: 978-1-53619-983-3 (eBook)

**Mesothelioma: Risk Factors, Treatment and Prognosis**
Albert K. Martin (Editor)
ISBN: 978-1-68507-075-5 (Softcover)
ISBN: 978-1-68507-134-9 (eBook)

**Combination Therapies and their Effectiveness in Breast Cancer Treatment**
Manzoor Ahmad Mir (Editor)
ISBN: 978-1-68507-195-0 (Hardcover)
ISBN: 978-1-68507-247-6 (eBook)

**Cancer and Pregnancy: A Practical Approach for the Gynecologist**
Elisa Picardo, Marco Mitidieri and Saverio Danese (Editors)
ISBN: 978-1-53619-844-7 (Hardcover)
ISBN: 978-1-53619-928-4 (eBook)

**Oral Squamous Cell Carcinoma: From Diagnosis to Treatment**
Matthew Rabin (Editor)
ISBN: 978-1-53619-895-9 (Hardcover)
ISBN: 978-1-53619-907-9 (eBook)

More information about this series can be found at
https://novapublishers.com/product-category/series/cancer-etiology-diagnosis-and-treatments/

**Katrin Sak**

# How Plant Flavonoids Affect the Outcome of Hormonal and Biological Cancer Therapies

## A Handbook for Doctors and Patients

nova
Medicine & Health
New York

DOI: https://doi.org/10.52305/HATJ3532



## Library of Congress Cataloging-in-Publication Data

ISBN: 978-1-68507-608-5

*Published by Nova Science Publishers, Inc. † New York*

*To the life.*
*To the amazing possibility to exist and experience.*

# Contents

# Preface

Cancer is a steadily increasing public health concern and severe socio-economic burden all over the world. Based on the current statistics of the WHO, almost 10 million people lost their lives due to malignant disorders in 2020, implying that one in every six deaths is due to cancer. In parallel, the global population of cancer survivors is also growing, propelled by advances in early detection, diagnosis and treatment methods, but also by demographic aging. More and more cancer patients today decide to use dietary supplements and herbal products in order to enhance their overall health, delay the progression of disease, augment the outcome of conventional therapies, mitigate diagnosis-related depression and anxiety, and alleviate drug-associated side effects, doing it mostly unbeknownst to their health care providers. Such over-the-counter supplements usually contain diverse flavonoids, such as catechins from green tea extracts, isoflavones from soy products, flavanones from citrus oils or silibinin from milk thistle seeds, just to name a few. A variety of flavonoid-rich products are often consumed also concurrently with standard cancer therapies, without anticipating and understanding the potential interactions between plant-derived bioactive flavonoids and clinically used anticancer drugs. In this book, diverse effects of these polyphenolic phytochemicals on hormonal and targeted biological cancer therapies are covered, being a reasoned follow-up to the two previous books *Plant Flavonoids Affect Cancer Chemotherapeutic Efficacy: A Handbook for Doctors and Patients* (2019) and *Dietary Flavonoids Interfere with Cancer Radiotherapy* (2019). Besides naturally occurring flavonoids, impact of flavonoid-rich plant extracts as well as semisynthetic derivatives on anticancer activities of co-administered hormonal and targeted drugs is thoroughly discussed, providing also some indicative recommendations to patients undergoing hormonal cancer therapies or targeted biological cancer therapies.

Unlike cytotoxic chemotherapeutics, the current knowledge about combinational effects between flavonoids and hormonal/biological drugs in the fight against different types of human malignancies is much less, basing mostly on preclinical findings. Such interactions are principally of three types: modulation of pharmacokinetic profile and bioavailability of the drug, augmentation of drug-induced anticancer activities through attacking different cell survival pathways and overcoming drug resistance, and protecting normal tissues from drug-elicited oxidative damage by flavonoids. In doing so, the co-effects are substantially dependent on doses and dosage regimens, molecular characteristics of malignant neoplasms, but above all on the structure of specific drugs and flavonoids. Ideally, synergistic interactions could allow to use lower drug doses for achieving anticancer responses, with lesser extent of adverse reactions. However, besides potentiation of therapeutic efficacy, in certain situations, concomitant use of drugs and flavonoids might lead also to antagonistic effects, ultimately reducing anticancer activities and stimulating malignant progression. The latter phenomenon is probably most critical, as these combinations never enter clinical trials for verification, but can still exist in patients and affect clinical outcomes.

Collectively, the data presented in this book clearly demonstrate that interactions between hormonal/biological cancer therapies and plant-derived flavonoids exist and can be strong enough to potentially impact the therapeutic outcomes. Therefore, we cannot consider flavonoids as placebos and ignore or underestimate their co-effects with hormonal and targeted cancer drugs, if we want to get the best clinical outcomes. Awareness of these interactions is important for making informed decisions by patients and their relatives, but also for counseling patients by physicians and nutritional oncologists, being probably especially valuable in the case of hormonal cancer drugs that are often prescribed for even up to ten years. On the other hand, taking account of rapid introduction of novel targeted drugs in both oncological and hematological practices over the past few decades, much more information is needed about potential interactions of these drugs with structurally diverse natural flavonoids, encouraging intensification of preclinical research. Besides identifying the most promising combinations for entering clinical trials and hopefully clinical use in the future, knowing co-effects between hormonal/targeted cancer drugs and plant-derived flavonoids might be useful also for avoiding consumption of contraindicated dietary supplements and herbal products by patients while receiving therapies. Moreover, unraveling molecular mechanisms under such interactions further confirms that successful fight against multifaceted and heterogenous machinery of cancer needs complex and combinational therapeutic strategies, blocking concurrently numerous signaling pathways important for survival of malignant cells. Eventually, it would be possible to make the current cancer treatment even more personalized, providing targeted nutritional recommendations for individual patients undergoing hormonal or biological cancer therapies, contributing to increase in clinical outcomes and improving quality of life of patients with different malignancies.

# About the Author

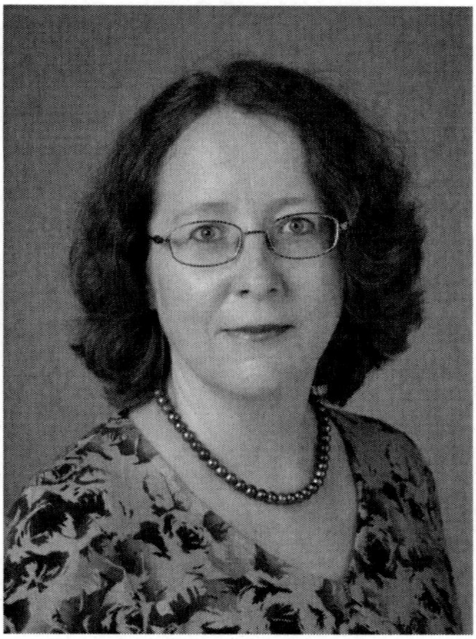

The author of this book, Dr. Katrin Sak, was born in Viljandi, Estonia, in 1975, as the daughter of schoolteachers. After studies in the University of Tartu, Estonia, she received a Bachelor`s degree (BSc) in Chemistry in 1996 and a Master's degree (MSc) in Bioorganic Chemistry in 1997. In 2001, she graduated with a Doctorate degree (PhD) in Bioorganic Chemistry. From 2001-2004, Dr. Sak did postdoctoral research at the Free University of Brussels, Belgium and in 2012, she acquired a diploma in cancer nutrition in the Health Schools Australia.

The major research topics of Dr. Sak involve different anticancer actions of plant-derived flavonoids in diverse malignant systems, affected molecular targets and modulated cellular signaling pathways, besides the metabolic bioconversion of these dietary polyphenols in the human body and bioactivities of various metabolites. In addition, the scientific activity of Dr.

Sak is focused on the interactions between natural flavonoids and traditional anticancer treatment modalities, including chemotherapy and radiotherapy, but also hormonal and targeted biological therapies.

Dr. Sak is the author of five international monographies *Flavonoids in the Fight against Upper Gastrointestinal Tract Cancers* (Nova Science Publishers, Inc., New York, 2018), *Plant Flavonoids Affect Cancer Chemotherapeutic Efficacy: A Handbook for Doctors and Patients* (Nova Science Publishers, Inc., New York, 2019), *Dietary Flavonoids Interfere with Cancer Radiotherapy* (Nova Science Publishers, Inc., New York, 2019), *Plant Flavonoids against Metastasis: New Concepts for Cancer Treatment* (Nova Science Publishers, Inc., New York, 2021) and *Combating Canine Cancers with Phytochemicals* (Nova Science Publishers, Inc., New York, 2021). She has published more than 100 articles in international peer-reviewed journals and numerous chapters in handbooks about nutraceuticals and cancer, is the author of the book *Food and Cancer* (in Estonian, 2013) and many popular-scientific articles published in the Estonian health journals.

Dr. Sak is an internationally renowned scientist whose work has been recognized by several prestigious organizations.

# Abbreviations

| | |
|---|---|
| $[^{18}F]FDG$ | 2-Deoxy-2-$[^{18}F]$fluoro-D-glucose |
| $[^{18}F]FLT$ | 3`-Deoxy-3`-$[^{18}F]$fluorothymidine |
| 4-HNE | 4-Hydroxy-2-nonenal |
| 4-OH-TAM | 4-Hydroxytamoxifen |
| 8-oxo-dG | 8-oxo-deoxyguanosine |
| $\gamma$-GT | Gamma glutamyl transferase |
| $\Delta\Psi m$ | Mitochondrial membrane potential |
| ABC | ATP-binding cassette |
| ABCG2 | ATP-binding cassette transporter G2 (=BCRB) |
| Abl | Abelson proto-oncogene |
| AI | Aromatase inhibitor |
| AKT | Protein kinase B |
| ALDH1 | Aldehyde dehydrogenase 1 |
| ALK | Anaplastic lymphoma kinase |
| ALL | Acute lymphocytic leukemia |
| ALP | Alkaline phosphatase |
| ALT | Alanine transaminase |
| AML | Acute myelogenous leukemia |
| AMP | Adenosine monophosphate |
| AMPK | AMP-activated protein kinase |
| AP-1 | Activator protein 1 |
| AR | Androgen receptor |
| AR-V7 | Androgen receptor splice variant 7 |
| AsA | Ascorbic acid |
| AST | Aspartate transaminase |
| ATF3 | Activating transcription factor 3 |
| ATP | Adenosine triphosphate |
| $AUC_{0-\infty}$ | Area under the plasma concentration-time curve from time zero to infinity |
| Bad | Bcl-2-associated agonist of cell death |

| | |
|---|---|
| Bak | Bcl-2 homologous antagonist/killer |
| BALP | Bone alkaline phosphatase |
| BaP | Benzo[a]pyrene |
| Bax | Bcl-2-associated X protein |
| Bcl-2 | B-cell lymphoma 2 |
| Bcl-xL | B-cell lymphoma-extra large |
| Bcr | Breakpoint cluster region gene |
| Bcr-Abl | Chimeric gene of Bcr and Abl |
| BCRP | Breast cancer resistance protein |
| Bid | BH3 interacting domain death agonist |
| Bim | Bcl-2-like protein 11 |
| BRAF | B-Raf proto-oncogene serine/ threonine-protein kinase |
| BTK | Bruton`s tyrosine kinase |
| bw | Body weight |
| CAT | Catalase |
| CCK-8 | Cell Counting Kit-8 |
| CCNE2 | Cyclin E2 |
| CD13 | Cluster of differentiation 13 |
| CD133 | Cluster of differentiation 133 |
| CD20 | Cluster of differentiation 20 |
| CD31 | Cluster of differentiation 31 |
| CD34 | Cluster of differentiation 34 |
| CD44 | Cluster of differentiation 44 |
| CD8α | Cluster of differentiation 8α |
| Cdc2 | Cell division control protein 2 |
| Cdc25A | Cell division cycle 25A |
| Cdk2 | Cyclin dependent kinase 2 |
| Cdk4 | Cyclin dependent kinase 4 |
| CDKN1A | Cyclin dependent kinase inhibitor 1A |
| c-FLIP | Cellular FLICE (FADD-like IL-1β-converting enzyme)-inhibitory protein |
| CHOP | CCAAT/enhancer binding protein homologous protein |
| CI | Combination index |
| cIAP1/2 | Cellular inhibitor of apoptosis proteins 1 and 2 |
| CL/F | Total body clearance |
| CLL | Chronic lymphocytic leukemia |
| $C_{max}$ | Peak plasma concentration |

| | |
|---|---|
| c-Met | Tyrosine-protein kinase Met |
| CML | Chronic myelogenous leukemia |
| COMT | Catechol-O-methyltransferase |
| COX-2 | Cyclooxygenase 2 |
| CREB | cAMP response element-binding protein |
| CS | Chitosan |
| CSC | Cancer stem cell |
| CV | Crystal violet |
| CXCL12 | CXC motif chemokine 12 (=stromal cell-derived factor 1) |
| CXCR7 | CXC chemokine receptor 7 |
| CYP | Cytochrome P450 |
| CYP19 | Cytochrome P450 19 (=aromatase) |
| CYP1A1 | Cytochrome P450 1A1 |
| CYP1A2 | Cytochrome P450 1A2 |
| CYP1B1 | Cytochrome P450 1B1 |
| CYP2C19 | Cytochrome P450 2C19 |
| CYP2C9 | Cytochrome P450 2C9 |
| CYP2D6 | Cytochrome P450 2D6 |
| CYP2E1 | Cytochrome P450 2E1 |
| CYP3A4 | Cytochrome P450 3A4 |
| CYR61 | Cysteine-rich angiogenic inducer 61 |
| cyt c | Cytochrome c |
| del | Deletion |
| DIABLO | Direct inhibitor of apoptosis-binding protein with low pI |
| DLBCL | Diffuse large B-cell lymphoma |
| DLT | Dose-limiting toxicity |
| DMBA | 7,12-Dimethylbenz[a]anthracene |
| DNMT | DNA methyltransferase |
| DR5 | Death receptor 5 |
| DRI | Dose-reduction index |
| E1 | Estrone |
| E2 | 17β-estradiol |
| EAT | Ehrlich ascites tumor |
| EBV | Epstein-Barr virus |
| ECG | Epicatechin 3-gallate |
| EGC | Epigallocatechin |
| EGCG | Epigallocatechin 3-gallate |

| | |
|---|---|
| EGF | Epidermal growth factor |
| EGFP | Enhanced green fluorescent protein |
| EGFR | Epidermal growth factor receptor (=HER1) |
| eIF2α | Eukaryotic initiation factor 2α |
| EML4 | Echinoderm microtubule-associated protein-like 4 |
| EMT | Epithelial-mesenchymal transition |
| EpCAM | Epithelial cell adhesion molecule |
| ER | Estrogen receptor |
| ERK1/2 | Extracellular signal-regulated kinases 1 and 2 (=p44/42 MAPK) |
| ERα | Estrogen receptor α (=ERα66) |
| ERα36 | Estrogen receptor α36 |
| ERβ | Estrogen receptor β |
| ESR1 | Estrogen receptor 1 |
| FDA | Food and Drug Administration |
| FGF2 | Fibroblast growth factor 2 |
| FGFR | Fibroblast growth factor receptor |
| FGFR2 | Fibroblast growth factor receptor 2 |
| FLT3 | FMS-like tyrosine kinase 3 |
| Foxo3a | Forkhead box O3a |
| Foxp3 | Forkhead box P3 |
| FSH | Follicle-stimulating hormone |
| G6-PD | Glucose-6-phosphate dehydrogenase |
| GADD34 | Growth arrest and DNA damage-inducible 34 |
| GADD45 | Growth arrest and DNA damage-inducible 45 |
| GAK | Cyclin G-associated kinase |
| GATA3 | GATA-binding protein 3 |
| GFP | Green fluorescent protein |
| Glut | Glucose transporter |
| GO | Graphene oxide |
| GPR30 | G protein-coupled receptor 30 |
| GPx | Glutathione peroxidase |
| GR | Glutathione reductase |
| GRP78 | Glucose-regulated protein 78 |
| GSH | Reduced glutathione |
| GSH-Px | Glutathione peroxidase |
| GSSG | Oxidized glutathione |
| GST | Glutathione-S-transferase |
| GTE | Green tea extract |

| | |
|---|---|
| $H_2O_2$ | Hydrogen peroxide |
| HCC | Hepatocellular carcinoma |
| HDAC | Histone deacetylase |
| HDL | High-density lipoprotein |
| HER2 | Human epidermal growth factor receptor-2 (also known as ErbB2) |
| HIF-1α | Hypoxia-inducible factor 1α |
| hnRNPA1 | Heterogeneous nuclear ribonucleoprotein A1 |
| HNSCC | Head and neck squamous cell carcinoma |
| HO-1 | Heme oxygenase-1 |
| HRT | Hormone replacement therapy |
| Hsp27 | Heat shock protein 27 |
| Hsp72 | Heat shock protein 72 |
| hTERT | Human telomerase reverse transcriptase |
| HUVEC | Human umbilical vein endothelial cell |
| i.g. | intragastric(ally) |
| i.p. | intraperitoneal(ly) |
| i.v. | intravenous(ly) |
| IAP | Inhibitor of apoptosis protein |
| $IC_{50}$ | Half maximal inhibitory concentration |
| ICI 182 780 | Fulvestrant |
| IKK | IκB kinase |
| IL-4 | Interleukin 4 |
| IL-6 | Interleukin 6 |
| IL-8 | Interleukin 8 |
| iNOS | Inducible nitric oxide synthase |
| $IP_3$ | Inositol 1,4,5-trisphosphate |
| IRS1 | Insulin receptor substrate-1 |
| IκBα | NF-κB inhibitor α |
| JAK1/2 | Janus kinases 1 and 2 |
| JNK1/2 | c-Jun N-terminal kinases 1 and 2 |
| KIT | Stem cell growth factor receptor |
| KLF4 | Krueppel-like factor 4 |
| KLK6 | Kallikrein 6 |
| KSHV | Kaposi`s sarcoma-associated herpesvirus |
| LC3 | Microtubule-associated protein 1A/1B light chain 3 |
| LDH | Lactate dehydrogenase |
| LDL | Low-density lipoprotein |
| LH | Luteinizing hormone |

| | |
|---|---|
| LPO | Lipid peroxidation |
| MAPK | Mitogen-activated protein kinase |
| Mcl-1 | Myeloid cell leukemia 1 |
| MCT1 | Monocarboxylate transporter 1 |
| MDA | Malondialdehyde |
| MDCK | Madin-Darby Canine Kidney |
| MDR | Multidrug resistance |
| MEK1 | Mitogen-activated protein kinase kinase 1 (=MAP2K1) |
| MEK2 | Mitogen-activated protein kinase kinase 2 (=MAP2K2) |
| MEK4 | Mitogen-activated protein kinase kinase 4 (=MAP2K4, =SEK1, =MKK4) |
| miR-1 | MicroRNA 1 |
| miR-148a | MicroRNA 148a |
| miR-200c | MicroRNA 200c |
| miR-21 | MicroRNA 21 |
| miR-34a | MicroRNA 34a |
| miR-379 | MicroRNA 379 |
| miR-8080 | MicroRNA 8080 |
| MMP-2 | Matrix metalloproteinase 2 |
| MMP-9 | Matrix metalloproteinase 9 |
| MMTV | Mouse mammary tumor virus |
| MnSOD | Manganese superoxide dismutase |
| MNU | N-methyl-N-nitrosourea |
| mRNA | Messenger RNA |
| MRP | Multidrug resistance protein |
| MRT | Mean resistance time |
| MTD | Maximum tolerated dose |
| mTOR | Mammalian target of rapamycin |
| mTORC1 | mTOR complex 1 |
| MTS | 3-(4,5-dimethylthiazol-2-yl)-5-(3-carboxymethoxyphenyl)-2-(4-sulfophenyl)-2H-tetrazolium |
| MTT | 3-(4,5-dimethylthiazol-2-yl)-2,5-diphenyltetrazolium bromide |
| MVD | Microvessel density |
| MWCNT | Multiwalled carbon nanotube |
| NC | Nanocapsule |

| | |
|---|---|
| NF-κB | Nuclear factor κB |
| NHL | Non-Hodgkin lymphoma |
| NMR | Nuclear magnetic resonance |
| NO | Nitric oxide |
| NOD | Non-obese diabetic |
| NOX2 | Nicotinamide adenine dinucleotide phosphate oxidase 2 |
| NP | Nanoparticle |
| NQO1 | NAD(P)H:quinone oxidoreductase 1 |
| Nrf2 | Nuclear factor erythroid 2-related factor 2 |
| NS | Nanosphere |
| NSCLC | Non-small cell lung cancer |
| OC | Osteocalcin |
| p.o. | per oral(ly) |
| P70S6K | Ribosomal protein S6 kinase beta-1 |
| PARP | Poly (ADP-ribose) polymerase |
| PC | Protein carbonyl |
| PCL | Polycaprolactone |
| PCNA | Proliferating cell nuclear antigen |
| PDGFR | Platelet-derived growth factor receptor |
| PD-L1 | Programmed death-ligand 1 |
| PEG | Polyethylene glycol |
| pEGFR | Phosphorylated EGFR |
| PFK | Phosphofructokinase |
| P-gp | P-glycoprotein |
| Ph | Philadelphia chromosome |
| PI3K | Phosphatidylinositol 3-kinase |
| PKCα | Protein kinase C α |
| PLGA | Poly (lactic-co-glycolic acid) |
| ppm | Parts per million |
| PR | Progesterone receptor |
| pRB | Retinoblastoma protein |
| PSA | Prostate specific antigen |
| PTEN | Phosphatase and tensin homolog |
| PTH | Parathyroid hormone |
| PVP | Polyvinylpyrrolidone |
| PXR | Pregnane X receptor |
| Raf | Rapidly accelerated fibrosarcoma |
| RB1 | Retinoblastoma gene |

| | |
|---|---|
| RCC | Renal cell carcinoma |
| ROS | Reactive oxygen species |
| ROS1 | c-ros oncogene 1 |
| RTK | Receptor tyrosine kinase |
| s.c. | subcutaneous(ly) |
| S6K | S6 kinase |
| SCC | Squamous cell carcinoma |
| SCID | Severe combined immunodeficient |
| SD | Sprague-Dawley |
| SERD | Selective estrogen receptor downregulator |
| SERM | Selective estrogen receptor modulator |
| SGOT | Serum glutamic oxaloacetic transaminase |
| SGPT | Serum glutamic pyruvic transaminase |
| SHP-1 | Src homology region 2 domain-containing phosphatase-1 |
| Sirt1 | Sirtuin 1 |
| Skp2 | S-phase kinase protein 2 |
| Slug | Zinc finger protein SNAI2 |
| Smac | Second mitochondria-derived activator of caspase |
| Snail | Zinc finger protein SNAI1 |
| SNEDDS | Self-nanoemulsifying drug delivery system |
| SOD | Superoxide dismutase |
| SOX2 | (Sex determining region Y)-box 2 |
| SPF | Specific-pathogen free |
| SRB | Sulforhodamine B |
| Stat3 | Signal transducer and activator of transcription 3 |
| Stat5 | Signal transducer and activator of transcription 5 |
| SULT1A1 | Sulfotransferase 1A1 |
| $t_{1/2}$ | Half-life |
| TAC | Total antioxidant capacity |
| TAM | Tamoxifen |
| TBARS | Thiobarbituric acid reactive substances |
| tBid | Truncated Bid |
| TEG | Tetraethylene glycol |
| TF-1 | Theaflavin |
| TF-2 | Mixture of theaflavin 3-gallate (TF-2a) and theaflavin 3`-gallate (TF-2b) |
| TF-3 | Theaflavin 3,3`-digallate |
| TG | Triglyceride |

| | |
|---|---|
| TGFβ | Transforming growth factor β |
| TIMP-2 | Tissue inhibitor of metalloproteinase 2 |
| TKI | Tyrosine kinase inhibitor |
| TLS | Tumor lysis syndrome |
| TNBC | Triple-negative breast cancer |
| TNFα | Tumor necrosis factor α |
| TRAP | Tartrate-resistant acid phosphatase |
| T-SH | Total thiols |
| TSP-1 | Thrombospondin-1 |
| TUNEL | Terminal deoxynucleotidyl transferase (TdT) dUTP Nick-End Labeling |
| Twist1 | Twist-related protein 1 |
| UGT | UDP-glucuronosyltransferase |
| uPA | Urokinase-type plasminogen activator |
| uPAR | Urokinase-type plasminogen activator receptor |
| UPR | Unfolded protein response |
| US | The United States |
| VEGF | Vascular endothelial growth factor |
| VEGF121 | Vascular endothelial growth factor 121 |
| VEGF165 | Vascular endothelial growth factor 165 |
| VEGFR | Vascular endothelial growth factor receptor |
| vs | versus |
| $V_z/F$ | Apparent volume of distribution |
| w | week |
| WHO | World Health Organization |
| WST-1 | Water soluble tetrazolium salt-1 |
| wt | wild-type |
| XIAP | X-linked inhibitor of apoptosis protein |
| XTT | 2,3-Bis-(2-methoxy-4-nitro-5-sulfophenyl)-2H-tetrazolium-5-carboxanilide |
| Zeb1 | Zinc finger E-box binding homeobox 1 (TCF8) |
| Zeb2 | Zinc finger E-box binding homeobox 2 (SIP1) |

# Chapter 1

# Cancer as an Increasing Public Health Concern All over the World

Cancer is an overwhelming health burden with a continuously increasing incidence rate all over the world. In fact, while there were an estimated 10.1 million new cancer cases and 6.2 million cancer-related deaths in 2000 [1]; in 2020, 19.3 million new cancer cases were diagnosed worldwide and almost 10.0 million people lost their lives to malignant diseases [2]. Moreover, it is expected that the global cancer burden will be 28.4 million new cases in 2040, if exposure to the risk factors associated with globalization and a growing economy will not decrease drastically [2]. These dismal numbers about continuous increase in cancer incidence over the last two decades are presented in Figure 1.1, compiled by the data of GLOBOCAN reports [1-5]. Currently, one out of five men and one out of six women develop cancer during their lifetime, and one out of eight men and one out of eleven women die from cancerous diseases [6]. The total number of cancer survivors within the 5-years of the diagnosis is estimated to be 43.8 million, growing along with continuous increase in cancer incidence and posing a great burden to healthcare systems globally [6]. The three most common cancer types include breast, lung and colorectal cancers in terms of incidence, accounting for about one-third of all new cancer cases diagnosed in the world, and ranking among the top five malignant tumors in terms of mortality [2]. Being a complex disease, cancer is induced by multiple interactive components, including genetic, environmental and lifestyle factors, among which many are avoidable, such as pollution, smoking, alcohol consumption, unhealthy dietary habits, obesity, low physical activity and changes in reproductive behavior like late age of first birth [7-9].

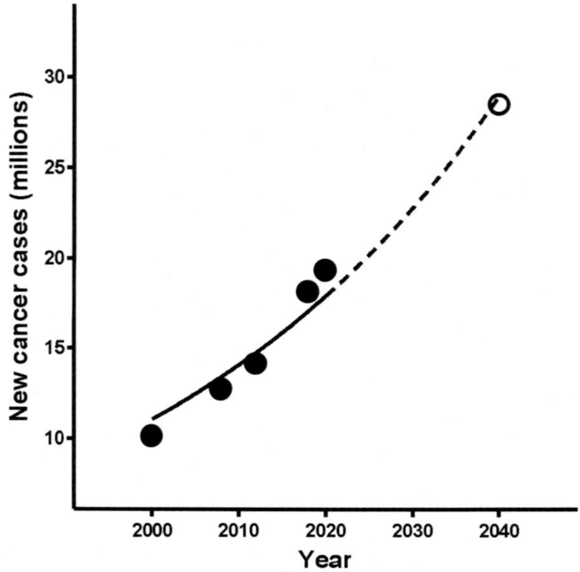


**Figure 1.1.** Continuous increase in the incidence of new cancer cases worldwide. Data taken from [1-5].

Cancer develops from normal cells that gain the ability to proliferate and grow uncontrollably. These cells can eventually become malignant, lose their function as healthy cells, and acquire the potential to spread into adjacent tissues and colonize distant organs [6, 10, 11]. Carcinogenesis is a complex process, advancing in time and space, and including initiation, promotion and progression phases [11]. Maintenance of abnormal growth as a net result of the balance between proliferation and elimination of tumor cells is the critical step in cancer initiation and progression [12, 13]. Cell growth, division and differentiation are driven by the cell cycle, being deregulated in tumor cells, and making cell cycle arrest a desirable target and an important mechanism for anticancer therapy [14-18]. However, cell cycle arrest alone can only induce stable disease without any tumor regression [19]. Apoptosis or programmed cell death-1 further plays a critical role in regulating cellular growth and survival through eliminating the unwanted cells and thereby balancing cell proliferation, being substantially suppressed in malignant cells [14, 20-22]. Apoptosis can occur either through mitochondrial-dependent (intrinsic) or death receptor-mediated (extrinsic) signaling pathway, leading to activation of initiator caspases (caspase-9, caspase-8) and executioner caspases (caspase-3), cleaving a number of nuclear and cytosolic targets, and ultimately resulting in cell destruction [14, 20, 22-24]. Mitochondrial apoptosis is mainly determined by the ratio of pro- (Bax) and antiapoptotic (Bcl-2) proteins that controls mitochondrial permeability and the release of cytochrome c to the cytosol [22, 25]. There are several good indicators for evaluation of apoptotic cell death, including the loss of mitochondrial membrane potential, but also a series of morphological features, such as cell shrinkage, membrane blebbing, chromatin condensation, nuclear fragmentation and apoptotic bodies [20, 26]. As malignant cells utilize a number of mechanisms to evade apoptosis and maintain their viability, induction of apoptosis is one of the major strategies for effective tumor regression by both traditional chemotherapeutic drugs as well as targeted anticancer therapies [19, 27-29]. Besides apoptosis, autophagy or programmed cell death-2 is another important cellular process to destroy cancer cells in response to severe cellular stresses [30, 31]. However, depending on the cellular context and the strength and duration of the stimulus, autophagy can also promote survival of tumor cells and maintain their functioning in unfavorable environmental conditions, allowing the cell to recover energy from damaged or unnecessary subcellular components [30, 31]. Therefore, manipulation with autophagy might be an additional approach to improve the antitumor efficacy of cancer therapeutics [30]. Another important hallmark of cancer, besides sustaining proliferative signaling, evading growth suppression and resisting cell death, is an altered cellular energetics with an increased metabolic rate. To cover the high energy requirements of tumors, cancer cells are dependent on aerobic glycolysis even under normoxic conditions, offering a selective advantage to rapidly growing malignant cells over normal differentiated cells [32]. Accordingly, glycolysis could be considered as a promising target for development of novel anticancer agents by depriving cancer cells from essential energy and substrates [32].

Not the primary tumor, but metastatic disease actually represents a major clinical challenge in the treatment of cancer. In fact, over 90% of cancer-related deaths are attributed to metastatic spread of primary neoplasms [33]. To acquire invasive capabilities, primary tumor cells undergo several molecular and morphological transformations collectively called the epithelial-mesenchymal transition (EMT) [14, 33]. During this process, tumor cells lose their epithelial characteristics and acquire mesenchymal phenotype to become migratory and invasive [33, 34]. Tumor cell dissemination starts with invasion of extracellular matrix by degrading the cellular membranes, facilitated through expression and activation of matrix metalloproteinases, followed by intravasation into blood vessels, extravasation at different target sites, and ultimately colonization of distant organs [20, 33, 35]. Therefore, upregulation of the EMT markers and proteolytic enzymes are generally related to poor clinical prognosis and high risk of metastasis [33]. Spread and growth of malignant cells is further promoted by formation of new blood vessels within the tumors, a process called angiogenesis [36, 37]. Accordingly, formation of tumor vasculature is considered as an additional prognostic indicator, representing also a promising target for the management of cancerous neoplasms [36]. Moreover, it is important to bear in mind that the complex carcinogenesis process occurs in tumor microenvironment where different cells, including tumor-associated macrophages, are present and contribute to proinflammatory milieu through producing many cytokines and interleukins, thereby further supporting progression and survival of malignant cells [7, 38]. The fight against cancer is even more complicated by the high genetic and biologic heterogeneity of tumoral tissues [17, 39]. One especially recalcitrant subset of cells within tumors, cancer stem cells, are believed to initiate and maintain malignant growth, causing relapses of disease over time [40]. Targeting these roots of cancer may be a promising new approach for improvement of cancer therapy [40, 41].

Current major strategies to control the malignant growth include chemotherapy, radiotherapy and surgery, whereas the best therapeutic regimen is typically decided by the type of cancer, its diagnostic stage and the overall health status of the patient [6, 7, 11]. Radiotherapy has been an effective tool for cancer treatment already for more than hundred years [42]. Chemotherapy has remained the front-line treatment for unresectable cancers since its advent in 1948, when antifolate aminopterin was first used in management of acute leukemia. Since then, a wide spectrum of structurally different chemotherapeutic agents has been developed and introduced into the clinical arsenal [8]. The first hormonal anticancer drug, tamoxifen, was approved as a palliative agent for the treatment of metastatic breast cancer in the end of 1977, being nowadays widely used against early and advanced estrogen receptor-positive breast cancers in both pre- and postmenopausal women [43, 44]. The new paradigm of targeted anticancer therapies started in 1997 with approval of the first monoclonal antibody rituximab for the treatment of relapsed or refractory non-Hodgkin lymphoma [44]. In the last two decades, the array of novel targeted biological therapies selectively directed at unique molecular alterations associated with specific cancer types, including both monoclonal antibodies and pharmacological inhibitors, has been essentially expanded, enhancing therapeutic efficacy and allowing more personalized approach for individual patients. Similar to conventional chemotherapy, targeted anticancer drugs eventually modulate crucial cellular processes, like growth inhibition, apoptosis promotion, metastasis restriction and angiogenesis suppression [45]. The timeline of the most important therapeutic breakthroughs occurred in the clinical management of malignancies is presented in Figure 1.2.

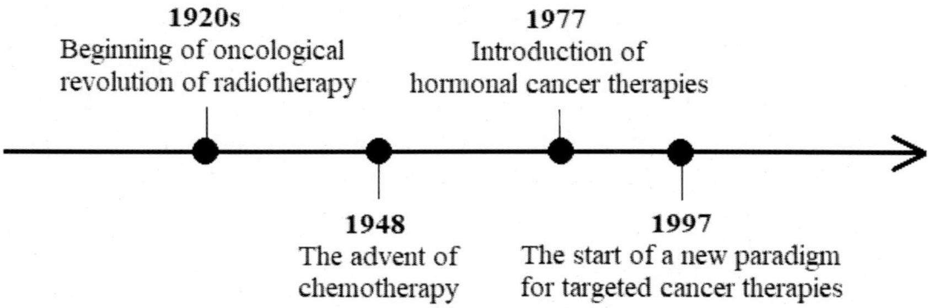


**Figure 1.2.** Simplified timeline of the most important therapeutic breakthroughs in cancer treatment. Data taken from [8, 42, 44].

Although the current therapeutic arsenal plays an important role in the overall treatment of most cancers, clinical success is still limited and the cure has not yet been realized due to two major obstacles [8, 46, 47]. Firstly, cancers either intrinsically possess or acquire over time the ability to bypass death-inducing effects of both cytotoxic agents as well as targeted therapies, representing the leading cause of cancer-related mortality [45, 48]. In fact, 90% of disease progression during and after anticancer therapy is related to drug resistance [45]. There are various complex molecular mechanisms under development of cancer drug resistance, including detoxification, activation of DNA repair process, modification of drug targets and evasion of drug-induced apoptotic pathways, besides an increased efflux of anticancer agents by ATP-binding cassette (ABC) transporters [6, 7, 49, 50]. Secondly, the foremost problem in anticancer drugs is their non-specific toxicity on normal healthy cells that is life-threatening and dose-limiting and causes persisting side effects [6, 8]. The most common adverse effects include illness, fatigue, nausea, vomiting, diarrhea, constipation, neuropathy, hair loss, trouble breathing and cardiotoxicity [6, 16]. Therefore, successful cancer therapy still presents one of the major medical challenges, demanding a continuous need for further improvements in therapeutic modalities [6]. An enhanced understanding of molecular mechanisms under carcinogenic processes provides a useful basis for novel drug discovery and development of more effective and technologically innovative therapeutic regimens [45]. As we know that cancer is a multifactorial disease and malignant tissue is highly heterogenic, its management also needs combined approaches, concomitantly affecting different molecular targets and modulating distinct cellular signaling pathways involved in cancer development and progression [11, 46, 51]. Co-administration of different antitumor drugs has indeed shown substantial therapeutic benefits with synergistic anticancer activities between two drugs; however, toxicities of these drugs might also be amplified [52]. Therefore, to overcome the pitfalls of current conventional approaches, combination of approved drugs with non-toxic bioactive adjuvants might present a promising new strategy to enhance therapeutic efficacy and clinical outcomes by retarding the development of resistance. Lowering the therapeutically effective doses further allows to reduce also systemic toxicity and intolerable adverse reactions, thereby improving the quality of life of cancer patients. Plant-derived flavonoids can be ideal candidates for potent adjuvant agents, being cheap, easily available and commonly safe, exerting themselves a wide variety of multitargeted anticancer activities. Further research in this field must be intensified in the near future, both in the level of preclinical *in vitro* and *in vivo* studies with immortalized cell lines, primary human cancer cells and appropriate animal models, as well as by initiating clinical trials with cancer patients.

## References

[1] Parkin DM, Bray F, Ferlay J, Pisani P. Estimating the world cancer burden: Globocan 2000. *Int J Cancer* 2001; 94: 153-6.

[2] Sung H, Ferlay J, Siegel RL, Laversanne M, Soerjomataram I, Jemal A, Bray F. Global cancer statistics 2020: GLOBOCAN estimates of incidence and mortality worldwide for 36 cancers in 185 countries. *CA Cancer J Clin* 2021; 71: 209-49.

[3] Ferlay J, Shin HR, Bray F, Forman D, Mathers C, Parkin DM. Estimates of worldwide burden of cancer in 2008: GLOBOCAN 2008. *Int J Cancer* 2010; 127: 2893-917.

[4] Ferlay J, Soerjomataram I, Dikshit R, Eser S, Mathers C, Rebelo M, Parkin DM, Forman D, Bray F. Cancer incidence and mortality worldwide: sources, methods and major patterns in GLOBOCAN 2012. *Int J Cancer* 2015; 136: E359-86.

[5] Ferlay J, Colombet M, Soerjomataram I, Mathers C, Parkin DM, Pineros M, Znaor A, Bray F. Estimating the global cancer incidence and mortality in 2018: GLOBOCAN sources and methods. *Int J Cancer* 2019; 144: 1941-53.

[6] Toric J, Markovic AK, Brala CJ, Barbaric M. Anticancer effects of olive oil polyphenols and their combinations with anticancer drugs. *Acta Pharm* 2019; 69: 461-82.

[7] Guneidy RA, Gad AM, Zaki ER, Ibrahim FM, Shokeer A. Antioxidant or pro-oxidant and glutathione transferase P1-1 inhibiting activities for Tamarindus indica seeds and their cytotoxic effect on MCF-7 cancer cell line. *J Genet Eng Biotechnol* 2020; 18: 74.

[8] Gaber M, Hany M, Mokhtar S, Helmy MW, Elkodairy KA, Elzoghby AO. Boronic-targeted albumin-shell oily-core nanocapsules for synergistic aromatase inhibitor/herbal breast cancer therapy. *Mater Sci Eng C Mater Biol Appl* 2019; 105: 110099.

[9] Daveri E, Adamo AM, Alfine E, Zhu W, Oteiza PI. Hexameric procyanidins inhibit colorectal cancer cell growth through both redox and non-redox regulation of the epidermal growth factor signaling pathway. *Redox Biol* 2021; 38: 101830.

[10] Li Y, Meeran SM, Patel SN, Chen H, Hardy TM, Tollefsbol TO. Epigenetic reactivation of estrogen receptor-alpha (ERalpha) by genistein enhances hormonal therapy sensitivity in ERalpha-negative breast cancer. *Mol Cancer* 2013; 12: 9.

[11] Memariani Z, Abbas SQ, Ul Hassan SS, Ahmadi A, Chabra A. Naringin and naringenin as anticancer agents and adjuvants in cancer combination therapy: Efficacy and molecular mechanisms of action, a comprehensive narrative review. *Pharmacol Res* 2021; 171: 105264.

[12] Bracke ME, Boterberg T, Depypere HT, Stove C, Leclercq G, Mareel MM. The citrus methoxyflavone tangeretin affects human cell-cell interactions. *Adv Exp Med Biol* 2002; 505: 135-9.

[13] Ruhul Amin AR, Khuri FR, Chen ZG, Shin DM. Synergistic growth inhibition of squamous cell carcinoma of the head and neck by erlotinib and epigallocatechin-3-gallate: the role of p53-dependent inhibition of nuclear factor-kappaB. *Cancer Prev Res* 2009; 2: 538-45.

[14] Xu Z, Zhao D, Zheng X, Huang B, Xia X, Pan X. Quercetin exerts bidirectional regulation effects on the efficacy of tamoxifen in estrogen receptor-positive breast cancer therapy: An in vitro study. *Environ Toxicol* 2020; 35: 1179-93.

[15] Kaushik S, Shyam H, Agarwal S, Sharma R, Nag TC, Dwivedi AK, Balapure AK. Genistein potentiates Centchroman induced

antineoplasticity in breast cancer via PI3K/Akt deactivation and ROS dependent induction of apoptosis. *Life Sci* 2019; 239: 117073.

[16] Jandial DD, Krill LS, Chen L, Wu C, Ke Y, Xie J, Hoang BH, Zi X. Induction of G2M arrest by flavokawain A, a kava chalcone, increases the responsiveness of HER2-overexpressing breast cancer cells to herceptin. *Molecules* 2017; 22: 462.

[17] Sirin N, Elmas L, Secme M, Dodurga Y. Investigation of possible effects of apigenin, sorafenib and combined applications on apoptosis and cell cycle in hepatocellular cancer cells. *Gene* 2020; 737: 144428.

[18] Tolomeo M, Grimaudo S, Di Cristina A, Pipitone RM, Dusonchet L, Meli M, Crosta L, Gebbia N, Invidiata FP, Titone L, Simoni D. Galangin increases the cytotoxic activity of imatinib mesylate in imatinib-sensitive and imatinib-resistant Bcr-Abl expressing leukemia cells. *Cancer Lett* 2008; 265: 289-97.

[19] Haque A, Rahman MA, Chen ZG, Saba NF, Khuri FR, Shin DM, Ruhul Amin AR. Combination of erlotinib and EGCG induces apoptosis of head and neck cancers through posttranscriptional regulation of Bim and Bcl-2. *Apoptosis* 2015; 20: 986-95.

[20] Xu Z, Huang B, Liu J, Wu X, Luo N, Wang X, Zheng X, Pan X. Combinatorial anti-proliferative effects of tamoxifen and naringenin: The role of four estrogen receptor subtypes. *Toxicology* 2018; 410: 231-46.

[21] Kaushik S, Shyam H, Sharma R, Balapure AK. Dietary isoflavone daidzein synergizes centchroman action via induction of apoptosis and inhibition of PI3K/Akt pathway in MCF-7/MDA MB-231 human breast cancer cells. *Phytomedicine* 2018; 40: 116-24.

[22] Youssef MM, Tolba MF, Badawy NN, Liu AW, El-Ahwany E, Khalifa AE, Zada S, Abdel-Naim AB. Novel combination of sorafenib and biochanin-A synergistically enhances the anti-proliferative and pro-apoptotic effects on hepatocellular carcinoma cells. *Sci Rep* 2016; 6: 30717.

[23] Charalambous C, Pitta CA, Constantinou AI. Equol enhances tamoxifen`s anti-tumor activity by induction of caspase-mediated apoptosis in MCF-7 breast cancer cells. *BMC Cancer* 2013; 13: 238.

[24] Yaacob NS, Nengsih A, Norazmi MN. Tualang honey promotes apoptotic cell death induced by tamoxifen in breast cancer cell lines. *Evid Based Complement Alternat Med* 2013; 2013: 989841.

[25] Roy Choudhury S, Karmakar S, Banik NL, Ray SK. Synergistic efficacy of sorafenib and genistein in growth inhibition by down regulating angiogenic and survival factors and increasing apoptosis through upregulation of p53 and p21 in malignant neuroblastoma cells having N-

Myc amplification or non-amplification. *Invest New Drugs* 2010; 28: 812-24.

[26] Jakubowicz-Gil J, Langner E, Badziul D, Wertel I, Rzeski W. Quercetin and sorafenib as a novel and effective couple in programmed cell death induction in human gliomas. *Neurotox Res* 2014; 26: 64-77.

[27] Mitchell C, Yacoub A, Hossein H, Martin AP, Bareford MD, Eulitt P, Yang C, Nephew KP, Dent P. Inhibition of MCL-1 in breast cancer cells promotes cell death in vitro and in vivo. *Cancer Biol Ther* 2010; 10: 903-17.

[28] Arya A, Khandelwal K, Ahmad H, Laxman TS, Sharma K, Mittapelly N, Agrawal S, Bhatta RS, Dwivedi AK. Co-delivery of hesperetin enhanced bicalutamide induced apoptosis by exploiting mitochondrial membrane potential via polymeric nanoparticles in a PC-3 cell line. *RSC Adv* 2016; 6: 5925.

[29] Pal HC, Baxter RD, Hunt KM, Agarwal J, Elmets CA, Athar M, Afaq F. Fisetin, a phytochemical, potentiates sorafenib-induced apoptosis and abrogates tumor growth in athymic nude mice implanted with BRAF-mutated melanoma cells. *Oncotarget* 2015; 6: 28296-311.

[30] Rong LW, Wang RX, Zheng XL, Feng XQ, Zhang L, Zhang L, Lin Y, Li ZP, Wang X. Combination of wogonin and sorafenib effectively kills human hepatocellular carcinoma cells through apoptosis potentiation and autophagy inhibition. *Oncol Lett* 2017; 13: 5028-34.

[31] Pons DG, Nadal-Serrano M, Torrens-Mas M, Oliver J, Roca P. The phytoestrogen genistein affects breast cancer cells treatment depending on the ERα/ERβ ratio. *J Cell Biochem* 2016; 117: 218-29.

[32] Li S, Wu L, Feng J, Li J, Liu T, Zhang R, Xu S, Cheng K, Zhou Y, Zhou S, Kong R, Chen K, Wang F, Xia Y, Lu J, Zhou Y, Dai W, Guo C. In vitro and in vivo study of epigallocatechin-3-gallate-induced apoptosis in aerobic glycolytic hepatocellular carcinoma cells involving inhibition of phosphofructokinase activity. *Sci Rep* 2016; 6: 28479.

[33] Pal HC, Diamond AC, Strickland LR, Kappes JC, Katiyar SK, Elmets CA, Athar M, Afaq F. Fisetin, a dietary flavonoid, augments the anti-invasive and anti-metastatic potential of sorafenib in melanoma. *Oncotarget* 2016; 7: 1227-41.

[34] Cufi S, Bonavia R, Vazquez-Martin A, Corominas-Faja B, Oliveras-Ferraros C, Cuyas E, Martin-Castillo B, Barrajon-Catalan E, Visa J, Segura-Carretero A, Bosch-Barrera J, Joven J, Micol V, Menendez JA. Silibinin meglumine, a water-soluble form of milk thistle silymarin, is an orally active anti-cancer agent that impedes the epithelial-to-mesenchymal transition (EMT) in EGFR-mutant non-small-cell lung carcinoma cells. *Food Chem Toxicol* 2013; 60: 360-8.

[35] Wu MH, Chiu YF, Wu WJ, Wu PL, Lin CY, Lin CL, Hsieh YH, Liu CJ. Synergistic antimetastatic effect of cotreatment with licochalcone A and sorafenib on human hepatocellular carcinoma cells through the inactivation of MKK4/JNK and uPA expression. *Environ Toxicol* 2018; 33: 1237-44.

[36] Ma ZS, Huynh TH, Ng CP, Do PT, Nguyen TH, Huynh H. Reduction of CWR22 prostate tumor xenograft growth by combined tamoxifen-quercetin treatment is associated with inhibition of angiogenesis and cellular proliferation. *Int J Oncol* 2004; 24: 1297-304.

[37] Wu XY, Xu H, Wu ZF, Chen C, Liu JY, Wu GN, Yao XQ, Liu FK, Li G, Shen L. Formononetin, a novel FGFR2 inhibitor, potently inhibits angiogenesis and tumor growth in preclinical models. *Oncotarget* 2015; 6: 44563-78.

[38] Quagliariello V, Iaffaioli RV, Armenia E, Clemente O, Barbarisi M, Nasti G, Berretta M, Ottaiano A, Barbarisi A. Hyaluronic acid nanohydrogel loaded with quercetin alone or in combination to a macrolide derivative of rapamycin RAD001 (everolimus) as a new treatment for hormone-responsive human breast cancer. *J Cell Physiol* 2017; 232: 2063-74.

[39] Park SJ, Kim MJ, Kim YK, Kim SM, Park JY, Myoung H. Combined cetuximab and genistein treatment shows additive anti-cancer effect on oral squamous cell carcinoma. *Cancer Lett* 2010; 292: 54-63.

[40] Zou H, Cao X, Xiao Q, Sheng X, Ren K, Quan M, Song Z, Li D, Zheng Y, Zeng W, Cao J, Peng Y. Synergistic inhibition of characteristics of liver cancer stem-like cells with a combination of sorafenib and 8-bromo-7-methoxychrysin in SMMC-7721 cell line. *Oncol Rep* 2016; 36: 1731-8.

[41] Corominas-Faja B, Oliveras-Ferraros C, Cuyas E, Segura-Carretero A, Joven J, Martin-Castillo B, Barrajon-Catalan E, Micol V, Bosch-Barrera J, Menendez JA. Stem cell-like ALDH(bright) cellular states in EGFR-mutant non-small cell lung cancer: a novel mechanism of acquired resistance to erlotinib targetable with the natural polyphenol silibinin. *Cell Cycle* 2013; 12: 3390-404.

[42] Thariat J, Hannoun-Levi JM, Sun Myint A, Vuong T, Gerard JP. Past, present, and future of radiotherapy for the benefit of patients. *Nat Rev Clin Oncol* 2013; 10: 52-60.

[43] Jordan VC. Tamoxifen as the first targeted long-term adjuvant therapy for breast cancer. *Endocr Relat Cancer* 2014; 21: R235-46.

[44] Santhosh S, Kumar P, Ramprasad V, Chaudhuri A. Evolution of targeted therapies in cancer: opportunities and challenges in the clinic. *Future Oncol* 2015; 11: 279-93.

[45] Liskova A, Samec M, Koklesova L, Brockmueller A, Zhai K, Abdellatif B, Siddiqui M, Biringer K, Kudela E, Pec M, Gadanec LK, Sudomova M,

Hassan STS, Zulli A, Shakibaei M, Giordano FA, Büsselberg D, Golubnitschaja O, Kubatka P. Flavonoids as an effective sensitizer for anti-cancer therapy: insights into multi-faceted mechanisms and applicability towards individualized patient profiles. *EPMA J* 2021; 12: 155-76.

[46] Sarkar FH, Li Y. Using chemopreventive agents to enhance the efficacy of cancer therapy. *Cancer Res* 2006; 66: 3347-50.

[47] Bae S, D`Cunha R, Shao J, An G. Effect of 5,7-dimethoxyflavone on Bcrp1-mediated transport of sorafenib in vitro and in vivo in mice. *Eur J Pharm Sci* 2018; 117: 27-34.

[48] Esmaeili MA. Combination of siRNA-directed gene silencing with epigallocatechin-3-gallate (EGCG) reverses drug resistance in human breast cancer cells. *J Chem Biol* 2015; 9: 41-52.

[49] Hyun HB, Moon JY, Cho SK. Quercetin suppresses CYR61-mediated multidrug resistance in human gastric adenocarcinoma AGS cells. *Molecules* 2018; 23: 209.

[50] Kumar M, Sharma G, Misra C, Kumar R, Singh B, Katare OP, Raza K. N-desmethyl tamoxifen and quercetin-loaded multiwalled CNTs: A synergistic approach to overcome MDR in cancer cells. *Mater Sci Eng C Mater Biol Appl* 2018; 89: 274-82.

[51] Wang C, Su L, Wu C, Wu J, Zhu C, Yuan G. RGD peptide targeted lipid-coated nanoparticles for combinatorial delivery of sorafenib and quercetin against hepatocellular carcinoma. *Drug Dev Ind Pharm* 2016; 42: 1938-44.

[52] Lockhart JN, Stevens DM, Beezer DB, Kravitz A, Harth E. Dual drug delivery of tamoxifen and quercetin: Regulated metabolism for anticancer treatment with nanosponges. *J Control Release* 2015; 220: 751-7.

# Chapter 2

# Anticancer Potential of Plant Flavonoids and Their Ability to Intervene in Conventional Cancer Therapies

Herbs and other plant-derived products have served as medicines in every culture throughout the human history [1]. Recently, increasing attention has been paid and research conducted for identifying novel therapeutic agents from herbal medicines and plant extracts as lead compounds for novel drug development, providing a valuable alternative or support to the current synthetic medicines [2-6]. The long-term history of human use indicates low toxicity and safety of plant-derived products that are typically also abundant and low-cost, besides exerting numerous important bioactivities [5, 7]. Accordingly, several well-known drugs in everyday clinical practice have been initially derived from plants, such as chemotherapeutics paclitaxel, vinblastine and vincristine [5, 8, 9].

## 2.1. Flavonoids as a Structurally Diverse Group of Plant Secondary Metabolites with Important Bioactivities in the Human Body

Flavonoids comprise a diverse group of low molecular weight polyphenolic compounds that are widely distributed in nature [10-12]. These compounds are biosynthesized in large quantities by various plants, serving as plant pigments and being responsible for much of the coloring in nature [7, 13, 14]. Flavonoids as secondary metabolites are present in different parts of plants, including roots, stems, flowers and fruits [12, 15]. As these phytochemicals occur ubiquitously in food plants, they constitute an integral part of the regular human diet [11]. Flavonoids can be indeed found in fruits, vegetables, berries, cereals, grains, seeds, spices, nuts, olive oil, tea, cocoa and coffee, but also in herbs and medicinal plants [15-19]. As a result, humans consume daily from 20 mg to 1 g of total flavonoids [16, 20, 21]. In addition to this, many dietary supplements also contain different flavonoids in their composition, essentially increasing the daily intake of these compounds [22]. Chemically, flavonoids are benzo-γ-pyrone derivatives, having fifteen-carbon skeletons that consist of two benzene rings connected through a pyrane ring [2, 17, 20]. The general backbone of flavonoids is presented in Figure 2.1. Variations in the substitution patterns of phenyl rings, i.e., hydroxyl or methoxyl groups, give rise to structural, biological and functional diversity of flavonoids [12, 14, 20, 23]. In general, while hydroxyl groups can increase solubility, methoxyl moieties enhance cell permeability [12]. Based on the nature of substitutions, their number and position at the basic skeleton, but also the degree of oxidation of the heterocyclic pyrane ring, flavonoids are divided into six major subgroups, i.e., flavanols or catechins, flavones, flavonols, flavanones, isoflavones and anthocyanidins [7, 14, 15, 17, 20]. High structural diversity of flavonoids provides a very broad spectrum of biological activities of these phytochemicals in the human body, exhibiting antioxidant, antiinflammatory, antiallergic, antiulcer, hepatoprotective, cardioprotective, nephroprotective, neuroprotective, analgesic, antiosteoporotic, antiatherosclerotic, antilipidemic, antithrombotic, antihypertensive, antihyperglycemic, antidiabetic, anti-aging, antifungal, antibacterial, antiviral, antimutagenic, anticarcinogenic and immunostimulatory activities [2, 10, 24-33]. Although these phytochemicals are not indispensable for normal functioning of the human body, they exert beneficial effects on health and contribute to prevention and treatment of several diseases [34, 35]. Collectively, flavonoids have been considered as "nature`s biological response modifiers" due to their inherent ability to modulate reactions of the body to various external stimuli, including carcinogens [24].

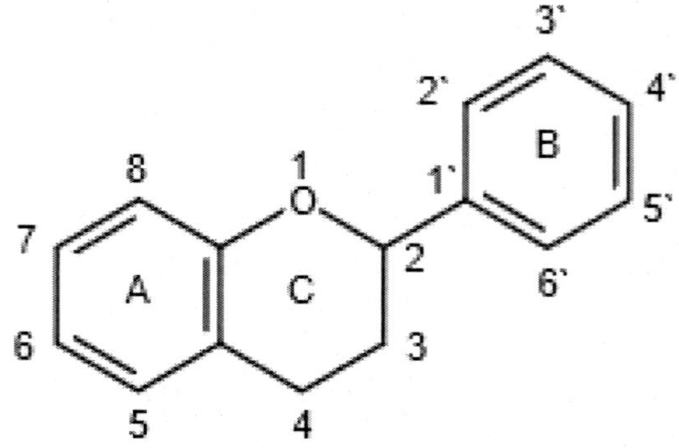


**Figure 2.1.** General structure of flavonoid backbone.

The structural formulas and the most common natural sources of flavonoids further covered in Chapters 3 and 4 of this book are presented in Table 2.1. If available, these data were derived from the USDA Database for the Flavonoid Content of Selected Foods [36] and the USDA Database for the Isoflavone Content of Selected Foods [37]. Two most well-known dietary sources of flavonoids are probably green tea and soy foods. The major flavanol present in green tea (brewed from the leaves of the plant *Camellia sinensis* (L.) Kuntze) is epigallocatechin 3-gallate (EGCG), accounting for more than 50% of the total polyphenol content, and reported to produce a number of positive health benefits due to its strong antioxidant properties. Other catechins found in green tea in lesser abundance include epigallocatechin (EGC), epicatechin 3-gallate (ECG) and epicatechin, all contributing to the beneficial effects ascribed to green tea products, promoted extensively for chemoprevention, cardioprotection, neuro-protection, glycemic control, weight loss and longevity [6, 11, 38-42]. The daily intake of EGCG in green tea in populations with high tea consumption (Korea, China, Japan) has been calculated to be even 500-700 mg [27]. For the manufacture of black tea, green tea polyphenols are oxidized during the fermentation process to form oligomeric flavanols, including different theaflavins [43]. Soybeans are the most significant source of isoflavones, intake of which is also geographically and culturally dependent [44-46]. For example, whereas the Japanese consumption of soy provides 20-35 mg isoflavones per day (being even more than 100 mg/day in about 5% of Japanese and Chinese older populations), the American and European diets provide on average only 1-3 mg (or even less than 1 mg) of soy isoflavones per day [45, 47, 48]. Due to its structural similarity to the female hormone 17β-estradiol and mimicking or modulating estrogen-like activities through binding to estrogen receptors, the predominant soy-derived isoflavone genistein has been used to relieve postmenopausal symptoms, besides reducing also cancer risk, maintaining cardiovascular health and enhancing bone density [44, 45, 49-54]. Another major phytoestrogen in soy products is daidzein, whereas its bioactive metabolite, equol, has been demonstrated to possess the greatest *in vitro* bioactivity and antioxidant activity among soy isoflavones. However, 30-50% of the adult population are not able to metabolize daidzein to equol because of the lack of equol-producing intestinal bacteria [55, 56]. Besides the dose, the stage of life during which isoflavones are consumed and the form that are ingested may also critically affect their biological responses [45, 57]. Another common natural source of flavonoids is various citrus fruits, such as grapefruits, oranges, pummelos, tangerines, bergamots, lemons and limes, that abundantly contain different flavanones in both aglycone (hesperetin and naringenin) as well as glycoside forms (hesperidin and naringin), but also several polymethoxylated flavones (tangeretin and nobiletin) [2, 16, 34, 58-64]. For example, the estimated concentrations of naringin in commercial grapefruit juices vary between 50-1200 mg/l [2, 65], while 20 ml of tangerine oil contains about 280 mg of tangeretin [66]. Most importantly, health benefits exerted by natural products can be typically not attributed to their single constituents, but are rather the sum or synergy of multiple bioactive components [67]. Furthermore, in addition to regular food sources, exposure to specific flavonoids occurs also through several over-the-counter dietary and herbal supplements that can be easily accessed at local grocery, pharmacy and health food stores, including highly concentrated green tea extracts (like Polyphenon E), soy isoflavone tablets, red clover extracts, citrus flavonoids tablets or silymarin herbal products, among others [4, 26, 40, 66, 68-72].

**Table 2.1.** Natural flavonoids studied in combinations with hormonal and targeted cancer therapies. Structural formulas and the most common natural sources

| Flavonoid | Structure | Natural sources | Ref. |
|---|---|---|---|
| FLAVANOLS | | | |
| (+)-Catechin | 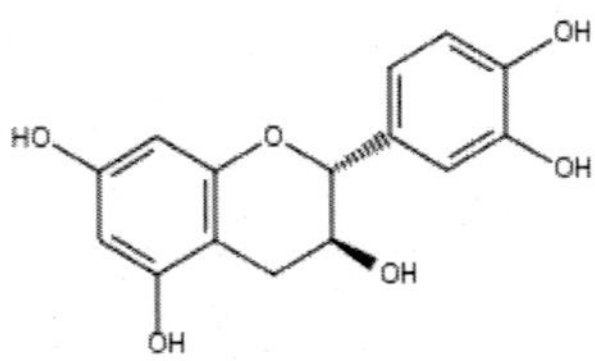 | Blueberries, cacao beans, grape seeds, green tea, cocoa powder, baking chocolate, carob flour, blackberries, cranberries, dark chocolate | [36] |
| (-)-Epicatechin | 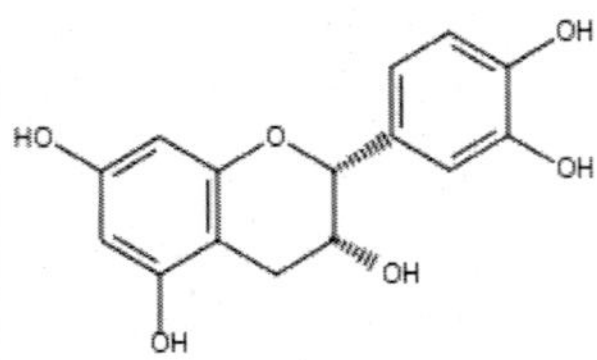 | Cocoa powder, baking chocolate, cacao beans, grape seeds, dark chocolate, black soybeans, broad beans seeds, apple skin, blueberries, green tea | [36] |

| Flavonoid | Structure | Natural sources | Ref. |
|---|---|---|---|
| (-)-Epigallocatechin (EGC) | 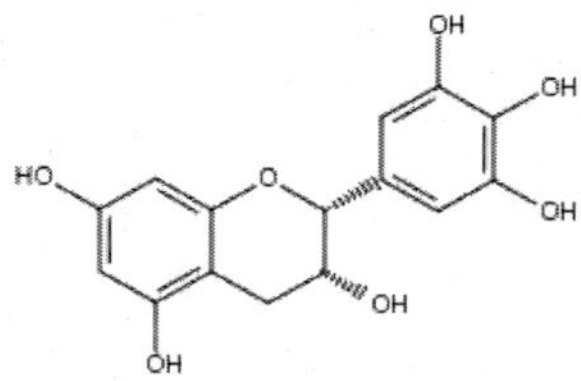 | Cacao beans, green tea, white tea, broad beans seeds, black diamond plums, black tea, oolong tea, marrowfat peas, pecan nuts | [36] |
| (-)-Epicatechin 3-gallate (ECG) | 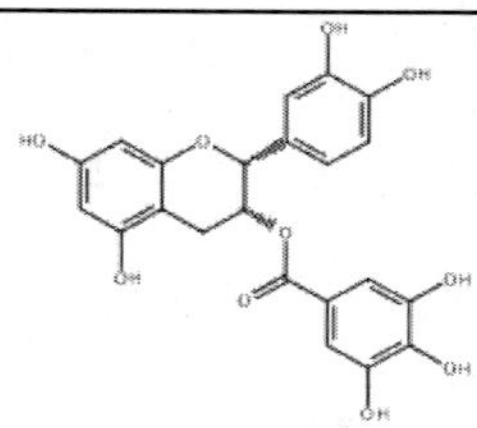 | Green tea, carob flour, white tea, oolong tea, black tea | [36] |
| (-)-Epigallocatechin 3-gallate (EGCG) | 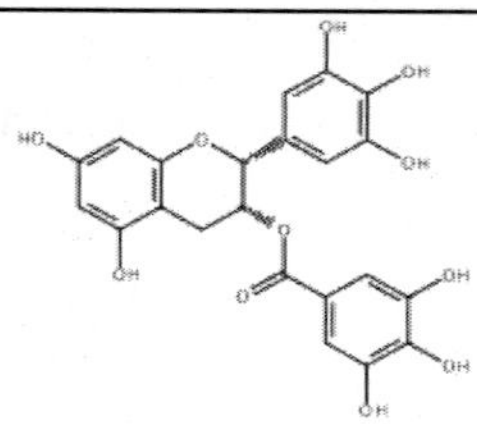 | Carob flour, green tea, white tea, oolong tea, black tea, fruit flavored tea | [36] |
| 2R,3R-6-methoxycarbonyl-gallocatechin-3-O-gallate | 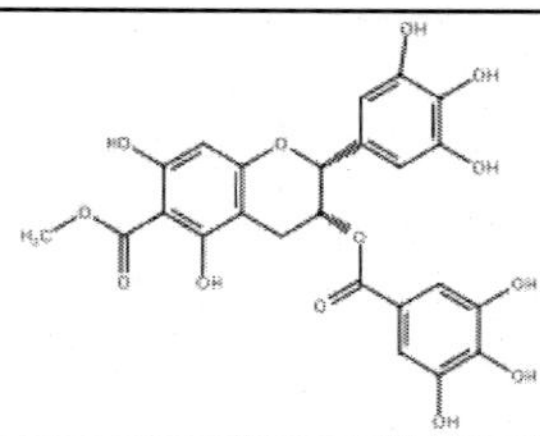 | Anhua dark tea | [6] |
| Theaflavin (TF-1) | 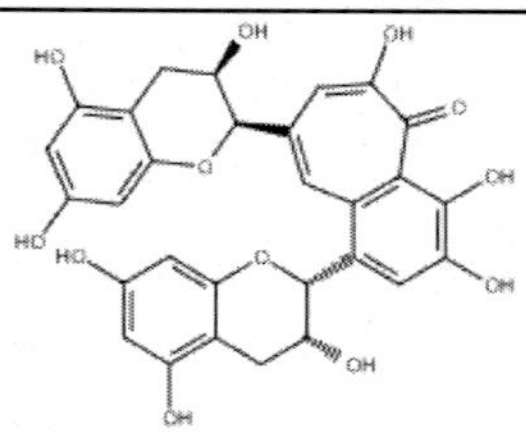 | Black tea, green tea | [36] |
| Theaflavin 3-gallate (TF-2a) | 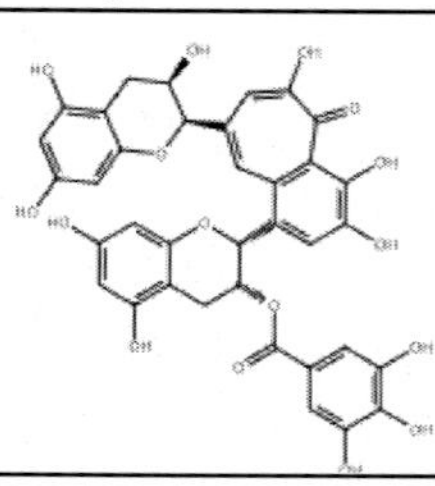 | Black tea, green tea | [43] |

**Table 2.1.** (Continued)

| Flavonoid | Structure | Natural sources | Ref. |
|---|---|---|---|
| Theaflavin 3`-gallate (TF-2b) | 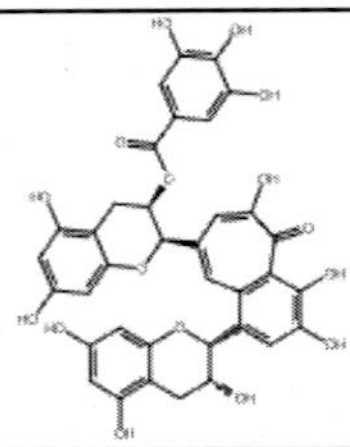 | Black tea, green tea | [36] |
| Theaflavin 3,3`-digallate (TF-3) | 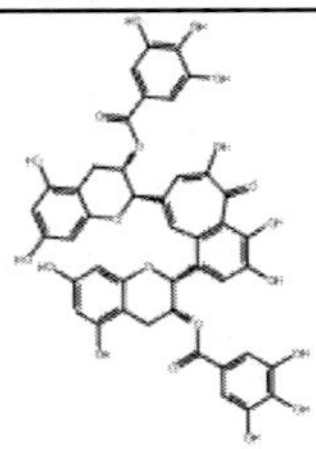 | Black tea, green tea | [36] |
| Hexameric proanthocyanidin | 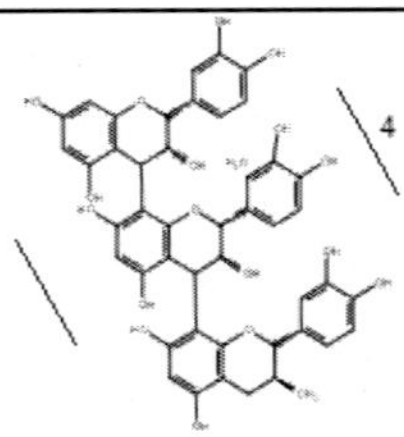 | Cinnamon, grape seeds, sorghum, baking chocolate, pinto and kidney and small red beans, pecans, grape juice, cranberries, hazelnuts, black plums | [73] |
| FLAVONES | | | |
| Chrysin | 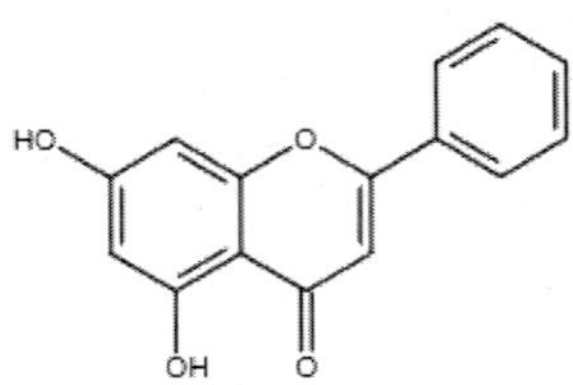 | Propolis | [74] |
| Baicalein | 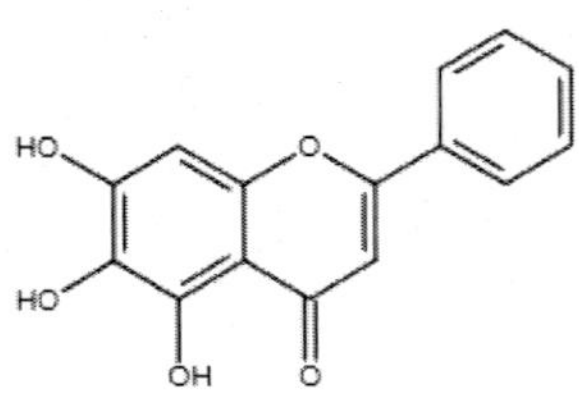 | Root of *Scutellaria baicalensis* Georgi | [13] |

| Flavonoid | Structure | Natural sources | Ref. |
|---|---|---|---|
| Apigenin | 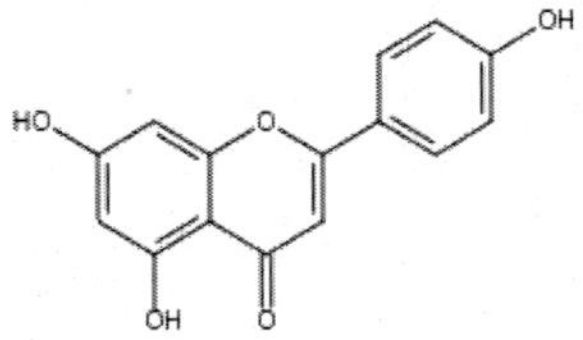 | Parsley, celery seeds, vine spinach, celery, kumquats, oregano, queen Anne`s lace, artichokes, juniper berries, peppermint | [36] |
| Luteolin | 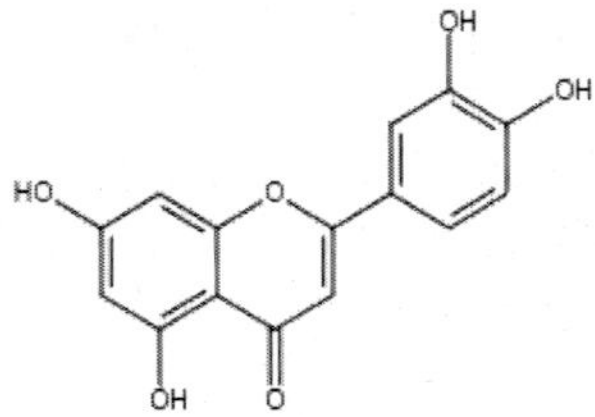 | Oregano, celery seeds, juniper berries, thyme, radicchio, celery, queen Anne`s lace, parsley, sage, peppermint | [36] |
| Tectochrysin | 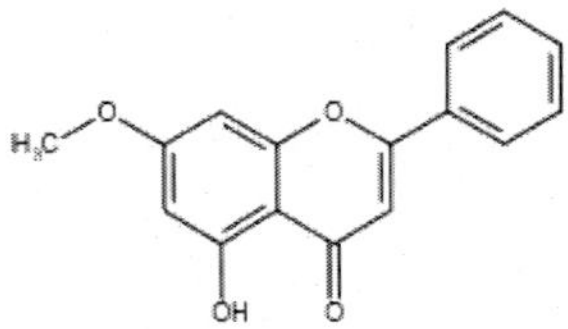 | *Alpinia oxyphylla* Miq. | [75] |
| Oroxylin A | 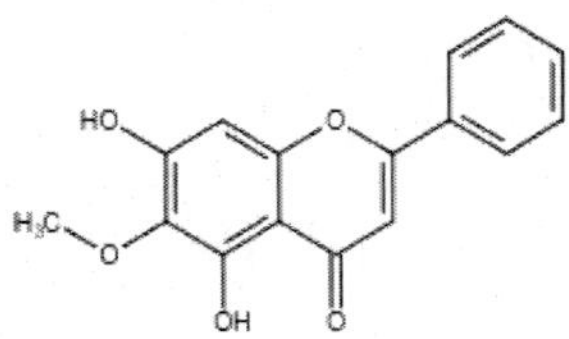 | Root of *Scutellaria baicalensis* Georgi | [76, 77] |
| Wogonin | 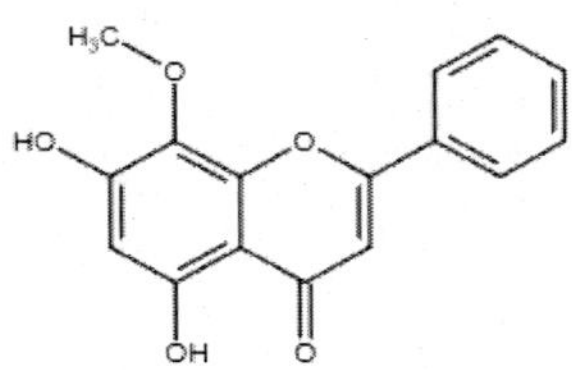 | Root of *Scutellaria baicalensis* Georgi | [78, 79] |
| Hispidulin | 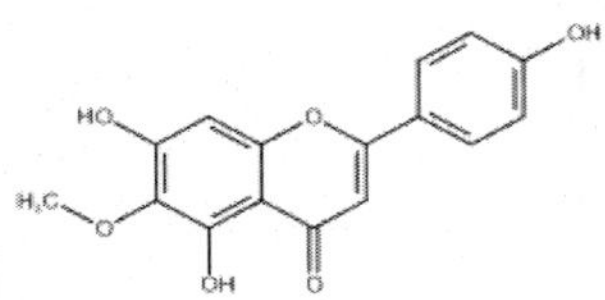 | Traditional Chinese medicinal herbs, such as *Saussurea involucrata* (Kar. & Kir.) Sch.Bip. | [33] |

**Table 2.1.** (Continued)

| Flavonoid | Structure | Natural sources | Ref. |
|---|---|---|---|
| 5,7-Dimethoxyflavone | 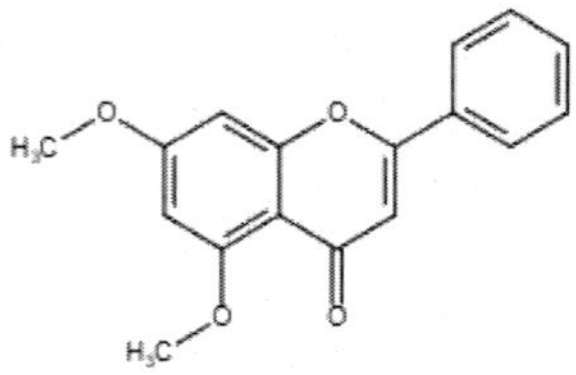 | *Kaempferia parviflora* Wall. ex Baker | [80] |
| 5-Desmethylsinensetin | 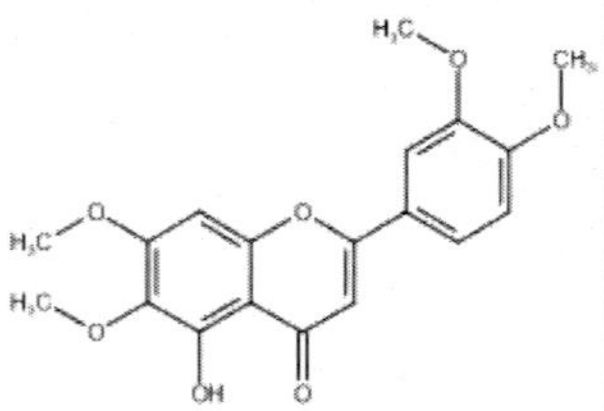 | *Stevia satureiifolia* var. *satureiifolia* extract | [81] |
| Tangeretin | 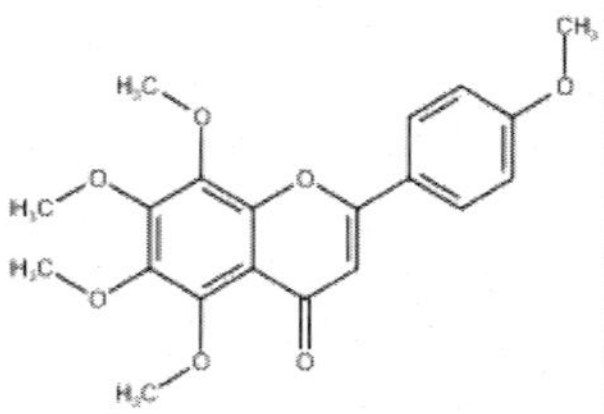 | Citrus fruits, such as tangerines, lemons, limes; peel oil of citrus fruits | [16, 59, 66] |
| 5,3`-Dihydroxy-3,6,7,8,4`-pentamethoxyflavone | 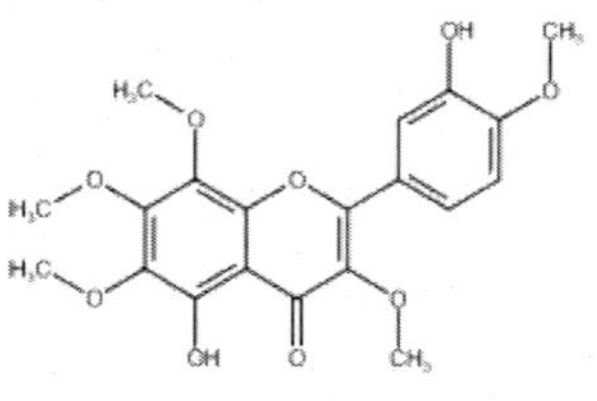 | Leaves of *Gardenia obtusifolia* Roxb. ex Hook.f. | [64] |
| Nobiletin | 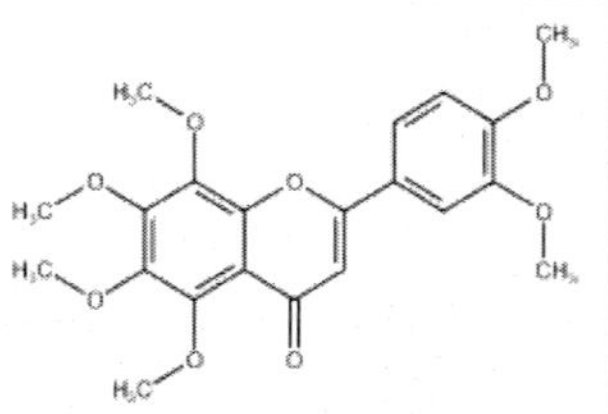 | Citrus fruits, such as tangerines, lemons, limes; oil of orange fruits | [16, 61, 63, 66] |

| Flavonoid | Structure | Natural sources | Ref. |
|---|---|---|---|
| Scutellarin | 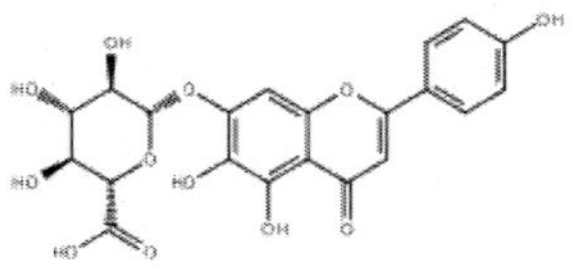 | *Erigeron breviscapus* (Vaniot) Hand-Mazz., genus *Scutellaria* | [82] |
| Vitexin | 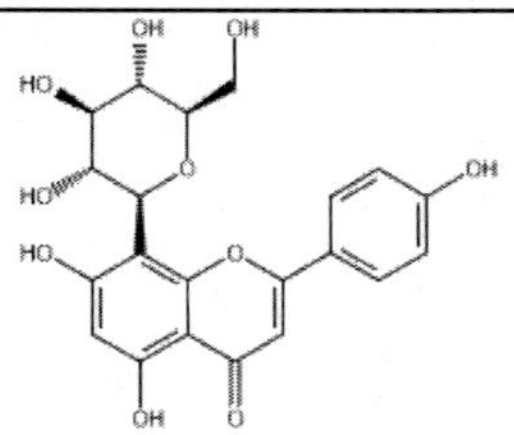 | Medicinal plants, such as hawthorn, pigeon pea, pearl millet, mung bean, mosses, bamboo, mimosa, wheat leaves, chaste tree | [83] |
| Amentoflavone (=bisapigenin) | 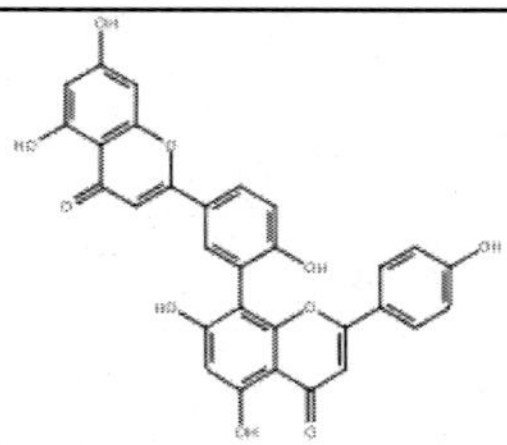 | *Scutellaria baicalensis* Georgi, *Selaginella tamariscina* (P. Beauv.) Spring | [84, 85] |
| FLAVONOLS | | | |
| 3-Hydroxyflavone | 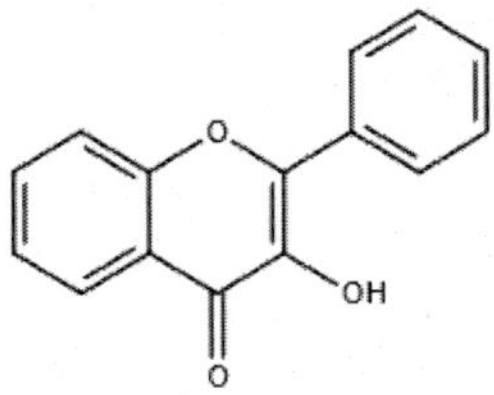 | Brassicas, tea, fenugreek, papaya | [86] |
| Galangin | 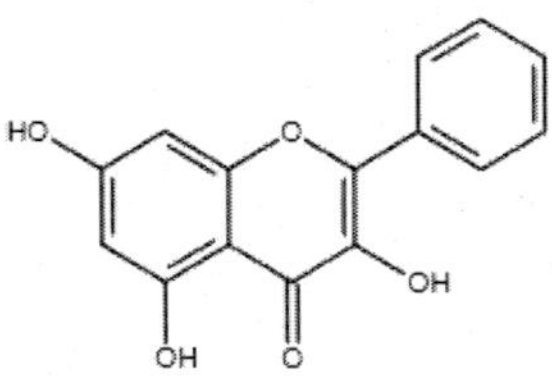 | Ginger, honey, propolis | [87] |
| Kaempferol | 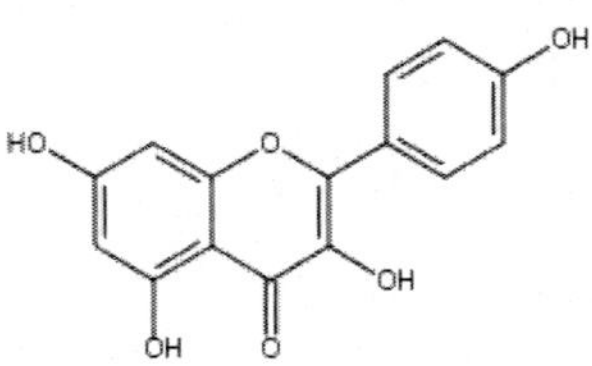 | Capers, saffron, kale, mustard greens, arugula, ginger, beans, onions, watercress, Chinese cabbage | [36] |

**Table 2.1.** (Continued)

| Flavonoid | Structure | Natural sources | Ref. |
|---|---|---|---|
| Fisetin | 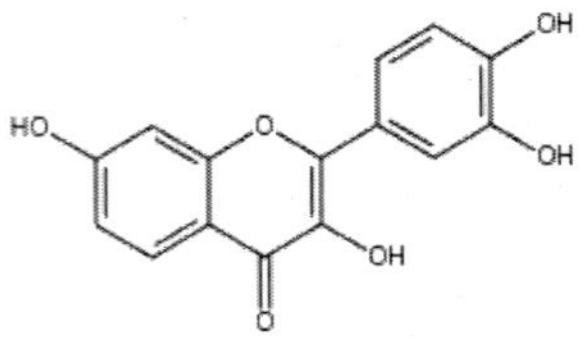 | Many plants, fruits and vegetables, such as parrot tree, honey locust, strawberries, apples, persimmons, grapes, onions and cucumbers | [32, 88] |
| Morin | 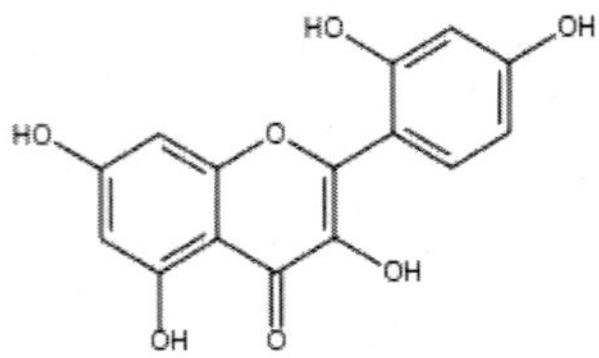 | Many herbs and fruits; mulberry figs and old fustic | [89, 90] |
| Quercetin | 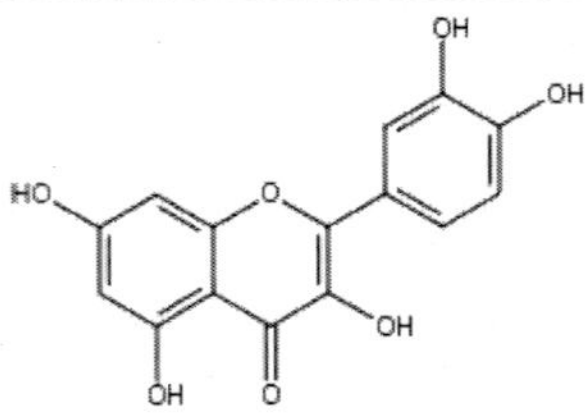 | Capers, lovage leaves, elderberry juice, dock, radish leaves, chokeberry juice, rocket, carob fiber, dill weed, coriander leaves | [36] |
| Myricetin | 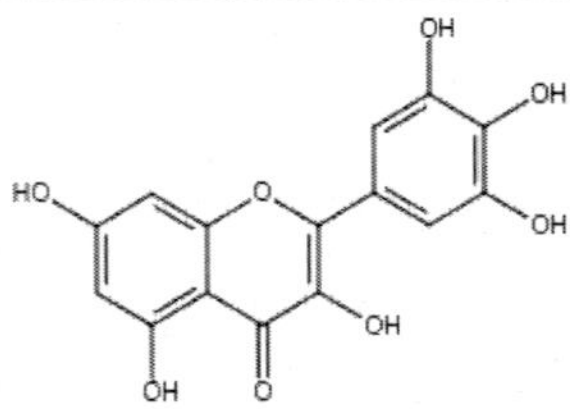 | Carob fiber, kibbles and flour, black currants juice concentrate and raw berries, fennel leaves, parsley, goji berries, bog whortleberries, cranberries and cranberry juice, dock, crowberries, sweet potato leaves | [36] |
| Rhamnetin | 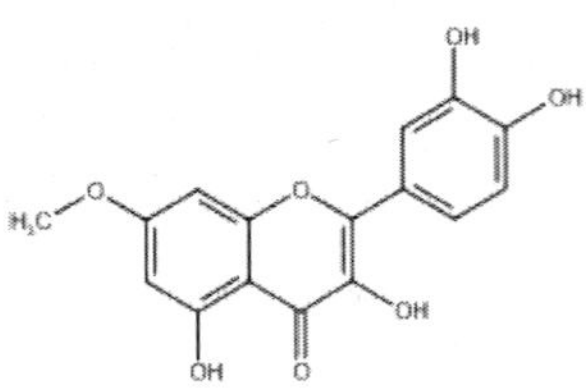 | Flowers, fruits and leaves of various plants, such as *Ginkgo biloba* L. and *Hippophae rhamnoides* L. | [91, 92] |

| Flavonoid | Structure | Natural sources | Ref. |
|---|---|---|---|
| 5,7-Dihydroxy-3,4`,6-trimethoxyflavone (=santin, =centauridin, =3-methylbetuletol) | 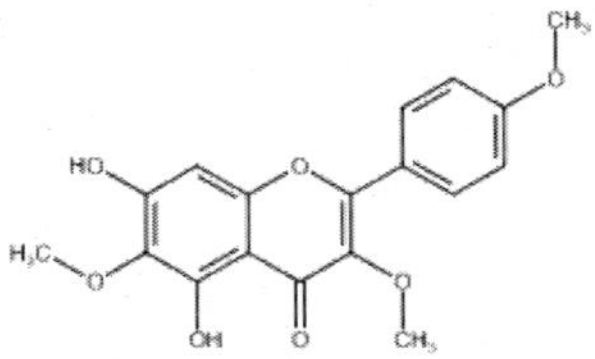 | *Gardenia oudiepe* Vieill. | [93] |
| 3`,5,7-Trihydroxy-3,4`,5`,6-tetramethoxyflavone | 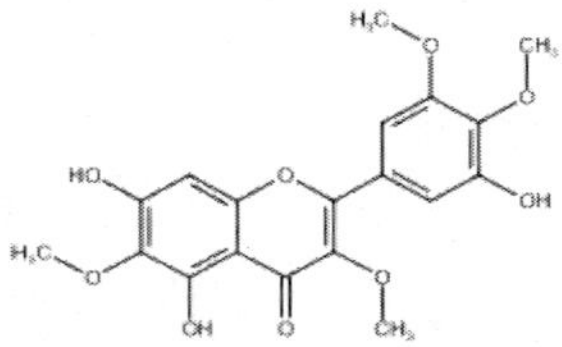 | *Gardenia oudiepe* Vieill. | [93] |
| Rutin | 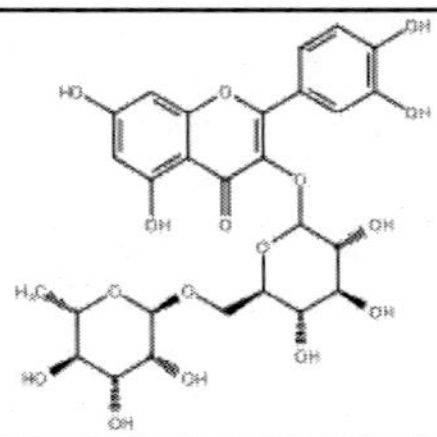 | Many plants, such as passion flower, buckwheat, tea and apple | [94] |
| Icariside II | 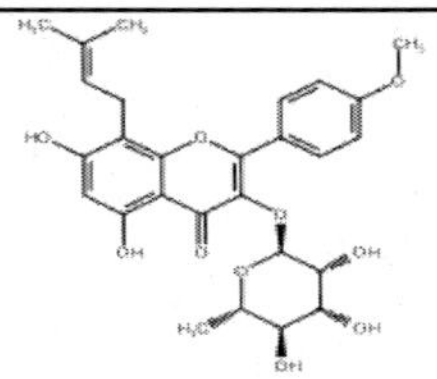 | Stems and leaves of *Epimedium koreanum* Nakai | [95] |
| FLAVANONES | | | |
| Naringenin | 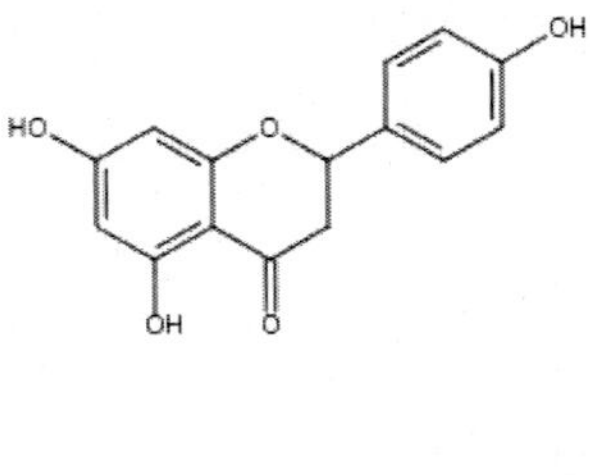 | Oregano, kumquats, grapefruits and grapefruit juice, tangelo juice, pummelo juice and pummelos, rosemary, yuzu, sour orange juice and oranges, artichokes, tangerines | [36] |
| Hesperetin | 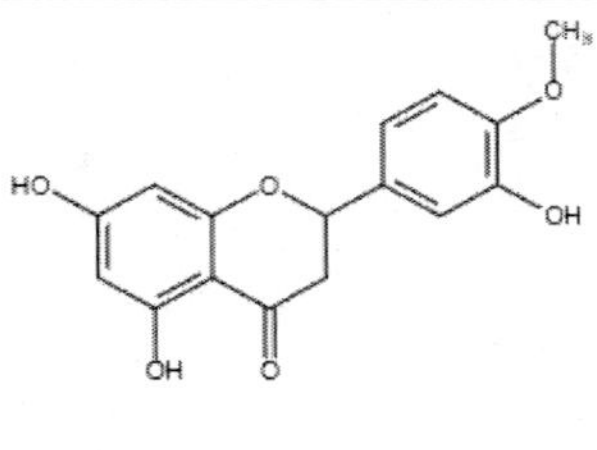 | Tangelo juice, limes and lime juice, yuzu, lemons and lemon juice, oranges and orange juice, tangerine juice and tangerines, tangor juice, peppermint, pummelo | [36] |

**Table 2.1.** (Continued)

| Flavonoid | Structure | Natural sources | Ref. |
|---|---|---|---|
| Naringin | 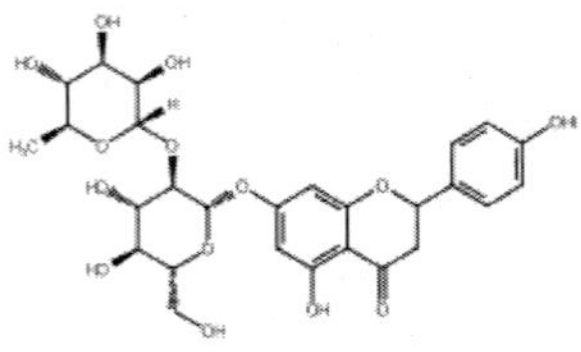 | Citrus fruits, such as grapefruits and grapefruit juice, oranges, pummelo; berries of black elderberry, fruits of *Grewia asiatica* L. | [2, 16, 65] |
| Hesperidin | 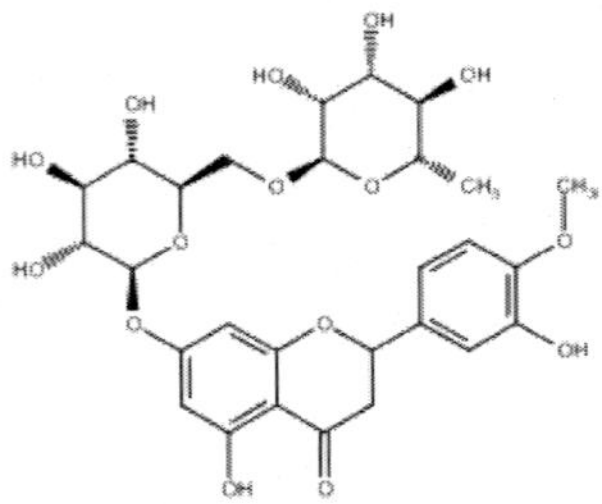 | Citrus fruits, such as oranges | [16, 58] |
| ISOFLAVONES | | | |
| Equol | 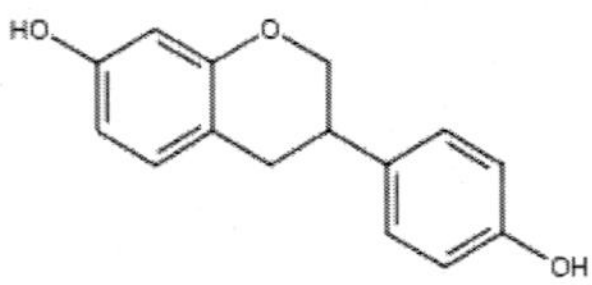 | A bioactive metabolite of daidzein, product of intestinal bacteria | [49, 55, 56] |
| Daidzein | 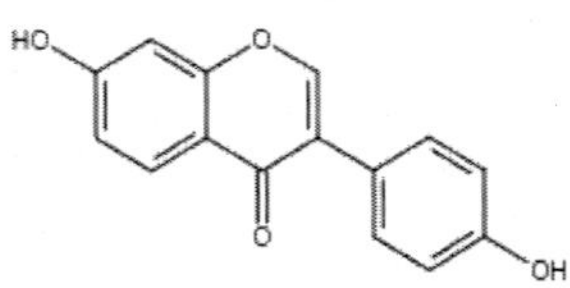 | Soybeans and soy products (soy flour, soy meal, soymilk, soy powder, soy protein, natto, tempeh, miso, tofu, soy paste) | [37] |
| Genistein | 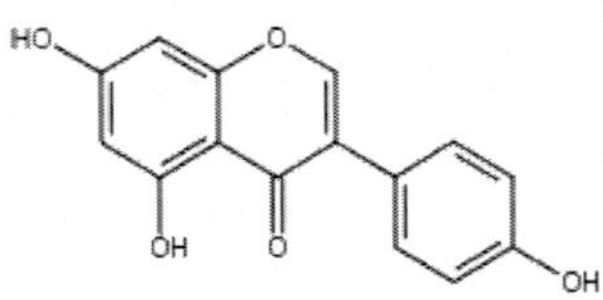 | Soybeans and soy products (soy meal, soymilk, soy flour, soy powder, soy protein, tofu, miso, tempeh, natto, soy paste) | [37] |

| Flavonoid | Structure | Natural sources | Ref. |
|---|---|---|---|
| Formononetin | 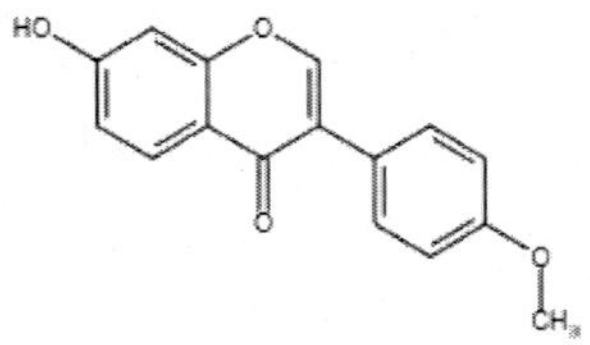 | Red clover, soybeans, clover sprouts, alfalfa seeds, pink and white beans, lima beans | [37] |
| Biochanin A | 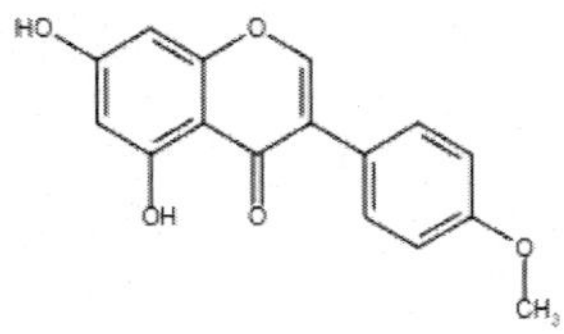 | Chickpeas, kala chana seeds, beans, clover sprouts, cowpeas, lima beans | [37] |
| Glabridin | 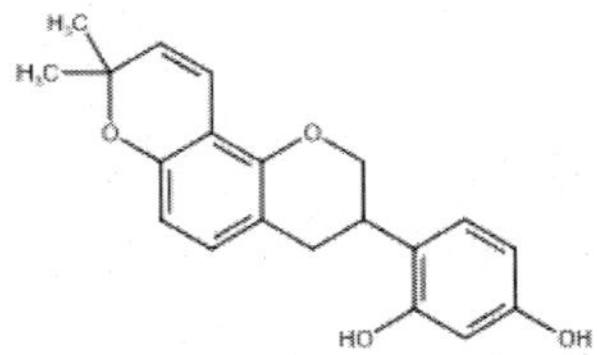 | Licorice roots | [96] |
| Daidzin | 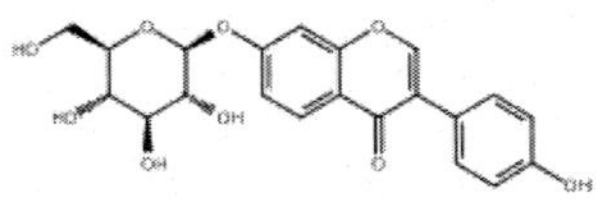 | Soybeans, *Pueraria lobata* (Willd.) Ohwi | [47, 97] |
| ANTHOCYANIDINS | | | |
| Delphinidin | 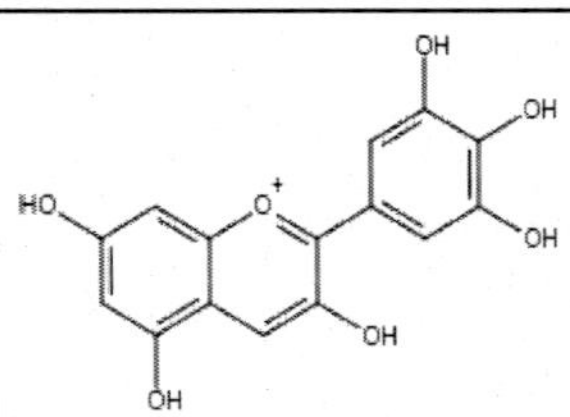 | Black currant juice and berries, bilberries, cowpeas, eggplant, grapes, maqui, serviceberries, blueberries, black beans, jambul | [36] |
| Cyanidin 3-glucoside (=chrysanthemin) | 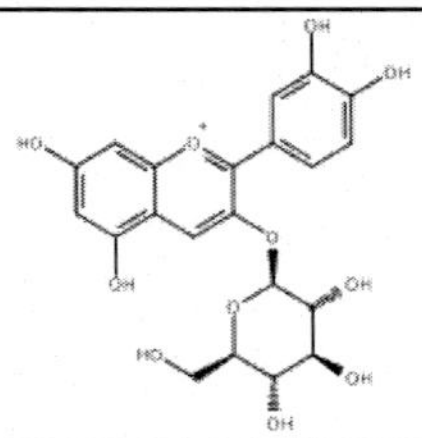 | Black rise | [98] |

**Table 2.1.** (Continued)

| Flavonoid | Structure | Natural sources | Ref. |
|---|---|---|---|
| Delphinidin 3-O-glucoside (=myrtillin) | 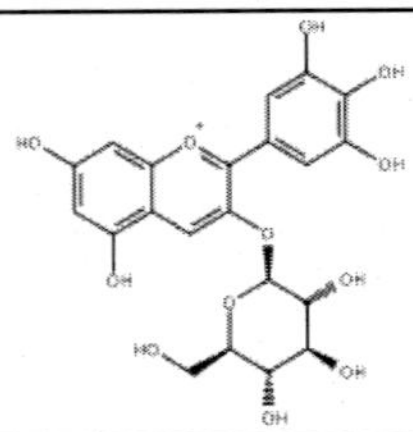 | Bilberry extract | [18] |
| FLAVANONOLS | | | |
| Ampelopsin (=dihydromyricetin) | 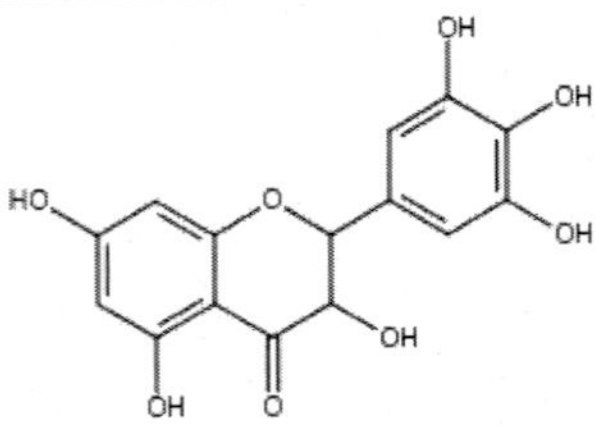 | *Ampelopsis grossedentata* (Hand.-Mazz) W.T.Wang | [99] |
| FLAVONOLIGNANS | | | |
| Silibinin | 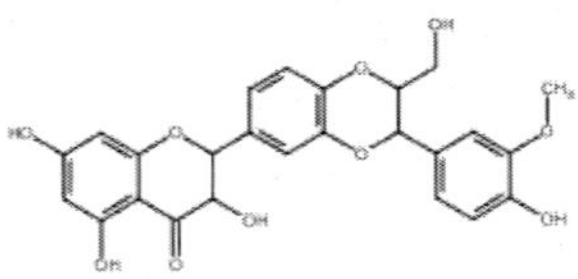 | Seeds of milk thistle (*Silybum marianum* (L.) Gaertn.) | [72, 100-103] |
| CHALCONES | | | |
| Phloretin | 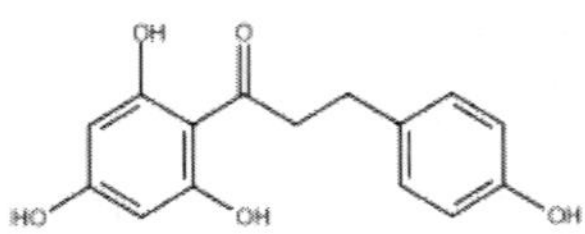 | Fruit, leaves and roots of apple tree | [104] |
| Butein | 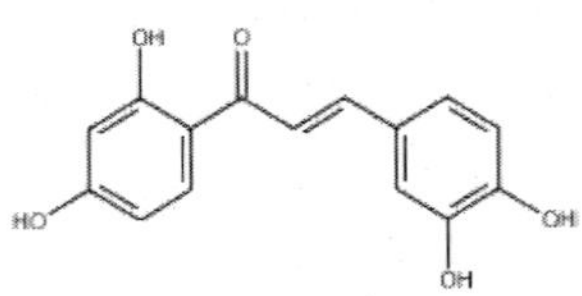 | Numerous plants, such as *Caragana jubata* (Pall.) Poir., *Rhus verniciflua* Stokes, stem bark of *Semecarpus anacardium* L.f. and heartwood of *Dalbergia odorifera* T. Chen | [105] |

| Flavonoid | Structure | Natural sources | Ref. |
|---|---|---|---|
| Licochalcone A | 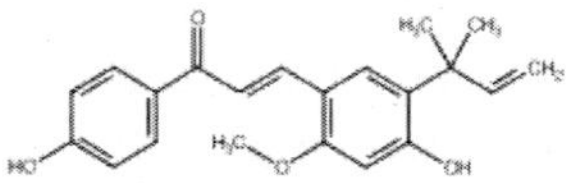 | Root of *Glycyrrhiza inflata* Batalin (licorice) | [106] |
| Flavokawain B | 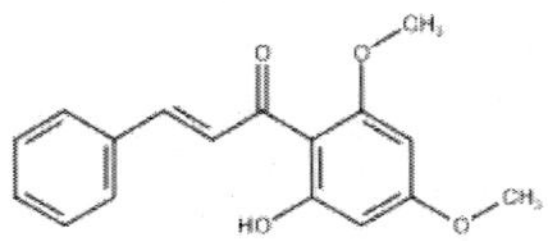 | Kava plant | [107] |
| Flavokawain A | 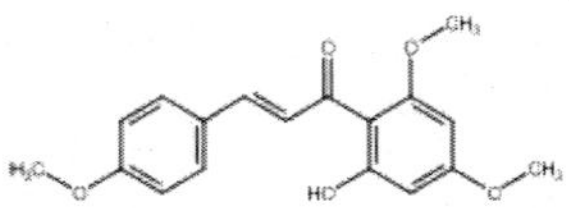 | Kava plant | [22] |
| Oxyfadichalcone C | 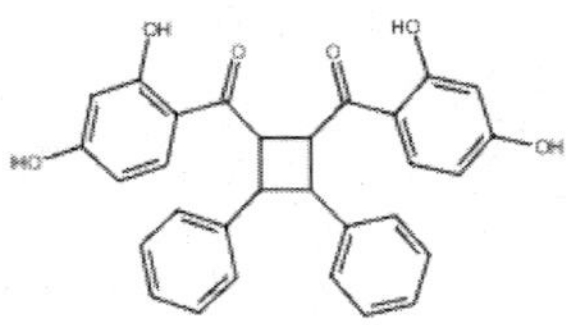 | Chinese traditional medicinal herbs *Oxytropis falcata* Bunge and *Oxytropis chilliophylla* Royle | [8] |

## 2.2. Anticancer Role of Flavonoids: Benefits, Bottlenecks and Solutions

Over the past few decades, plant-derived flavonoids have been demonstrated to exert potent anticancer activities, inhibiting, reversing or retarding multistep carcinogenesis [17, 67, 108]. Numerous *in vitro* and *in vivo* preclinical studies have indeed shown that structurally diverse flavonoids suppress the development, growth and progression of various cancers, in the models of both solid tumors as well as hematological malignancies [29, 32, 54, 109-113]. In doing so, flavonoids can arrest cell cycle, inhibit proliferation, induce differentiation, alter cell metabolism, promote apoptosis, and restrict migration and invasion of cancerous cells, besides suppressing also angiogenesis, mitigating inflammatory tumor microenvironment and stimulating the host immunity [15, 35, 114, 115]. These effects are achieved through intervention in a variety of cellular mechanisms and modulation of diverse signaling pathways associated with neoplastic transformation and malignant progression, by attacking multiple molecular targets [3, 7, 17, 34, 116, 117]. This multitarget action may provide a great advantage to several flavonoids against multifaceted machinery of cancers, especially as compared to synthetic drugs that are primarily focused on modulating single cellular events [114, 118-120]. At that, therapeutic efficacy of flavonoids has been shown to be greatly related to their structure, as the number of hydroxyl groups in phenyl rings and the presence of the 2,3-double bond in pyrane ring play an important role in cytotoxicity of these phytochemicals [29, 121] (Figure 2.1). In many cases, however, the exact molecular mechanisms underlying anticancer activities of flavonoids have still remained unresolved [46, 90, 104, 122]. Most importantly, flavonoids generally exert their anticarcinogenic properties without causing apparent toxicities to normal healthy cells, displaying a high safety profile and low adverse side effects [2, 3, 11, 14, 17, 19, 58, 104, 111, 123]. Such well tolerability is in good correlation with a long history of the human use of flavonoid-rich natural products either as food items or medicinal herbs [102, 103]. Therefore, flavonoids might be beneficial in the treatment of malignant disorders, having a great potential to be developed as novel anticancer drugs.

Nevertheless, despite a huge amount of promising preclinical research, clinical studies evaluating anticancer action of flavonoids in the human body have remained scarce and clinical application of these compounds is still limited [12, 17]. The main reason for this is the fact that pharmacologically active doses are usually not achievable in circulation by dietary intake of flavonoid-rich natural products, due to low water solubility, poor absorption, and extensive phase I and phase II bioconversion of these phytochemicals in the intestinal wall and the liver [25, 39, 40, 50, 101, 124-127]. As a result, many glucuronidated, sulfated and methylated metabolites enter systemic circulation and reach target tissues, bioactivities of which are greatly unknown [2]. In addition, there is a large interindividual variability in flavonoid metabolism, depending primarily on gut microflora and genetic polymorphisms in metabolizing enzymes [46, 56, 128, 129]. Accordingly, oral bioavailability of flavonoids in humans has been shown to be very low, being only 0.1-1.1% for EGCG [127], less than 2% for quercetin [12, 124, 126], around 15% for pure naringenin [2] and about 5-9% for naringin [2].

The conjugates and unabsorbed flavonoids are further metabolized by microbes to yield phenolic catabolites, which are excreted from the body in the urine and feces [2]. As a consequence of poor bioavailability, plasma concentrations of flavonoids attained after oral intake are usually remarkably lower than the levels shown to be required for biological responses in preclinical studies. For example, EGCG concentrations after oral administration of green tea (three tea bags containing 213 mg of EGCG) and green tea supplements (three capsules containing 193 mg of EGCG) in men were found to be 80 nM and 150 nM, respectively, whereas the maximal plasma levels of total flavanols (EGCG, ECG, EGC and epicatechin) after oral administration of green tea reached only 1.2 μM [127]. Similarly, total plasma concentrations of isoflavones have been reported to reach low micromolar range (1-5 μM), following to consumption of soy-rich diets [47, 50, 52]. The circulating concentrations of genistein in humans consuming high soy diets, typical for Asian countries, usually remain about 0.5 μM, while being only 7-18 nM in people depending on standard Western diets [130-132]. Actually, maximum plasma levels after consuming 50 mg of pure genistein or daidzein were reported to be 1.26 μM and 0.76 μM [133]. The peak serum levels of quercetin were shown to be 0.8 μM after an onion meal [21]. Plasma concentrations of naringenin in healthy volunteers were measured to be 0.6 μM and 6.0 μM after consumption of orange or grapefruit juices (8 ml/kg), respectively [2]. Hence, such poor bioavailability of flavonoids demands high dosage to overcome their subtherapeutic levels in circulation [134]. Plasma levels can be indeed risen upon supplement intake, reaching 3 μM EGCG in people taking 800 mg of EGCG supplements after fasting [135] or 10 μM genistein after moderate intake of soy isoflavone supplements [50, 130] or even up to 27 μM genistein after administration of high doses (300-600 mg) of soy extracts daily [130, 136]. Moreover, it is possible that tissue levels of flavonoids at their actual sites of action might be significantly higher than their concentrations in the plasma [128, 137].

Innovative methods are of great significance to enhance oral bioavailability of flavonoids, thereby increasing also the potential for their clinical applicability in future. One possibility to improve bioavailability of flavonoids includes delivering these bioactive plant metabolites on different nanosized carriers, such as polymeric matrices, lipid-based vehicles, micelles or inclusion complexes [2, 12, 101, 127, 138]. In general, a vehicle should encapsulate and retain the bioactive agent by protecting it from oxidative and enzymatic environment, escape the immune system, prolong the circulation time and then release the agent in the targeted diseased organs, while reducing residual toxicity and off-target accumulation [125, 134, 139]. Site specific or organ targeting action of nanocarriers can be further amplified through conjugating certain ligands to the surface of nanoparticles, such as monoclonal antibodies, folic acid, biotin, oligopeptides and hyaluronic acid, employing as tumor-specific guiding moieties. Target molecules for these ligands are indeed frequently overexpressed in cancerous cells [125, 139, 140]. Moreover, dual loading of bioactive compounds into nanoformulations has also drawn considerable attention in the recent years, with the aim to improve therapeutic benefits of anticancer agents by delivering them in different synergistic combinations to the same tumor cell [124]. Another attractive option to overcome low bioavailability of flavonoids is designing of pro-drugs and derivatives of these phytochemicals with better physicochemical and pharmacokinetic properties [127, 141]. Hence, the development of novel analogs of flavonoids has gained a lot of attention in the past few years, as a result of which a novel chemically modified form of EGCG with added peracetate protections to its reactive hydroxyl groups was shown to possess higher bioavailability, stability and anticancer activities [6, 127, 142]. Furthermore, bioavailability of specific flavonoids can be improved also by their co-administration with other natural compounds, as has been demonstrated for EGCG when given with black pepper-derived piperine to mice [127].

## 2.3. Interactions between Flavonoids and Anticancer Drugs: Novel Perspectives in Cancer Therapy

Because of various reported health benefits, the consumption of over-the-counter flavonoid-rich dietary supplements and herbal products has been growing increasingly during the past decade [25, 49, 143]. Based on different estimations, more than half of cancer survivors have taken dietary supplements and herbal remedies with the aim to enhance their overall health, support conventional therapy and combat cancer more effectively, but also to alleviate drugs-related adverse side effects, such as menopausal symptoms, and mitigate depression and anxiety associated with diagnosis and classical treatments [51, 68, 144]. Moreover, a lot of cancer patients use such supplements concurrently with conventional anticancer drugs, although the possible interactions between flavonoids and drugs are still largely unknown [20]. As some anticancer drugs, such as hormonal therapies, are often prescribed for taking over a long period (even up to ten years) and are associated with several side effects that substantially impair quality of life, many patients decide to simultaneously consume diverse natural supplements, mostly without the knowledge of their health care providers. However, this can potentially lead to compromising the drug safety and efficacy [40, 49, 68].

Although relatively little is still known, naturally occurring flavonoids may cause clinically relevant interactions with cancer drugs, affecting the drug activities through multiple mechanisms [29, 70]. In general, the concurrent use of flavonoids-rich dietary and herbal supplements with conventional medications can mimic, enhance or reduce the activities of either component, resulting in flavonoid-drug interactions with both additive, synergistic as well as antagonistic outcomes [7, 70]. The possible adverse interactions are probably most disturbing and cautionary, representing a significant clinical concern [38, 40]. In principle, flavonoids can influence the therapeutic efficacy of cancer drugs in three major ways (Figure 2.2). Firstly, the presence of flavonoids may cause altered pharmacokinetics of co-administered oral anticancer drugs through various mechanisms, including modulation of different phase I enzymes (cytochrome P450 (CYP) enzymes) and phase II enzymes, as well as intestinal and hepatic uptake and efflux transporters [25, 38, 40, 70, 143, 145-147]. Hence, pharmacokinetic drug-flavonoid interaction can occur in the intestinal, hepatic, biliary and renal systems, leading to alterations in absorption, metabolism, distribution and excretion processes of drugs [25, 38, 70]. Over the past years, a number of preclinical studies on rat model have been performed to unravel the molecular mechanisms under pharmacokinetic interactions between different anticancer drugs and structurally diverse flavonoids [25]. As a result, several flavonoids have been demonstrated to be able to modulate metabolic conversion and transport of orally administered anticancer drugs, ultimately leading to increase or decrease in their plasma levels and altered exposure to malignant tissues [25, 143, 145]. Therefore, opportunities exist for combining anticancer drugs with specific flavonoids for enhancing bioavailability of the drug, resulting in reduction of dosages and improving the therapeutic index [25, 147]. Without doubt, more preclinical investigations are needed on pharmacokinetic interactions between different flavonoids (flavonoid-containing natural products and dietary supplements) and anticancer drugs, not only to select the most appropriate combinations for further clinical trials and potential therapeutic use, but also for preventing possible adverse reactions [70].

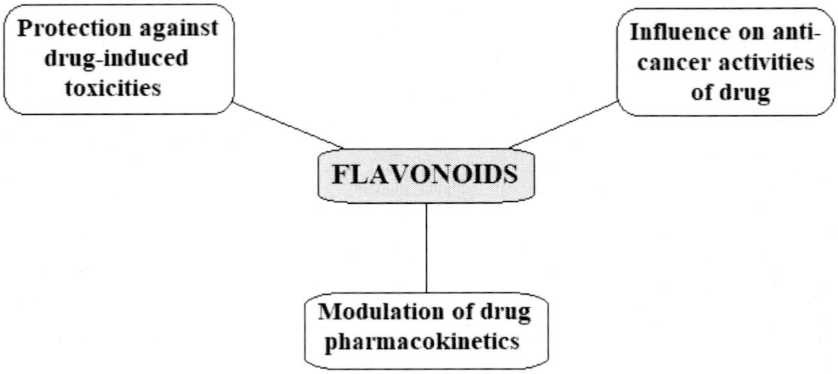


**Figure 2.2.** Spectrum of the effects of flavonoids on conventional anticancer drugs.

Secondly, numerous preclinical studies have recently demonstrated that flavonoids can improve the therapeutic efficacy of anticancer drugs in a variety of human cancers, by acting themselves as antitumoral agents and inhibiting malignant growth and progression through attacking different targets and regulating multiple signal transduction pathways [3, 17, 29, 78, 148-151]. Potentiation of antiproliferative and cytotoxic effects of anticancer drugs may be regulated by diverse mechanisms, including prooxidant properties of flavonoids, but also intervening in the cell cycle and modulating apoptotic and autophagic processes [7]. Moreover, flavonoids might sensitize malignant cells to conventional drugs also by suppressing survival cascades activated via compensatory feedback mechanisms in response to the drugs, resulting in reversal of resistance to therapeutic agents [115, 148]. Multidrug resistance phenomenon can be overcome by flavonoids also through downregulation of ATP-binding cassette (ABC) transporters, such as P-gp or BCRP, and inhibition of the efflux of drugs, thereby increasing their retention time in tumoral cells and improving treatment success [25, 131, 152, 153]. Furthermore, augmentation of therapeutic efficacy of anticancer drugs can allow to reduce the drug doses, leading to decrease in toxicities on normal healthy cells and controlling undesirable side effects [14, 139, 154, 155]. Nevertheless, although combination of drugs and flavonoids may lead to additive and synergistic outcomes against various cancer types, in certain situations, antagonistic interactions may also appear, leading to impairment of the drug efficacy and showing that caution must be exercised when flavonoid-rich dietary supplements or herbal products are consumed concurrently with conventional anticancer drugs [3, 7, 116, 149, 151]. Therefore, much more studies with cancer cell lines *in vitro* and animal tumor models *in vivo* are required to investigate the molecular mechanisms underlying interactions between anticancer drugs and flavonoids, in order to ultimately convert them into effective clinical practice [7, 148].

Thirdly, besides reducing the spectrum of drug-related adverse effects through lowering the therapeutically effective doses in combinational therapies, flavonoids can also directly protect normal tissues against anticancer drug-induced toxicities, due to their strong antioxidant potential [148, 156]. There is growing evidence that anticancer drug-elicited tissue damage is associated with free radical injury and oxidative stress, being characterized by altered non-enzymatic and enzymatic antioxidant systems and/or increased lipid peroxidation [10]. Naturally occurring flavonoids might play important roles in the protection against oxidative damage caused by conventional anticancer therapies, especially by preventing the drug-induced hepatotoxicity and cardiotoxicity [4, 101, 124, 157].

Collectively, based on the huge amount of promising preclinical studies, there is a growing interest in exploring the novel opportunities to combine conventional anticancer drugs with specific plant-derived flavonoids for application in the clinical practice in future. Such combinational approach might bring current cancer therapy to even more personalized level to improve treatment success of individual patients. However, more research is still needed to unravel precise molecular mechanisms behind the multifaceted interactions between anticancer drugs and flavonoids, to prevent possible adverse reactions and further augment the therapeutic benefit. In doing so, *in vitro* studies remain the mainstay of the initial evaluation of promising combinations, due to easy operation, high throughput nature and relatively low costs of these investigations, providing valuable input for further *in vivo* research and ultimately establishing a good basis for designing of clinical trials.

The two following chapters of this book are devoted to diverse interactions between hormonal cancer therapies and plant-derived flavonoids (Chapter 3), and targeted biological therapies and flavonoids (Chapter 4).

## References

[1] Tu SH, Ho CT, Liu MF, Huang CS, Chang HW, Chang CH, Wu CH, Ho YS. Luteolin sensitises drug-resistant human breast cancer cells to

tamoxifen via the inhibition of cyclin E2 expression. *Food Chem* 2013; 141: 1553-61.

[2] Memariani Z, Abbas SQ, UI Hassan SS, Ahmadi A, Chabra A. Naringin and naringenin as anticancer agents and adjuvants in cancer combination therapy: Efficacy and molecular mechanisms of action, a comprehensive narrative review. *Pharmacol Res* 2021; 171: 105264.

[3] Lewandowska U, Gorlach S, Owczarek K, Hrabec E, Szewczyk K. Synergistic interactions between anticancer chemotherapeutics and phenolic compounds and anticancer synergy between polyphenols. *Postepy Hig Med Dosw* 2014; 68: 528-40.

[4] El-Beshbishy HA. Hepatoprotective effect of green tea (Camellia sinensis) extract against tamoxifen-induced liver injury in rats. *J Biochem Mol Biol* 2005; 38: 563-70.

[5] Yaacob NS, Nengsih A, Norazmi MN. Tualang honey promotes apoptotic cell death induced by tamoxifen in breast cancer cell lines. *Evid Based Complement Alternat Med* 2013; 2013: 989841.

[6] Liu J, Zhong T, Yi P, Fan C, Zhang Z, Liang G, Xu Y, Fan Y. A new epigallocatechin gallate derivative isolated from Anhua dark tea sensitizes the chemosensitivity of gefitinib via the suppression of PI3K/mTOR and epithelial-mesenchymal transition. *Fitoterapia* 2020; 143: 104590.

[7] Guneidy RA, Gad AM, Zaki ER, Ibrahim FM, Shokeer A. Antioxidant or pro-oxidant and glutathione transferase P1-1 inhibiting activities for Tamarindus indica seeds and their cytotoxic effect on MCF-7 cancer cell line. *J Genet Eng Biotechnol* 2020; 18: 74.

[8] Peng X, Wang Z, Liu Y, Peng X, Liu Y, Zhu S, Zhang Z, Qiu Y, Jin M, Wang R, Zhang Q, Kong D. Oxyfadichalcone C inhibits melanoma A375 cell proliferation and metastasis via suppressing PI3K/Akt and MAPK/ERK pathways. *Life Sci* 2018; 206: 35-44.

[9] Demain AL, Vaishnav P. Natural products for cancer chemotherapy. *Microb Biotechnol* 2011; 4: 687-99.

[10] Parvez S, Tabassum H, Rehman H, Banerjee BD, Athar M, Raisuddin S. Catechin prevents tamoxifen-induced oxidative stress and biochemical perturbations in mice. *Toxicology* 2006; 225: 109-18.

[11] Esmaeili MA. Combination of siRNA-directed gene silencing with epigallocatechin-3-gallate (EGCG) reverses drug resistance in human breast cancer cells. *J Chem Biol* 2015; 9: 41-52.

[12] Hyun HB, Moon JY, Cho SK. Quercetin suppresses CYR61-mediated multidrug resistance in human gastric adenocarcinoma AGS cells. *Molecules* 2018; 23: 209.

[13] Li C, Kim M, Choi H, Choi J. Effects of baicalein on the pharmacokinetics of tamoxifen and its main metabolite, 4-hydroxytamoxifen, in rats: possible role of cytochrome P450 3A4 and P-glycoprotein inhibition by baicalein. *Arch Pharm Res* 2011; 34: 1965-72.

[14] Kim JH, Song M, Kang GH, Lee ER, Choi HY, Lee C, Kim JH, Kim Y, Koo BN, Cho SG. Combined treatment of 3-hydroxyflavone and imatinib mesylate increases apoptotic cell death of imatinib mesylate-resistant leukemia cells. *Leuk Res* 2012; 36: 1157-64.

[15] Sanaei M, Kavoosi F, Atashpour S, Haghighat S. Effects of genistein and synergistic action in combination with tamoxifen on the HepG2 human hepatocellular carcinoma cell line. *Asian Pac J Cancer Prev* 2017; 18: 2381-5.

[16] Guthrie N, Carroll KK. Inhibition of mammary cancer by citrus flavonoids. *Adv Exp Med Biol* 1998; 439: 227-36.

[17] Liskova A, Samec M, Koklesova L, Brockmueller A, Zhai K, Abdellatif B, Siddiqui M, Biringer K, Kudela E, Pec M, Gadanec LK, Sudomova M, Hassan STS, Zulli A, Shakibaei M, Giordano FA, Büsselberg D. Golubnitschaja O, Kubatka P. Flavonoids as an effective sensitizer for anti-cancer therapy: insights into multi-faceted mechanisms and applicability towards individualized patient profiles. *EPMA J* 2021; 12: 155-76.

[18] Aichinger G, Pahlke G, Nagel LJ, Berger W, Marko D. Bilberry extract, its major polyphenolic compounds, and the soy isoflavone genistein antagonize the cytostatic drug erlotinib in human epithelial cells. *Food Funct* 2016; 7: 3628-36.

[19] Tolomeo M, Grimaudo S, Di Cristina A, Pipitone RM, Dusonchet L, Meli M, Crosta L, Gebbia N, Invidiata FP, Titone L, Simoni D. Galangin increases the cytotoxic activity of imatinib mesylate in imatinib-sensitive and imatinib-resistant Bcr-Abl expressing leukemia cells. *Cancer Lett* 2008; 265: 289-97.

[20] Jia L, Liu FT. Why bortezomib cannot go with 'green'? *Cancer Biol Med* 2013; 10: 206-13.

[21] Liu FT, Agrawal SG, Movasaghi Z, Wyatt PB, Rehman IU, Gribben JG, Newland AC, Jia L. Dietary flavonoids inhibit the anticancer effects of the proteasome inhibitor bortezomib. *Blood* 2008; 112: 3835-46.

[22] Jandial DD, Krill LS, Chen L, Wu C, Ke Y, Xie J, Hoang BH, Zi X. Induction of G2M arrest by flavokawain A, a kava chalcone, increases the responsiveness of HER2-overexpressing breast cancer cells to herceptin. *Molecules* 2017; 22: 462.

[23] Selim ME, Aleisa NA, Daghestani MH. Evaluation of the possible protective role of quercetin on letrozole-induced testicular injury in male albino rats. *Ultrastruct Pathol* 2013; 37: 204-17.

[24] Li C, Lim SC, Kim J, Choi JS. Effects of myricetin, an anticancer compound, on the bioavailability and pharmacokinetics of tamoxifen and its main metabolite, 4-hydroxytamoxifen, in rats. *Eur J Drug Metab Pharmacokinet* 2011; 36: 175-82.

[25] Srinivas NR. Recent trends in preclinical drug-drug interaction studies of flavonoids – Review of case studies, issues and perspectives. *Phytother Res* 2015; 29: 1679-91.

[26] Singh SP, Wahajuddin, Ali MM, Kohli K, Jain GK. Liquid chromatography-mass spectrometry method for the quantification of tamoxifen and its metabolite 4-hydroxytamoxifen in rat plasma: application to interaction study with biochanin A (an isoflavone). *J Chromatogr B Analyt Technol Biomed Life Sci* 2011; 879: 2845-51.

[27] Shin SC, Choi JS. Effects of epigallocatechin gallate on the oral bioavailability and pharmacokinetics of tamoxifen and its main metabolite, 4-hydroxytamoxifen, in rats. *Anticancer Drugs* 2009; 20: 584-8.

[28] Tanos V, Brzezinski A, Drize O, Strauss N, Peretz T. Synergistic inhibitory effects of genistein and tamoxifen on human dysplastic and malignant epithelial breast cells in vitro. *Eur J Obstet Gynecol Reprod Biol* 2002; 102: 188-94.

[29] Danisman Kalindemirtas F, Birman H, Candöken E, Bilgis Gazioglu S, Melikoglu G, Kuruca S. Cytotoxic effects of some flavonoids and imatinib on the K562 chronic myeloid leukemia cell line: Data analysis using the combination index method. *Balkan Med J* 2019; 36: 96-105.

[30] Glynn SJ, Gaffney KJ, Sainz MA, Louie SG, Petasis NA. Molecular characterization of the boron adducts of the proteasome inhibitor bortezomib with epigallocatechin-3-gallate and related polyphenols. *Org Biomol Chem* 2015; 13: 3887-99.

[31] Galal AAA, Mohamed AA, Khater SI, Metwally MMM. Beneficial role of biochanin A on cutaneous and renal tissues of ovariectomized rats treated with anastrozole. *Life Sci* 2018; 201: 9-16.

[32] Zhang L, Huang Y, Zhuo W, Zhu Y, Zhu B, Chen Z. Fisetin, a dietary phytochemical, overcomes Erlotinib-resistance of lung adenocarcinoma cells through inhibition of MAPK and AKT pathways. *Am J Transl Res* 2016; 8: 4857-68.

[33] Gao H, Jiang Q, Han Y, Peng J, Wang C. Hispidulin potentiates the antitumor effect of sunitinib against human renal cell carcinoma in laboratory models. *Cell Biochem Biophys* 2015; 71: 757-64.

[34] Xu Z, Huang B, Liu J, Wu X, Luo N, Wang X, Zheng X, Pan X. Combinatorial anti-proliferative effects of tamoxifen and naringenin: The role of four estrogen receptor subtypes. *Toxicology* 2018; 410: 231-46.

[35] Xu Z, Zhao D, Zheng X, Huang B, Xia X, Pan X. Quercetin exerts bidirectional regulation effects on the efficacy of tamoxifen in estrogen receptor-positive breast cancer therapy: An in vitro study. *Environ Toxicol* 2020; 35: 1179-93.

[36] Bhagwat S, Haytowitz DB. USDA Database for the Flavonoid Content of Selected Foods. Release 3.2 (November 2015). Nutrient Data Laboratory, Beltsville Human Nutrition Research Center, ARS, USDA, 2016. https://doi.org/10.15482/USDA.ADC/1324465.

[37] Bhagwat S, Haytowitz DB. USDA Database for the Isoflavone Content of Selected Foods, Release 2.1 (November 2015). Nutrient Data Laboratory, Beltsville Human Nutrition Research Center, ARS, USDA, 2015. https://doi.org/10.15482/USDA.ADC/1324538.

[38] Albassam AA, Markowitz JS. An appraisal of drug-drug interactions with green tea (Camellia sinensis). *Planta Med* 2017; 83: 496-508.

[39] Yiannakopoulou EC. Interaction of green tea catechins with breast cancer endocrine treatment: a systematic review. *Pharmacology* 2014; 94: 245-8.

[40] Tian DD, Kellogg JJ, Okut N, Oberlies NH, Cech NB, Shen DD, McCune JS, Paine MF. Identification of intestinal UDP-glucuronosyltransferase inhibitors in green tea (Camellia sinensis) using a biochemometric approach: Application to raloxifene as a test drug via in vitro to in vivo extrapolation. *Drug Metab Dispos* 2018; 46: 552-60.

[41] Ge J, Tan BX, Chen Y, Yang L, Peng XC, Li HZ, Lin HJ, Zhao Y, Wei M, Cheng K, Li LH, Dong H, Gao F, He JP, Wu Y, Qiu M, Zhao YL, Su JM, Hou JM, Liu JY. Interaction of green tea polyphenol epigallocatechin-3-gallate with sunitinib: potential risk of diminished sunitinib bioavailability. *J Mol Med* 2011; 89: 595-602.

[42] Modernelli A, Naponelli V, Giovanna Troglio M, Bonacini M, Ramazzina I, Bettuzzi S, Rizzi F. EGCG antagonizes bortezomib cytotoxicity in prostate cancer cells by an autophagic mechanism. *Sci Rep* 2015; 5: 15270.

[43] Way TD, Lee HH, Kao MC, Lin JK. Black tea polyphenol theaflavins inhibit aromatase activity and attenuate tamoxifen resistance in HER2/neu-transfected human breast cancer cells through tyrosine kinase suppression. *Eur J Cancer* 2004; 40: 2165-74.

[44] Du M, Yang X, Hartman JA, Cooke PS, Doerge DR, Ju YH, Helferich WG. Low-dose dietary genistein negates the therapeutic effect of tamoxifen in athymic nude mice. *Carcinogenesis* 2012; 33: 895-901.

[45] Liu B, Edgerton S, Yang X, Kim A, Ordonez-Ercan D, Mason T, Alvarez K, McKimmey C, Liu N, Thor A. Low-dose dietary phytoestrogen abrogates tamoxifen-associated mammary tumor prevention. *Cancer Res* 2005; 65: 879-86.

[46] Guha N, Kwan ML, Quesenberry Jr CP, Weltzien EK, Castillo AL, Caan BJ. Soy isoflavones and risk of cancer recurrence in a cohort of breast cancer survivors: the Life After Cancer Epidemiology study. *Breast Cancer Res Treat* 2009; 118: 395-405.

[47] Messina MJ, Wood CE. Soy isoflavones, estrogen therapy, and breast cancer risk: analysis and commentary. *Nutr J* 2008; 7: 17.

[48] Magee PJ, Rowland I. Soy products in the management of breast cancer. *Curr Opin Clin Nutr Metab Care* 2012; 15: 586-91.

[49] Constantinou AI, White BE, Tonetti D, Yang Y, Liang W, Li W, van Breemen RB. The soy isoflavone daidzein improves the capacity of tamoxifen to prevent mammary tumours. *Eur J Cancer* 2005; 41: 647-54.

[50] Chen J, Halls SC, Alfaro JF, Zhou Z, Hu M. Potential beneficial metabolic interactions between tamoxifen and isoflavones via cytochrome P450-mediated pathways in female rat liver microsomes. *Pharm Res* 2004; 21: 2095-104.

[51] Ju YH, Doerge DR, Allred KF, Allred CD, Helferich WG. Dietary genistein negates the inhibitory effect of tamoxifen on growth of estrogen-dependent human breast cancer (MCF-7) cells implanted in athymic mice. *Cancer Res* 2002; 62: 2474-7.

[52] Jones JL, Daley BJ, Enderson BL, Zhou JR, Karlstad MD. Genistein inhibits tamoxifen effects on cell proliferation and cell cycle arrest in T47D breast cancer cells. *Am Surg* 2002; 68: 575-8.

[53] Zhang X, Cook KL, Warri A, Cruz IM, Rosim M, Riskin J, Helferich W, Doerge D, Clarke R, Hilakivi-Clarke L. Lifetime genistein intake increases the response of mammary tumors to tamoxifen in rats. *Clin Cancer Res* 2017; 23: 814-24.

[54] Honndorf VS, Wiehr S, Rolle AM, Schmitt J, Kreft L, Quintanilla-Martinez L, Kohlhofer U, Reischl G, Maurer A, Boldt K, Schwarz M, Schmidt H, Pichler BJ. Preclinical evaluation of the anti-tumor effects of the natural isoflavone genistein in two xenograft mouse models monitored by [18F]FDG, [18F]FLT, and [64Cu]NODAGA-cetuximab small animal PET. *Oncotarget* 2016; 7: 28247-61.

[55] Charalambous C, Pitta CA, Constantinou AI. Equol enhances tamoxifen`s anti-tumor activity by induction of caspase-mediated apoptosis in MCF-7 breast cancer cells. *BMC Cancer* 2013; 13: 238.

[56] Hatono M, Ikeda H, Suzuki Y, Kajiwara Y, Kawada K, Tsukioki T, Kochi M, Suzawa K, Iwamoto T, Yamamoto H, Shien T, Yamane M,

Taira N, Doihara H, Toyooka S. Effect of isoflavones on breast cancer cell development and their impact on breast cancer treatments. *Breast Cancer Res Treat* 2021; 185: 307-16.

[57] Ju YH, Doerge DR, Woodling KA, Hartman JA, Kwak J, Helferich WG. Dietary genistein negates the inhibitory effect of letrozole on the growth or aromatase-expressing estrogen-dependent human breast cancer cells (MCF-7Ca) in vivo. *Carcinogenesis* 2008; 29: 2162-8.

[58] Khamis AAA, Ali EMM, El-Moneim MAA, Abd-Alhaseeb MM, El-Magd MA, Salim EI. Hesperidin, piperine and bee venom synergistically potentiate the anticancer effect of tamoxifen against breast cancer cells. *Biomed Pharmacother* 2018; 105: 1335-43.

[59] Bracke ME, Boterberg T, Depypere HT, Stove C, Leclercq G, Mareel MM. The citrus methoxyflavone tangeretin affects human cell-cell interactions. *Adv Exp Med Biol* 2002; 505: 135-9.

[60] Gaber M, Hany M, Mokhtar S, Helmy MW, Elkodairy KA, Elzoghby AO. Boronic-targeted albumin-shell oily-core nanocapsules for synergistic aromatase inhibitor/herbal breast cancer therapy. *Mater Sci Eng C Mater Biol Appl* 2019; 105: 110099.

[61] Rahideh ST, Keramatipour M, Nourbakhsh M, Koohdani F, Hoseini M, Shidfar F. The effects of nobiletin, hesperetin, and letrozole in a combination on the activity and expression of aromatase in breast cancer cells. *Cell Mol Biol* 2017; 63: 9-13.

[62] Arya A, Khandelwal K, Singh A, Ahmad H, Agrawal S, Khatik R, Mittapelly N, Dwivedi AK. Validation of RP-HPLC method for simultaneous quantification of bicalutamide and hesperetin in polycaprolactone-bicalutamide-hesperetin-chitosan nanoparticles. *J Chromatogr Sci* 2015; 53: 1485-90.

[63] Yen JH, Lin CY, Chuang CH, Chin HK, Wu MJ, Chen PY. Nobiletin promotes megakaryocytic differentiation through the MAPK/ERK-dependent EGR1 expression and exerts anti-leukemic effects in human chronic myeloid leukemia (CML) K562 cells. *Cells* 2020; 9: 877.

[64] Phromnoi K, Prasad S, Gupta SC, Kannappan R, Reuter S, Limtrakul P, Aggarwal BB. Dihydroxypentamethoxyflavone down-regulates constitutive and inducible signal transducers and activators of transcription-3 through the induction of tyrosine phosphatase SHP-1. *Mol Pharmacol* 2011; 80: 889-99.

[65] Choi JS, Kang KW. Enhanced tamoxifen bioavailability after oral administration of tamoxifen in rats pretreated with naringin. *Arch Pharm Res* 2008; 31: 1631-6.

[66] Bracke ME, Depypere HT, Boterberg T, Van Marck VL, Vennekens KM, Vanluchene E, Nuytinck M, Serreyn R, Mareel MM. Influence of

tangeretin on tamoxifen`s therapeutic benefit in mammary cancer. *J Natl Cancer Inst* 1999; 91: 354-9.

[67] Sartippour MR, Pietras R, Marquez-Garban DC, Chen HW, Heber D, Henning SM, Sartippour G, Zhang L, Lu M, Weinberg O, Rao JY, Brooks MN. The combination of green tea and tamoxifen is effective against breast cancer. *Carcinogenesis* 2006; 27: 2424-33.

[68] Golden EB, Lam PY, Kardosh A, Gaffney KJ, Cadenas E, Louie SG, Petasis NA, Chen TC, Schönthal AH. Green tea polyphenols block the anticancer effects of bortezomib and other boronic acid-based proteasome inhibitors. *Blood* 2009; 113: 5927-37.

[69] Shah JJ, Kuhn DJ, Orlowski RZ. Bortezomib and EGCG: no green tea for you? *Blood* 2009; 113: 5695-6.

[70] Singh SP, Wahajuddin, Raju KS, Ali MM, Kohli K, Jain GK. Reduced bioavailability of tamoxifen and its metabolite 4-hydroxytamoxifen after oral administration with biochanin A (an isoflavone) in rats. *Phytother Res* 2012; 26: 303-7.

[71] This P, Magdelenat H. Phytoestrogens and adjuvant endocrine treatment of breast cancer. *J Clin Oncol* 2000; 18: 2792-3.

[72] Kim CS, Choi SJ, Park CY, Li C, Choi JS. Effects of silybinin on the pharmacokinetics of tamoxifen and its active metabolite, 4-hydroxytamoxifen in rats. *Anticancer Res* 2010; 30: 79-85.

[73] Gu L, Kelm MA, Hammerstone JF, Beecher G, Holden J, Haytowitz D, Gebhardt S, Prior RL. Concentrations of proanthocyanidins in common foods and estimations of normal consumption. *J Nutr* 2004; 134: 613-7.

[74] Wei CT, Chen LC, Hsiang YP, Hung YJ, Chien PH, Pan HL, Chen YJ. Chrysin-induced ERK1/2 phosphorylation enhances the sensitivity of human hepatocellular carcinoma cells to sorafenib. *Anticancer Res* 2019; 39: 695-701.

[75] Park MH, Hong JE, Hwang CJ, Choi M, Choi JS, An YJ, Son DJ, Hong JT. Synergistic inhibitory effect of cetuximab and tectochrysin on human colon cancer cell growth via inhibition of EGFR signal. *Arch Pharm Res* 2016; 39: 721-9.

[76] Li X, Miao H, Zhang Y, Li W, Li Z, Zhou Y, Zhao L, Guo Q. Bone marrow microenvironment confers imatinib resistance to chronic myelogenous leukemia and oroxylin A reverses the resistance by suppressing Stat3 pathway. *Arch Toxicol* 2015; 89: 121-36.

[77] Li W, Ding Q, Ding Y, Lu L, Wang X, Zhang Y, Zhang X, Guo Q, Zhao L. Oroxylin A reverses the drug resistance of chronic myelogenous leukemia cells to imatinib through CXCL12/CXCR7 axis in bone marrow microenvironment. *Mol Carcinog* 2017; 56: 863-76.

[78] Rong LW, Wang RX, Zheng XL, Feng XQ, Zhang L, Zhang L, Lin Y, Li ZP, Wang X. Combination of wogonin and sorafenib effectively kills human hepatocellular carcinoma cells through apoptosis potentiation and autophagy inhibition. *Oncol Lett* 2017; 13: 5028-34.

[79] Xu X, Zhang X, Liu Y, Yang L, Huang S, Lu L, Wang S, Guo Q, Zhao L. BM microenvironmental protection of CML cells from imatinib through Stat5/NF-κB signaling and reversal by Wogonin. *Oncotarget* 2016; 7: 24436-54.

[80] Bae S, D`Cunha R, Shao J, An G. Effect of 5,7-dimethoxyflavone on Bcrp1-mediated transport of sorafenib in vitro and in vivo in mice. *Eur J Pharm Sci* 2018; 117: 27-34.

[81] Beer MF, Frank FM, German Elso O, Ernesto Bivona A, Cerny N, Giberti G, Luis Malchiodi E, Susana Martino V, Alonso MR, Patricia Sülsen V, Cazorla SI. Trypanocidal and leishmanicidal activities of flavonoids isolated from Stevia satureiifolia var. satureiifolia. *Pharm Biol* 2016; 54: 2188-95.

[82] Chledzik S, Strawa J, Matuszek K, Nazaruk J. Pharmacological effects of scutellarin, an active component of genus Scutellaria and Erigeron: A systematic review. *Am J Chin Med* 2018; 46: 319-37.

[83] Lee JH, Mohan CD, Shanmugam MK, Rangappa S, Sethi G, Siveen KS, Chinnathambi A, Alahmadi TA, Alharbi SA, Basappa S, Rangappa KS, Ahn KS. Vitexin abrogates invasion and survival of hepatocellular carcinoma cells through targeting STAT3 signaling pathway. *Biochimie* 2020; 175: 58-68.

[84] Tsai JJ, Hsu FT, Pan PJ, Chen CW, Kuo YC. Amentoflavone enhances the therapeutic efficacy of sorafenib by inhibiting anti-apoptotic potential and potentiating apoptosis in hepatocellular carcinoma in vivo. *Anticancer Res* 2018; 38: 2119-25.

[85] Chen WL, Hsieh CL, Chen JH, Huang CS, Chen WT, Kuo YC, Chen CY, Hsu FT. Amentoflavone enhances sorafenib-induced apoptosis through extrinsic and intrinsic pathways in sorafenib-resistant hepatocellular carcinoma SK-Hep1 cells in vitro. *Oncol Lett* 2017; 14: 3229-34.

[86] Satchanska G. Antimicrobial activity of natural polyphenols. *Acta Microbiol Bulg* 2020; 36: 132-8.

[87] Chaihongsa N, Maneesai P, Sangartit W, Potue P, Bunbupha S, Pakdeechote P. Galangin alleviates vascular dysfunction and remodelling through modulation of the TNF-R1, p-NF-κB and VCAM-1 pathways in hypertensive rats. *Life Sci* 2021; 285: 119965.

[88] Pal HC, Baxter RD, Hunt KM, Agarwal J, Elmets CA, Athar M, Afaq F. Fisetin, a phytochemical, potentiates sorafenib-induced apoptosis and

abrogates tumor growth in athymic nude mice implanted with BRAF-mutated melanoma cells. *Oncotarget* 2015; 6: 28296-311.

[89] Shin SC, Piao YJ, Choi JS. Effects of morin on the bioavailability of tamoxifen and its main metabolite, 4-hydroxytamoxifen, in rats. *In Vivo* 2008; 22: 391-5.

[90] Gupta SC, Phromnoi K, Aggarwal BB. Morin inhibits STAT3 tyrosine 705 phosphorylation in tumor cells through activation of protein tyrosine phosphatase SHP1. *Biochem Pharmacol* 2013; 85: 898-912.

[91] Li B, Feng F, Jia H, Jiang Q, Cao S, Wei L, Zhang Y, Lu J. Rhamnetin decelerates the elimination and enhances the antitumor effect of the molecular-targeting agent sorafenib in hepatocellular carcinoma cells via the miR-148a/PXR axis. *Food Funct* 2021; 12: 2404-17.

[92] Jia H, Yang Q, Wang T, Cao Y, Jiang QY, Ma HD, Sun HW, Hou MX, Yang YP, Feng F. Rhamnetin induces sensitization of hepatocellular carcinoma cells to a small molecular kinase inhibitor or chemotherapeutic agents. *Biochim Biophys Acta* 2016; 1860: 1417-30.

[93] Goncalves de Oliveira-Junior R, Marcoult-Freville N, Prunier G, Beaugeard L, Beserra de Alencar Filho E, Simoes Mourao ED, Michel S, Quintans-Junior LJ, Guedes da Silva Almeida JR, Grougnet R, Picot L. Polymethoxyflavones from Gardenia oudiepe (Rubiaceae) induce cytoskeleton disruption-mediated apoptosis and sensitize BRAF-mutated melanoma cells to chemotherapy. *Chem Biol Interact* 2020; 325: 109109.

[94] Ganeshpurkar A, Saluja AK. The pharmacological potential of rutin. *Saudi Pharm J* 2017; 25: 149-64.

[95] Kim SH, Ahn KS, Jeong SJ, Kwon TR, Jung JH, Yun SM, Han I, Lee SG, Kim DK, Kang M, Chen CY, Lee JW, Kim SH. Janus activated kinase 2/signal transducer and activator of transcription 3 pathway mediates icariside II-induced apoptosis in U266 multiple myeloma cells. *Eur J Pharmacol* 2011; 654: 10-6.

[96] Jen SH, Wei MP, Yin AC. The combinatory effects of glabridin and tamoxifen on Ishikawa and MCF-7 cell lines. *Nat Prod Commun* 2015; 10: 1573-6.

[97] Yang MH, Jung SH, Chinnathambi A, Alahmadi TA, Alharbi SA, Sethi G, Ahn KS. Attenuation of STAT3 signaling cascade by daidzin can enhance the apoptotic potential of bortezomib against multiple myeloma. *Biomolecules* 2020; 10: 23.

[98] Liu W, Xu J, Liu Y, Yu X, Tang X, Wang Z, Li X. Anthocyanins potentiate the activity of trastuzumab in human epidermal growth factor receptor 2-positive breast cancer cells in vitro and in vivo. *Mol Med Rep* 2014; 10: 1921-6.

[99] Hong SW, Park NS, Noh MH, Shim JA, Ahn BN, Kim YS, Kim D, Lee HK, Hur DY. Combination treatment with erlotinib and ampelopsin overcomes erlotinib resistance in NSCLC cells via the Nox2-ROS-Bim pathway. *Lung Cancer* 2017; 106: 115-24.

[100] Cufi S, Bonavia R, Vazquez-Martin A, Oliveras-Ferraros C, Corominas-Faja B, Cuyas E, Martin-Castillo B, Barrajon-Catalan E, Visa J, Segura-Carretero A, Joven J, Bosch-Barrera J, Micol V, Menendez JA. Silibinin suppresses EMT-driven erlotinib resistance by reversing the high miR-21/low miR-200c signature in vivo. *Sci Rep* 2013; 3: 2459.

[101] Cufi S, Bonavia R, Vazquez-Martin A, Corominas-Faja B, Oliveras-Ferraros C, Cuyas E, Martin-Castillo B, Barrajon-Catalan E, Visa J, Segura-Carretero A, Bosch-Barrera J, Joven J, Micol V, Menendez JA. Silibinin meglumine, a water-soluble form of milk thistle silymarin, is an orally active anti-cancer agent that impedes the epithelial-to-mesenchymal transition (EMT) in EGFR-mutant non-small-cell lung carcinoma cells. *Food Chem Toxicol* 2013; 60: 360-8.

[102] Rho JK, Choi YJ, Jeon BS, Choi SJ, Cheon GJ, Woo SK, Kim HR, Kim CH, Choi CM, Lee JC. Combined treatment with silibinin and epidermal growth factor receptor tyrosine kinase inhibitors overcomes drug resistance caused by T790M mutation. *Mol Cancer Ther* 2010; 9: 3233-43.

[103] Mao J, Yang H, Cui T, Pan P, Kabir N, Chen D, Ma J, Chen X, Chen Y, Yang Y. Combined treatment with sorafenib and silibinin synergistically targets both HCC cells and cancer stem cells by enhanced inhibition of the phosphorylation of STAT3/ERK/AKT. *Eur J Pharmacol* 2018; 832: 39-49.

[104] Saraswati S, Alhaider A, Abdelgadir AM, Tanwer P, Korashy HM. Phloretin attenuates STAT-3 activity and overcomes sorafenib resistance targeting SHP-1-mediated inhibition of STAT3 and Akt/VEGFR2 pathway in hepatocellular carcinoma. *Cell Commun Signal* 2019; 17: 127.

[105] Pandey MK, Sung B, Ahn KS, Aggarwal BB. Butein suppresses constitutive and inducible signal transducer and activator of transcription (STAT) 3 activation and STAT3-regulated gene products through the induction of a protein tyrosine phosphatase SHP-1. *Mol Pharmacol* 2009; 75: 525-33.

[106] Wu MH, Chiu YF, Wu WJ, Wu PL, Lin CY, Lin CL, Hsieh YH, Liu CJ. Synergistic antimetastatic effect of cotreatment with licochalcone A and sorafenib on human hepatocellular carcinoma cells through the inactivation of MKK4/JNK and uPA expression. *Environ Toxicol* 2018; 33: 1237-44.

[107] Li X, Pham V, Tippin M, Fu D, Rendon R, Song L, Uchio E, Hoang BH, Zi X. Flavokawain B targets protein neddylation for enhancing the anti-prostate cancer effect of Bortezomib via Skp2 degradation. *Cell Commun Signal* 2019; 17: 25.

[108] Fujiki H, Suganuma M, Kurusu M, Okabe S, Imayoshi Y, Taniguchi S, Yoshida T. New TNF-alpha releasing inhibitors as cancer preventive agents from traditional herbal medicine and combination cancer prevention study with EGCG and sulindac or tamoxifen. *Mutat Res* 2003; 523-524: 119-25.

[109] Sakata M, Ikeda T, Imoto S, Jinno H, Kitagawa Y. Prevention of mammary carcinogenesis in C3H/OuJ mice by green tea and tamoxifen. *Asian Pac J Cancer Prev* 2011; 12: 567-71.

[110] Ruhul Amin AR, Khuri FR, Chen ZG, Shin DM. Synergistic growth inhibition of squamous cell carcinoma of the head and neck by erlotinib and epigallocatechin-3-gallate: the role of p53-dependent inhibition of nuclear factor-kappaB. *Cancer Prev Res* 2009; 2: 538-45.

[111] Zhang Z, Guo Y, Chen M, Chen F, Liu B, Shen C. Kaempferol potentiates the sensitivity of pancreatic cancer cells to erlotinib via inhibition of the PI3K/AKT signaling pathway and epidermal growth factor receptor. *Inflammopharmacology* 2021; 29: 1587-601.

[112] Gu HR, Park SC, Choi SJ, Lee JC, Kim YC, Han CJ, Kim J, Yang KY, Kim YJ, Noh GY, No SH, Jeong JH. Combined treatment with silibinin and either sorafenib or gefitinib enhances their growth-inhibiting effects in hepatocellular carcinoma cells. *Clin Mol Hepatol* 2015; 21: 49-59.

[113] Ambrosio R, Ombra MN, Gridelli C, Picariello G, DI Stasio M, Volpe MG. Isoflavone extracts enhance the effect of epidermal growth factor receptor inhibitors in NSCLC cell lines. *Anticancer Res* 2016; 36: 5827-33.

[114] Shervington A, Pawar V, Menon S, Thakkar D, Patel R. The sensitization of glioma cells to cisplatin and tamoxifen by the use of catechin. *Mol Biol Rep* 2009; 36: 1181-6.

[115] Sirin N, Elmas L, Secme M, Dodurga Y. Investigation of possible effects of apigenin, sorafenib and combined applications on apoptosis and cell cycle in hepatocellular cancer cells. *Gene* 2020; 737: 144428.

[116] Milligan SA, Burke P, Coleman DT, Bigelow RL, Steffan JJ, Carroll JL, Williams BJ, Cardelli JA. The green tea polyphenol EGCG potentiates the antiproliferative activity of c-Met and epidermal growth factor receptor inhibitors in non-small cell lung cancer cells. *Clin Cancer Res* 2009; 15: 4885-94.

[117] Wu Z, Xu B, Yu Z, He Q, Hu Z, Zhou S, Chen M, Zhu L. Trifolium flavonoids overcome gefitinib resistance of non-small-cell lung cancer

cell by suppressing ERK and STAT3 signaling pathways. *Biomed Res Int* 2020; 2020: 2491304.

[118] Hatkevich T, Ramos J, Santos-Sanchez I, Patel YM. A naringenin-tamoxifen combination impairs cell proliferation and survival of MCF-7 breast cancer cells. *Exp Cell Res* 2014; 327: 331-9.

[119] Tiwari H, Karki N, Pal M, Basak S, Verma RK, Bal R, Kandpal ND, Bisht G, Sahoo NG. Functionalized graphene oxide as a nanocarrier for dual drug delivery applications: The synergistic effect of quercetin and gefitinib against ovarian cancer cells. *Colloids Surf B Biointerfaces* 2019; 178: 452-9.

[120] Granato M, Rizzello C, Gilardini Montani MS, Cuomo L, Vitillo M, Santarelli R, Gonnella R, D`Orazi G, Faggioni A, Cirone M. Quercetin induces apoptosis and autophagy in primary effusion lymphoma cells by inhibiting PI3K/AKT/mTOR and STAT3 signaling pathways. *J Nutr Biochem* 2017; 41: 124-36.

[121] Rahideh ST, Shidfar F, Nourbakhsh M, Hoseini M, Koohdani F, Entezam M, Keramatipour M. The individual or combinational effects of Hesperetin and Letrozole on the activity and expression of aromatase in MCF-7 cells. *Cell Mol Biol* 2016; 62: 38-43.

[122] Shen F, Xue X, Weber G. Tamoxifen and genistein synergistically down-regulate signal transduction and proliferation in estrogen receptor-negative human breast carcinoma MDA-MB-435 cells. *Anticancer Res* 1999; 19: 1657-62.

[123] Zhu K, Wang W. Green tea polyphenol EGCG suppresses osteosarcoma cell growth through upregulating miR-1. *Tumour Biol* 2016; 37: 4373-82.

[124] Jain AK, Thanki K, Jain S. Co-encapsulation of tamoxifen and quercetin in polymeric nanoparticles: implications on oral bioavailability, antitumor efficacy, and drug-induced toxicity. *Mol Pharm* 2013; 10: 3459-74.

[125] El-Lakany SA, Elgindy NA, Helmy MW, Abu-Serie MM, Elzoghby AO. Lactoferrin-decorated vs PEGylated zein nanospheres for combined aromatase inhibitor and herbal therapy of breast cancer. *Expert Opin Drug Deliv* 2018; 15: 835-50.

[126] Shen Y, TanTai J. Co-delivery anticancer drug nanoparticles for synergistic therapy against lung cancer cells. *Drug Des Devel Ther* 2020; 14: 4503-10.

[127] Le CT, Leenders WPJ, Molenaar RJ, van Noorden CJF. Effects of the green tea polyphenol epigallocatechin-3-gallate on glioma: A critical evaluation of the literature. *Nutr Cancer* 2018; 70: 317-33.

[128] van Duursen MB, Smeets EE, Rijk JC, Nijmeijer SM, van den Berg M. Phytoestrogens in menopausal supplements induce ER-dependent cell

proliferation and overcome breast cancer treatment in an in vitro breast cancer model. *Toxicol Appl Pharmacol* 2013; 269: 132-40.

[129] Tonetti DA, Zhang Y, Zhao H, Lim SB, Constantinou AI. The effect of the phytoestrogens genistein, daidzein, and equol on the growth of tamoxifen-resistant T47D/PKC alpha. *Nutr Cancer* 2007; 58: 222-9.

[130] Lattrich C, Lubig J, Springwald A, Goerse R, Ortmann O, Treeck O. Additive effects of trastuzumab and genistein on human breast cancer cells. *Anticancer Drugs* 2011; 22: 253-61.

[131] Rigalli JP, Ciriaci N, Arias A, Ceballos MP, Villanueva SS, Luquita MG, Mottino AD, Ghanem CI, Catania VA, Ruiz ML. Regulation of multidrug resistance proteins by genistein in a hepatocarcinoma cell line: impact on sorafenib cytotoxicity. *PLoS One* 2015; 10: e0119502.

[132] Ferrari SM, Antonelli A, Guidi P, Bernardeschi M, Scarcelli V, Fallahi P, Frenzilli G. Genotoxicity evaluation of the soybean isoflavone genistein in human papillary thyroid cancer cells. Study of its potential use in thyroid cancer therapy. *Nutr Cancer* 2019; 71: 1335-44.

[133] Limer JL, Parkes AT, Speirs V. Differential response to phytoestrogens in endocrine sensitive and resistant breast cancer cells in vitro. *Int J Cancer* 2006; 119: 515-21.

[134] Arya A, Khandelwal K, Ahmad H, Laxman TS, Sharma K, Mittapelly N, Agrawal S, Bhatta RS, Dwivedi AK. Co-delivery of hesperetin enhanced bicalutamide induced apoptosis by exploiting mitochondrial membrane potential via polymeric nanoparticles in a PC-3 cell line. *RSC Adv* 2016; 6: 5925.

[135] Bannerman B, Xu L, Jones M, Tsu C, Yu J, Hales P, Monbaliu J, Fleming P, Dick L, Manfredi M, Claiborne C, Bolen J, Kupperman E, Berger A. Preclinical evaluation of the antitumor activity of bortezomib in combination with vitamin C or with epigallocatechin gallate, a component of green tea. *Cancer Chemother Pharmacol* 2011; 68: 1145-54.

[136] Li Y, Meeran SM, Patel SN, Chen H, Hardy TM, Tollefsbol TO. Epigenetic reactivation of estrogen receptor-α (ERα) by genistein enhances hormonal therapy sensitivity in ERα-negative breast cancer. *Mol Cancer* 2013; 12: 9.

[137] Castillo-Pichardo L, Dharmawardhane SF. Grape polyphenols inhibit Akt/mammalian target of rapamycin signaling and potentiate the effects of gefitinib in breast cancer. *Nutr Cancer* 2012; 64: 1058-69.

[138] Lockhart JN, Stevens DM, Beezer DB, Kravitz A, Harth E. Dual drug delivery of tamoxifen and quercetin: Regulated metabolism for anticancer treatment with nanosponges. *J Control Release* 2015; 220: 751-7.

[139] Quagliariello V, Iaffaioli RV, Armenia E, Clemente O, Barbarisi M, Nasti G, Berretta M, Ottaiano A, Barbarisi A. Hyaluronic acid nanohydrogel loaded with quercetin alone or in combination to a macrolide derivative of rapamycin RAD001 (Everolimus) as a new treatment for hormone-responsive human breast cancer. *J Cell Physiol* 2017; 232: 2063-74.

[140] Parashar P, Tripathi CB, Arya M, Kanoujia J, Singh M, Yadav A, Kumar A, Guleria A, Saraf SA. Biotinylated naringenin intensified anticancer effect of gefitinib in urethane-induced lung cancer in rats: favourable modulation of apoptotic regulators and serum metabolomics. *Artif Cells Nanomed Biotechnol* 2018; 46Suppl3: S598-610.

[141] Tummala R, Lou W, Gao AC, Nadiminty N. Quercetin targets hnRNPA1 to overcome enzalutamide resistance in prostate cancer cells. *Mol Cancer Ther* 2017; 16: 2770-9.

[142] Iwasaki R, Ito K, Ishida T, Hamanoue M, Adachi S, Watanabe T, Sato Y. Catechin, green tea component, causes caspase-independent necrosis-like cell death in chronic myelogenous leukemia. *Cancer Sci* 2009; 100: 349-56.

[143] Wang Z, Wang L, Xia MM, Sun W, Huang CK, Cui X, Hu GX, Lian QQ, Wang ZS. Pharmacokinetics interaction between imatinib and genistein in rats. *Biomed Res Int* 2015; 2015: 368976.

[144] Li H, Wu C, Liu Y, Zhang S, Gao X. Baihe Zhimu formula attenuates the efficacy of tamoxifen against breast cancer in mice through modulation of CYP450 enzymes. *BMC Complement Altern Med* 2019; 19: 240.

[145] Liu XY, Xu T, Li WS, Luo J, Geng PW, Wang L, Xia MM, Chen MC, Yu L, Hu GX. The effect of apigenin on pharmacokinetics of imatinib and its metabolite N-desmethyl imatinib in rats. *Biomed Res Int* 2013; 2013: 789184.

[146] Wang L, Wang Z, Xia MM, Wang YY, Wang HY, Hu GX. Inhibitory effect of silybin on pharmacokinetics of imatinib in vivo and in vitro. *Can J Physiol Pharmacol* 2014; 92: 961-4.

[147] Liu J, Liu H, Zeng Q. The effect of naringenin on the pharmacokinetics of ibrutinib in rat: A drug-drug interaction study. *Biomed Chromatogr* 2019; 33: e4507.

[148] Sarkar FH, Li Y. Using chemopreventive agents to enhance the efficacy of cancer therapy. *Cancer Res* 2006; 66: 3347-50.

[149] Toric J, Markovic AK, Brala CJ, Barbaric M. Anticancer effects of olive oil polyphenols and their combinations with anticancer drugs. *Acta Pharm* 2019; 69: 461-82.

[150] Kaushik S, Shyam H, Agarwal S, Sharma R, Nag TC, Dwivedi AK, Balapure AK. Genistein potentiates Centchroman induced

antineoplasticity in breast cancer via PI3K/Akt deactivation and ROS dependent induction of apoptosis. *Life Sci* 2019; 239: 117073.

[151] Guney Eskiler G, Deveci AO, Bilir C, Kaleli S. Synergistic effects of nobiletin and sorafenib combination on metastatic prostate cancer cells. *Nutr Cancer* 2019; 71: 1299-312.

[152] Kumar M, Sharma G, Misra C, Kumar R, Singh B, Katare OP, Raza K. N-desmethyl tamoxifen and quercetin-loaded multiwalled CNTs: A synergistic approach to overcome MDR in cancer cells. *Mater Sci Eng C Mater Biol Appl* 2018; 89: 274-82.

[153] Nair B, Anto RJ, Sabitha M, Nath LR. Kaempferol-mediated sensitization enhances chemotherapeutic efficacy of sorafenib against hepatocellular carcinoma: An in silico and in vitro approach. *Adv Pharm Bull* 2020; 10: 472-6.

[154] Kaushik S, Shyam H, Sharma R, Balapure AK. Genistein synergizes centchroman action in human breast cancer cells. *Indian J Pharmacol* 2016; 48: 637-42.

[155] Suganuma M, Saha A, Fujiki H. New cancer treatment strategy using combination of green tea catechins and anticancer drugs. *Cancer Sci* 2011; 102: 317-23.

[156] Tabassum H, Parvez S, Rehman H, Banerjee BD, Raisuddin S. Catechin as an antioxidant in liver mitochondrial toxicity: Inhibition of tamoxifen-induced protein oxidation and lipid peroxidation. *J Biochem Mol Toxicol* 2007; 21: 110-7.

[157] Kumarappan C, Vijayakumar M, Thilagam E, Balamurugan M, Thiagarajan M, Senthil S, Das SC, Mandal SC. Protective and curative effects of polyphenolic extracts from Ichnocarpus frutescense leaves on experimental hepatotoxicity by carbon tetrachloride and tamoxifen. *Ann Hepatol* 2011; 10: 63-72.

# Chapter 3

# Plant Flavonoids Affect the Outcome of Hormonal Cancer Therapies

Hormones help certain types of cancers to grow. Malignant neoplasms in breast and prostate are the most well-characterized tumors, development and growth of which are controlled by the endocrine system. Hormonal therapy is recommended to slow the growth of these cancers and stop their spreading. In general, hormonal therapy blocks the body from making certain hormones or keeps them from working in the way that they usually do. Historically, the Scottish surgeon George Thomas Beatson observed the disturbance of breast functions in suckling rabbits after removing their ovaries already in the end of the 19th century, leading to oophorectomy as the first systemic therapy for breast cancer patients and laying foundation for the modern hormonal cancer therapies. However, it still took more than 60 years before tamoxifen as the first adjuvant agent for ovarian ablation was discovered [1]. To date, the spectrum of hormonal therapeutics available for treatment of hormone-dependent breast and prostate tumors has been substantially expanded (Figure 3.1).

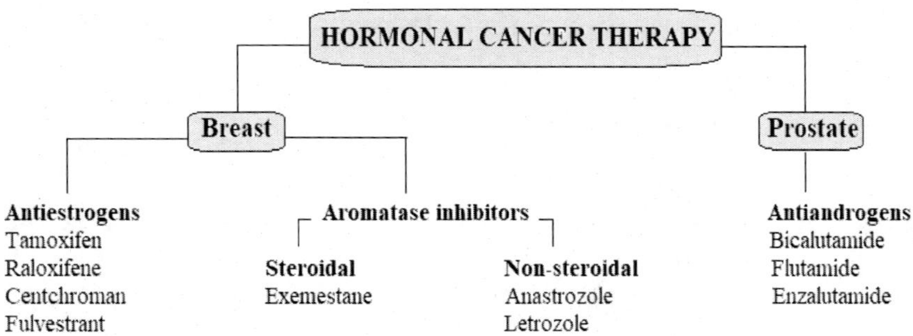


**Figure 3.1.** Hormonal cancer therapies studied in combination with flavonoids.

## 3.1. Interfering of Flavonoids with Hormonal Breast Cancer Therapies

### 3.1.1. Breast Cancer as a Hormone-Dependent Tumor

Breast cancer is the most common cancer type and the leading cause of cancer-related mortality in women worldwide, with more than 2.26 million new cases and almost 685,000 new deaths annually [2]. In 2020, breast cancer accounted for 11.7% of all diagnosed cancer cases in both sexes and constituted 24.5% of all malignant neoplasms among women [2]. Despite improvements in our understanding of biological mechanisms and behavior of these tumors, as well as advancements in diagnostic and treatment modalities, the incidence and mortality rates of breast cancer are continuing to rise in both industrialized and developing countries, putting it at the top of all life-threatening diseases in women [3-5]. Although progress in screening methods can explain the increased rate of diagnoses to some extent, this situation mainly reflects a growing exposure to risk factors, representing an important ongoing public health concern [3, 6]. Therefore, a high priority must be placed on development of more effective therapeutic options with minimal adverse effects to improve prognosis and prolong survival of breast cancer patients.

The etiopathogenesis of breast cancer is multifactorial and complex, comprising genetic, environmental and hormonal components [7]. The most commonly mentioned risk factors include age, obesity, sedentary lifestyle and higher socio-economic status, genetic predisposition and family history, previous breast cancer or non-cancerous diseases, and activities of endogenous and exogenous estrogens [7, 8]. Incidence rate of breast cancer increases with age, whereas more than 75% of cases are diagnosed in postmenopausal women over the age of 50 [9, 10]. Breast cancer incidence is raised also by higher doses and prolonged duration of estrogen exposure, including greater lifelong exposure to ovarian estrogen derived from early menarche, nulliparity and late menopause. On the other hand, oophorectomy decreases the susceptibility to developing breast cancer in premenopausal women [11-13]. Among postmenopausal women, both obesity and alcohol intake are described to result in higher levels of endogenous estrogen, being associated with increased breast cancer risk [12, 13]. Although the extent to which postmenopausal exogenous estrogen exposure affects breast carcinogenesis has remained less clear, long-term use of hormone replacement therapy (HRT) for relieving menopausal symptoms has been associated with an elevated risk [10, 12, 14]. In fact, the incidence rate of hormone-dependent breast cancer cases was significantly reduced after the drop of HRT use that began in 2002, especially among women aged 50-69 years [10, 15]. The possible effects of xenoestrogens found in environment or food products on breast cancer risk have also remained rather uncertain [7]. However, whereas in general, formation of 70% of malignant tumors is related to environmental factors, in the case of breast cancer this percentage has been shown to reach 90-95% [7]. Based on epidemiological evidence, the risk of breast cancer varies substantially throughout the world. Rates tend to be the highest among women in the United States and Western Europe, and the lowest in Asian countries [8]. This difference cannot be explained by genetic factors as incidence of breast cancer of Asian women typically approaches that of American women after several generations of residence in the United States [3, 8, 16]. Indeed, Asian women born in the West have similar incidence rates of breast cancer to those women residing in the same regions, suggesting that direct environmental influences, including diet and nutrition, play a pivotal role in breast carcinogenesis [5, 8]. The lower incidence of breast cancer in Asia has been related to 10-50 times higher consumption of phytoestrogens-containing soy and soy products in Eastern countries as compared to people living in Western areas [17-20]. Therefore, soybean food might have protective action against development and progression of malignancies in the breast tissue, and these beneficial effects appear to depend on time point in life when exposure to soy begins [13, 16, 20].

In addition to their activities in proper tissue development and regulating many physiological functions, endogenous estrogens are believed to play a key role in breast carcinogenesis [7, 21]. Estrogens can stimulate proliferation and facilitate the growth of cancer cells via binding to estrogen receptors (ERs), whereas altered expression of ERs and aberrant activation of their signaling pathways are critical for the initiation, promotion and progression of malignant neoplasms in breast [7, 22]. About 60-70% of all breast cancers contain ERs, being ER-positive and growing in response to estrogens [23-26]. There are two types of ERs, ERα and ERβ, both of which are nuclear receptors functioning as ligand-activated transcription factors and regulating the expression of their various target genes [7, 8, 26]. However, these two receptors may exhibit opposite effects on proliferation of mammary gland cells: whereas ERβ isoform is shown to exert proapoptotic activities, ERα stimulates estrogen-induced carcinogenic effects and promotes unlimited and uncontrolled cell proliferation playing a crucial role in the pathogenesis of breast cancer [7, 20, 27]. In addition to ER-dependent mechanisms, estrogens can exert their carcinogenic effects also by ER-independent pathways, involving the production of toxic and highly reactive metabolites (catechol estrogens) that damage vital biomolecules [28, 29]. Another important predictor for breast cancer prognosis is the status of human epidermal growth factor receptor-2 (HER2 or ErbB2). Overexpression of this tyrosine kinase receptor is detected in approximately 30% of human invasive breast cancers and correlates with more aggressive and chemoresistant tumors, higher histological grade and worse clinical outcome [11, 30-32]. Although HER2 overexpression is generally related to ER negativity, about one-third of HER2-altered malignancies co-express ERs. These tumors are termed luminal type B breast cancers, and comprise 10-20% of all cases [32]. In more detail, according to the expression of ERs, progesterone receptors (PRs) and HER2, breast cancers can be subclassified into three major subtypes: ER+/PR+/HER2- (the most frequently diagnosed type, in about 70% of cases, known also as luminal type A tumor), HER2+ tumors (ER+/PR+/HER2+ as luminal type B and ER-/PR-/HER2+ tumor, occurring in 15-20% of cases), and triple-negative breast cancer (lacking expression of any of these receptors and accounting for about 15% of all breast cancer cases) [7, 32, 33].

As human breast cancer is generally a heterogenous disease, its clinical treatment largely depends on distinct molecular alterations [20]. The principal strategies for breast cancer therapy involve surgical resection in combination with pre- or postoperative chemotherapy, and/or radiotherapy [7, 20, 24]. In addition, since over 60% of breast tumors express ERs, targeting these receptors and their signaling pathway by adjuvant hormonal therapies is common for patients with ER+ cancers, with the aim to reduce the estrogens-stimulated malignant growth, prevent the risk of recurrence and metastasis, and prolong patients` survival [14, 20, 26, 34]. Therefore, ER expression has been used as a marker of probable clinical responsiveness of cancerous cells to antiestrogenic agents [11, 31, 35]. Drugs used in the treatment of estrogen-dependent breast tumors involve selective estrogen receptor modulators (SERMs), selective estrogen receptor downregulators (SERDs) and aromatase inhibitors (AIs) [7] (Figure 3.1). For many years, tamoxifen has been considered as the gold standard for the treatment of estrogen-dependent breast cancers in both premenopausal and postmenopausal women [7, 36]. This most widely prescribed SERM-type compound binds to ER on breast cancer cells, blocks their stimulation by estrogens and inhibits proliferative ability [7, 11, 37]. However, in some other tissues, such as skeletal cells, tamoxifen can behave as an agonist, mimicking the action of estrogens [7]. A newer generation SERM, raloxifene, has been shown to be effective for the treatment of invasive hormone-dependent breast cancers [35]. Another antiestrogen, fulvestrant, acts as a SERD-type agent eliminating the effects of estrogens through ER degradation and, unlike tamoxifen, is not able to exert any agonistic activities [7]. Alternatively, suppression of the action of estrogens on malignant cells can be achieved also by drugs that block production of estrogens in the body [7]. The aromatase enzyme, i.e., CYP19 (cytochrome P450 19), that converts androgens (androstenedione, testosterone) to estrogens (estrone, estradiol), regulates the availability of endogenous estrogens to support the growth of hormone-dependent breast cancers [13, 30]. Overexpression of this enzyme in breast cancer tissues can substantially affect tumor progression and maintenance [30, 38]. Aromatase inhibitors (AIs), both steroidal (exemestane) as well as non-steroidal (anastrozole, letrozole), suppress the activity of aromatase enzyme and reduce the synthesis of estrogens, and are used in postmenopausal women in whom estrogens are mostly produced in peripheral tissues (adipose tissue, skin, liver) [7, 30]. Therefore, as the treatment of estrogen-dependent breast cancers in premenopausal women mainly includes the use of tamoxifen for 5-10 years, in postmenopausal women, both tamoxifen and AIs are applied, also for a total of 5-10 years [7, 10, 20]. Furthermore, tamoxifen can be administered also prophylactically to women at high risk of breast cancer for prevention of developing ER+ tumors [3, 20, 39].

Although hormonal therapies are highly effective in preventing and treating ER+ breast cancers, resistance to these treatments still poses a significant clinical challenge. In fact, nearly 40% of breast cancers do not respond to the treatment with tamoxifen despite the expression of ERs in malignant cells, exhibiting de novo resistance [18, 36]. Moreover, the positive response to this antiestrogen is usually of short duration, as most tumors eventually acquire resistance to tamoxifen within 2-5 years and recur [18, 36, 40]. Factors determining the responsiveness to hormonal therapy have remained largely unknown [18]. However, several studies have reported that co-expression of HER2 in breast cancer cells is associated with a reduced response of ER+ tumors to hormonal therapies, such as tamoxifen, being a major therapeutic problem [30, 32]. Simultaneous targeting of these receptors and their signaling pathways might be necessary to potentiate prevention of breast cancer development and progression [36]. Moreover, most of breast tumors are heterogenous consisting of ER+ as well as ER-cells, highlighting the need to develop therapies that concurrently block the growth of both hormone-dependent as well as -independent cancers [41, 42]. In addition, a 5-year (or even 10-year) course of tamoxifen has become associated with numerous serious side effects and health complications [4, 40, 43]. These data clearly demonstrate that alternative interventions are needed to supplement the arsenal of current therapeutic regimens [40, 43]. Modulation of tamoxifen sensitivity by natural products that prevent resistance and reduce adverse effects, while augmenting therapeutic efficacy would be highly desired [4, 36]. There are indeed reasons to believe that multiple agents might be more effective than single drugs in the treatment of breast cancer [40, 43, 44]. Development of such novel multi-therapeutic approaches definitely premises a detail molecular understanding of the cellular mechanisms involved in breast cancer formation and progression [45].

It is well known that the use of both antiestrogens as well as AIs can substantially deteriorate the quality of life of breast cancer patients leading to the onset of menopausal symptoms, such as hot flashes, vaginal dryness and weight gain, but also joint and muscle pain, sleeping disorders, anxiety and mood swings, and skin aging. These bothersome symptoms are the result of a decrease in endogenous estrogen supply [10, 37, 46-48]. In a recent report, it was estimated that 72% of tamoxifen users experience disruptive hot flashes [49]. The patients suffering from such complaints may not be able to continue with these therapies, and seek alternative options to control and relieve menopausal symptoms [37, 46]. As many oncologists do not recommend HRT to breast cancer patients due to the concern that it may increase the risk of tumor recurrence, women often decide to increase their intake of dietary phytoestrogens, either through food products or health supplements that are commonly freely available on the market [9, 10, 37, 49, 50]. In fact, 28-91% of breast cancer patients use one or more complementary dietary supplements without the knowledge of their physicians, believing that constituents of products with natural origin are generally regarded safe [9-11, 37, 50]. Phytoestrogens are plant-derived bioactive phenolic substances, with soy and flax considered the richest sources [7, 49]. Soy isoflavones are similar in their chemical structure to 17β-estradiol, can bind to ERs and exert weak but substantial estrogenic properties [10, 12, 39, 49]. Their effects in the human body depend largely on the doses and time of exposure, concentrations of endogenous estrogens, and individual characteristics [18, 49, 51]. Genistein is the major soy isoflavone, and is detected in substantial amounts in the breast tissue after dietary intake of soy products, increasing the total content of estrogen-like agents in the body [37]. Moreover, serum concentrations of isoflavones following to intake of a high-soy meal can reach low micromolar levels, exceeding postmenopausal estrogen concentrations even by 1000-fold [12]. However, the knowledge on how soy isoflavones interact with hormonal cancer therapies in women who are either at high risk of developing breast cancer or in those who are being treated for breast cancer is still rather unclear and controversial [39, 50]. If these phytochemicals negate the beneficial effects of tamoxifen, their simultaneous intake may result in undesirable outcome for breast cancer patients, posing a potential risk and representing an important clinical and toxicological issue [9, 10, 15]. Several laboratorial studies conducted with ER+ breast cancer cells *in vitro* or experimental animals *in vivo* have indeed described the overwhelming effects of soy isoflavones on tumor-repressive action of tamoxifen and AIs, promoting thus the tumor growth [16, 18, 37, 52, 53]. In other rodent cancer models, however, soy isoflavones have been found to enhance the antitumor action of tamoxifen [21, 52, 54, 55]. Furthermore, analysis of epidemiological studies has concluded that soy foods consumed at the levels comparable to Asian populations do not appear to interfere with tamoxifen or AI treatment [37]. Therefore, it is highly important to unravel this issue before advocating safe use or, on the contrary, warning against consuming soy isoflavones in breast cancer survivors receiving adjuvant hormonal therapies. Currently, many women are still confused whether to incorporate soy into their diet, and also health professionals lack a common understanding whether to advice their patients to consume soy items or not [12, 18, 54, 56].

In addition to early menopausal complications, almost 10% of breast cancer patients experience major depressive disorder that often remains underrecognized and undertreated [57]. These women may also try to self-medicate with herbal remedies and natural supplements containing a variety of bioactive flavonoids [57]. Potential impact of these polyphenolic components on the efficacy of antiestrogens and AIs is largely unknown and definitely needs further investigations. In the subsections 3.1.2 and 3.1.3, the current knowledge about interactions of diverse plant flavonoids with antiestrogens (tamoxifen, raloxifene, centchroman, fulvestrant) and AIs (exemestane, anastrozole, letrozole) are compiled and analyzed, highlighting the most important conclusions with dietary recommendations to breast cancer patients in the subsection 3.1.4.

### 3.1.2. Influence of Flavonoids on Therapeutic Action of Antiestrogens

#### *3.1.2.1. Tamoxifen*

Tamoxifen is considered the gold standard for the treatment of both early and advanced ER+ breast cancers in pre- and postmenopausal women, already since 1973 [5, 7, 25, 58] (Figure 3.2). This non-steroidal SERM-type antiestrogen acts through binding to ERs on malignant cells, blocks their stimulation by estrogens and inhibits proliferation, thus helping maintain disease-free status and increasing overall survival in breast cancer survivors [7, 45, 57]. It is estimated that administration of tamoxifen can decrease the annual recurrence rate by almost half and cancer-related mortality by about one-third in women with ER+ breast tumors [53, 57]. However, in some other tissues, such as skeleton, cardiovascular system and endometrium, this drug behaves as an agonist and mimics the effects of endogenous estrogens [7, 28, 59]. To get the best antineoplastic effects and therapeutic outcomes, adjuvant tamoxifen (routinely used at a dose of 20 mg/day) should be given for a long time, i.e., 5-10 years [4, 7]. In addition, besides being the agent of choice for the treatment, tamoxifen has been approved also for prevention of breast cancer in women at high risk for the disease, to reduce the incidence of both invasive and non-invasive primary mammary tumors [60-62]. Moreover, a number of recent studies have suggested that antitumor action of tamoxifen can involve also ER-independent signaling pathways, increasing oxidative stress by generating reactive oxygen species (ROS) and promoting apoptosis. Tamoxifen can indeed diminish mitochondrial functionality and induce cytotoxic responses in ER- breast cancer cells [17, 45, 63]. However, these effects generally occur at considerably higher doses, creating opportunities for combinational strategies with potentiating agents and providing novel targets for the treatment of human breast cancers [63, 64].

Orally administered tamoxifen undergoes extensive hepatic metabolism and subsequent biliary excretion of its metabolites [58, 65, 66] (Figure 3.3). Accordingly, the oral bioavailability of tamoxifen is poor (10-20%), limiting the availability of free drug in the site of malignancy [67]. Moreover, interindividual variation in the plasma levels of tamoxifen and its metabolites is large, being affected by several factors, including the age, menopausal status, body size and the use of hypertensive medications [52]. In humans, the major route of tamoxifen biotransformation proceeds via cytochrome P450 (CYP) 3A4-catalyzed N-demethylation [58, 65]. Formation of the minor metabolite, 4-hydroxytamoxifen (4-OH-TAM), is catalyzed mainly by CYP2D6, but also CYP2C9, CYP2E1 and CYP3A4 enzymes [58, 65, 66, 68]. Although the plasma and tumor concentrations of 4-OH-TAM constitute only about 2% of those of the parent compound, this metabolite is reported to be 30- to 100-fold more potent than tamoxifen at inhibiting ERs and suppressing estrogen-dependent cell proliferation [58, 65, 66]. The secondary metabolite, endoxifen, exhibits similar potency to 4-OH-TAM [59, 65]. Therefore, tamoxifen is referred to as a prodrug that requires metabolic activation before exerting antineoplastic effects [27, 57, 65]. As this antiestrogen has no access to the first-pass metabolism for cancerous cells in culture, most *in vitro* studies are performed with 4-OH-TAM as a model compound [27]. In addition, tamoxifen and its metabolites are also substrates for P-glycoprotein (P-gp) that colocalizes with CYP3A4 in the polarized epithelial cells of the intestine, liver and kidney and mediates the efflux of foreign agents into the intestinal lumen, bile and urine, thus regulating the bioavailability of orally ingested drug [58, 65, 66, 68]. Considering a substantial overlap in substrate specificity between CYP3A4 and P-gp, modulators of P-gp and CYP3A4 might affect the oral bioavailability of tamoxifen [58, 59, 65].

| Hormonal Breast Cancer Therapies | |
|---|---|
| Antiestrogens | |
| 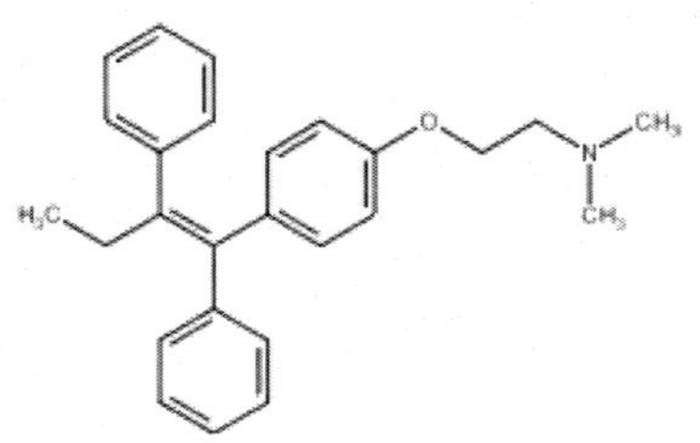 Tamoxifen (SERM) | 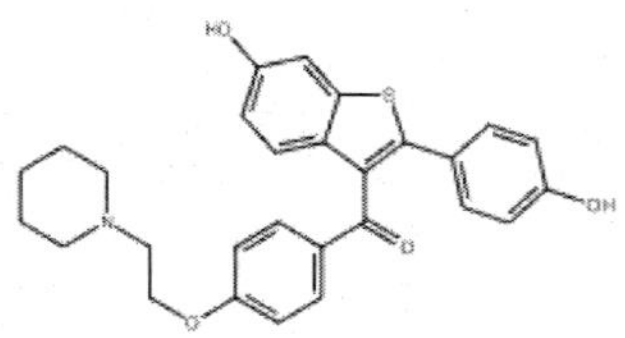 Raloxifene (SERM) |
| 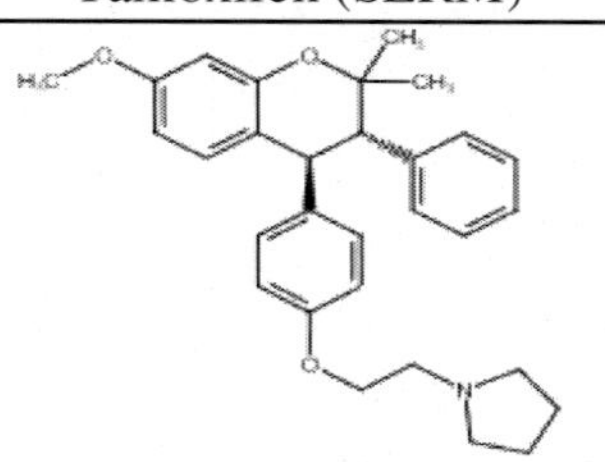 Centchroman (SERM) | 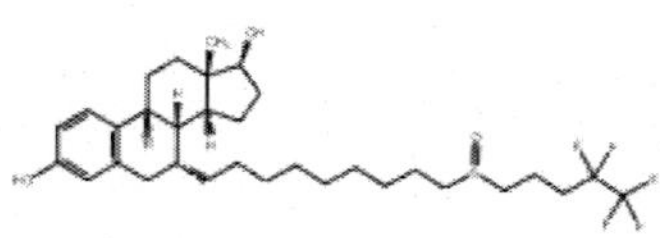 Fulvestrant (SERD) |

**Figure 3.2.** (Continued).

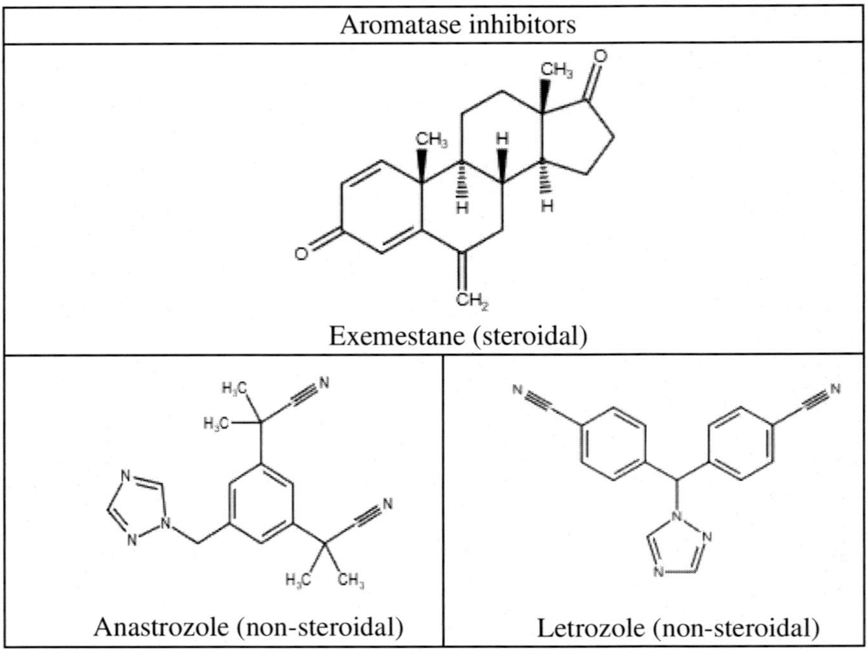


**Figure 3.2.** Structural formulas of hormonal breast cancer therapies studied in combination with flavonoids.

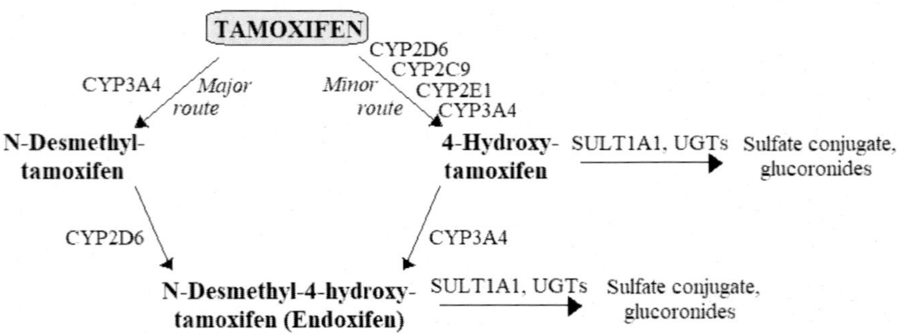


**Figure 3.3.** Metabolic conversion of tamoxifen in the human body.

Despite beneficial role of tamoxifen in the fight against breast cancer, its long-lasting use produces numerous severe side effects, such as an increased risk of endometrial cancer and uterine sarcoma, liver damage and thromboembolic events (multiple vein thrombosis, pulmonary embolism, stroke) [4, 53, 67, 69]. Besides formation of DNA adducts, tissue-specific proliferative effects of tamoxifen and its metabolites may contribute to the increased incidence of endometrial cancer [25, 53, 70]. Tamoxifen has been described to be a hepatocarcinogen also in rats via generating DNA adducts and causing oxidative liver damage [71-73]. Additionally, over 40% of patients with ER+ breast tumors fail to respond to tamoxifen treatment, limiting clinical efficacy of this adjuvant drug and representing a critical problem in hormonal therapy [36, 45, 74]. Moreover, the positive response is usually of short duration, while most tumors eventually develop tamoxifen resistance [36]. Tamoxifen resistance, however, can often lead to relapse, metastases and death [34, 74]. In fact, it is estimated that about one-third of breast cancer patients treated with tamoxifen for five years have recurrent disease within 15 years [25]. Although the underlying molecular mechanisms are complex, overexpression of HER2 has been shown to play a major role in tamoxifen resistance in hormone-dependent breast tumors, while suppression of HER2 expression enhances the responsiveness to tamoxifen [34, 36]. Furthermore, it has been reported that ER+ mammary neoplasms with acquired tamoxifen resistance may be not only unresponsive to this SERM, but can demonstrate also tamoxifen-stimulated growth while retaining ER expression [34, 74]. Another major cause of resistance to hormonal therapy is suggested to involve downregulation or loss of ERs expression, and alterations of their signaling pathways [34, 75]. Therefore, novel safe and efficient modalities are urgently needed to increase the responsiveness of ER+ breast tumors to tamoxifen treatment, thereby augmenting its antitumor efficacy and minimizing adverse side effects [36, 45, 74]. Development of combination therapies with natural anticancer agents, especially plant-derived flavonoids, is one of the developmental trends and promising strategies to achieve this goal and improve clinical outcome of breast cancer patients.

#### *3.1.2.1.1. Effects of Flavonoids on Pharmacokinetics of Tamoxifen*

Some patients with ER+ breast cancer who receive tamoxifen treatment could get therapeutic benefit from natural supplements that influence the first-pass metabolism of this antiestrogen drug [57]. Although the knowledge about such interactions *in vivo* is still rather scarce, plant-derived flavonoids that act as dual inhibitors of CYP3A4 and P-gp might contribute to the substantial alterations in pharmacokinetic fate of tamoxifen and its metabolites as substrates for these proteins [59, 65, 76]. The results of such studies are compiled in Table 3.1 and discussed more thoroughly in the current subsection.

**Table 3.1.** Effects of flavonoids on pharmacokinetic parameters of tamoxifen (TAM) and its major active metabolite 4-hydroxytamoxifen (4-OH-TAM) (highlighted rows indicate undesired negative effects on bioavailability)

| Flavonoid and its dosage | Tamoxifen and its dosage | Biological system | Effects | Purported mechanism | Ref. |
|---|---|---|---|---|---|
| FLAVANOLS | | | | | |
| EGCG; 3 or 10 mg/kg, intragastrically through a feeding tube | TAM; 10 mg/kg, intragastrically through a feeding tube | Male Sprague-Dawley rats | Increase in $AUC_{0-\infty}$ and $C_{max}$ of TAM | | [77] |
| EGCG; 0.5, 3 or 10 mg/kg, intragastrically using a feeding tube, 30 min before TAM | TAM; 10 mg/kg, intragastrically using a feeding tube | Male Sprague-Dawley rats | Increase in $AUC_{0-\infty}$ and $C_{max}$, enhancement of bioavailability of TAM. Increase in $AUC_{0-\infty}$ of 4-OH-TAM (at 10 mg/kg EGCG). Reduction of metabolite-parent ratio | Decrease in first-pass metabolism of TAM by inhibition of P-gp and CYP3A4 | [78] |
| FLAVONES | | | | | |
| Baicalein; 0.5, 3 or 10 mg/kg, intragastrically using a feeding tube, 30 min before TAM | TAM; 10 mg/kg, intragastrically using a feeding tube | Male Sprague-Dawley rats | Increase in $AUC_{0-\infty}$ and $C_{max}$, decrease in CL/F, enhancement of oral bioavailability of TAM. Reduction of metabolite-parent AUC ratio | Inhibition of CYP3A4-mediated TAM metabolism and P-gp activity | [79] |
| FLAVONOLS | | | | | |
| Kaempferol; 2.5 or 10 mg/kg, intragastrically using a feeding tube, 30 min before TAM | TAM; 10 mg/kg, intragastrically using a feeding tube | Male Sprague-Dawley rats | Increase in $AUC_{0-\infty}$ and $C_{max}$, enhancement of bioavailability of TAM. No effect on pharmacokinetic parameters of 4-OH-TAM. No effect on metabolite ratio | Inhibition of P-gp and CYP3A | [80] |
| Morin; 3 or 10 mg/kg, intragastrically, 30 min before TAM | TAM; 10 mg/kg, intragastrically using a feeding tube | Male Sprague-Dawley rats | Increase in $AUC_{0-\infty}$ and $C_{max}$, decrease in CL/F, enhancement of oral bioavailability of TAM. Increase in $AUC_{0-\infty}$ of 4-OH-TAM. No significant effect on metabolite-parent ratio | Decrease in the first-pass metabolism of TAM (inhibition of CYP3A and P-gp) | [65] |

| Flavonoid and its dosage | Tamoxifen and its dosage | Biological system | Effects | Purported mechanism | Ref. |
|---|---|---|---|---|---|
| Myricetin; 2 or 8 mg/kg, intragastrically, 30 min before TAM | TAM; 10 mg/kg, intragastrically using a feeding tube | Male Sprague-Dawley rats | Increase in $AUC_{0\text{-}\infty}$ and $C_{max}$, enhancement of oral bioavailability of TAM. Reduction of metabolite-parent AUC ratio | Inhibition of CYP3A4- and CYP2C9-mediated metabolism of TAM; inhibition of P-gp pump | [58] |
| Quercetin; 2.5 or 7.5 mg/kg, oral administration | TAM; 10 mg/kg, oral administration | Female Sprague-Dawley rats | Increase in $AUC_{0\text{-}\infty}$ and $C_{max}$, enhancement of oral bioavailability of TAM. Increase in $AUC_{0\text{-}\infty}$ of 4-OH-TAM. Reduction of metabolite-parent AUC ratio | Inhibition of MDR transporters efflux and CYP3A4-mediated metabolism of TAM | [68] |
| FLAVANONES | | | | | |
| Naringin; 1.5, 7.5 or 15 mg/kg, oral administration, 30 min before TAM | TAM; 10 mg/kg, oral administration | Female Sprague-Dawley rats | Increase in $AUC_{0\text{-}\infty}$ and $C_{max}$, enhancement of oral bioavailability of TAM. Increase in $AUC_{0\text{-}\infty}$ of 4-OH-TAM. Reduction of metabolite-parent AUC ratio | Inhibition of CYP3A4 and P-gp | [66] |
| ISOFLAVONES | | | | | |
| Biochanin A; 5, 10 or 20 mg/kg, oral administration, 10 min before TAM | TAM; 10 mg/kg, oral administration | Female Sprague-Dawley rats | No effect on pharmacokinetics of TAM and formation of 4-OH-TAM. Decrease in $C_{max}$ of 4-OH-TAM | | [81] |
| Biochanin A; 100 mg/kg, oral administration, 10 min before TAM | TAM; 10 mg/kg, oral administration | Female Sprague-Dawley rats | Decrease in $AUC_{0\text{-}\infty}$ and $C_{max}$, reduction of bioavailability of TAM and 4-OH-TAM. No effect on 4-OH-TAM formation | | [60] |
| FLAVONOLIGNANS | | | | | |
| Silibinin; 2.5 or 10 mg/kg, intragastrically using a feeding tube, 30 min before TAM | TAM; 10 mg/kg, intragastrically using a feeding tube | Male Sprague-Dawley rats | Increase in $AUC_{0\text{-}\infty}$ and $C_{max}$, enhancement of oral bioavailability of TAM. Increase in $AUC_{0\text{-}\infty}$ of 4-OH-TAM. Reduction of metabolite-parent ratio (at 10 mg/kg) | Promotion of intestinal absorption and reduction of first-pass metabolism of TAM | [59] |

Experiments with male Sprague-Dawley rats have recently shown that oral coadministration of tamoxifen with green tea flavanol EGCG leads to an improved drug bioavailability, with significant increases in the area under the plasma concentration-time curve ($AUC_{0-\infty}$) and the peak plasma concentration ($C_{max}$) of tamoxifen [77, 78]. Rats are considered preferable rodent animal models for investigation of tamoxifen pharmacokinetics, as the potent metabolite 4-OH-TAM is presented in lower concentrations in both rats and humans, but in higher doses in mice [68]. Although EGCG elevated $AUC_{0-\infty}$ also of 4-OH-TAM, the metabolite-parent ratio of 4-OH-TAM was significantly decreased [78]. The increased plasma concentrations of tamoxifen were likely due to the reduction of its first-pass metabolism in the intestine and liver by inhibition of CYP3A4 and P-gp in the presence of EGCG [77, 78]. Pharmacokinetic parameters of orally administered tamoxifen were shown to be considerably altered also by some other flavonoids. Concomitant administration of tamoxifen with flavone baicalein resulted in a significant elevation of $AUC_{0-\infty}$ and $C_{max}$ of the drug in male rats, with a decrease in the total body clearance (CL/F). Consequently, oral bioavailability of tamoxifen was substantially enhanced. The formation of 4-OH-TAM was also affected by baicalein, as the metabolite-parent ratio was significantly reduced. Improved bioavailability of tamoxifen in the presence of baicalein was attributed to suppression of the CYP3A4-catalyzed drug metabolism in the small intestine and liver, inhibition of the P-gp-mediated efflux in the small intestine, and reduction of total body clearance by baicalein [79]. In addition, flavonol kaempferol increased $AUC_{0-\infty}$ and $C_{max}$ of tamoxifen when administered concomitantly to male rats, leading to enhanced oral bioavailability of the drug. These modulating effects were again due to the inhibition of CYP3A and P-gp activities by kaempferol. However, kaempferol was unable to alter the pharmacokinetic parameters of the major active metabolite of tamoxifen, 4-OH-TAM, as well as exerted no significant influence on the metabolite ratio [80]. The presence of another flavonol, morin, significantly reduced CL/F, while increasing $AUC_{0-\infty}$ and $C_{max}$ of tamoxifen in male rats. As a consequence, oral bioavailability of this antiestrogen was considerably improved by morin through suppressing the first-pass metabolism of tamoxifen in the intestine and liver. Although this flavonol could increase $AUC_{0-\infty}$ also for 4-OH-TAM, the metabolite-parent ratio was still not altered significantly with the combination treatment [65]. Similarly, $AUC_{0-\infty}$ and $C_{max}$ of oral tamoxifen were elevated in the presence of flavonol myricetin, leading to increase in the drug bioavailability in rats. This was accompanied by impact on the production of 4-OH-TAM, manifested as decrease in the metabolite-parent ratio. The enhanced bioavailability of tamoxifen was mainly explained by inhibiting CYP3A4- and CYP2C9-mediated drug metabolism in the small intestine and liver, besides reduction of P-gp efflux pump activity in the small intestine by myricetin [58]. Moreover, coadministration of tamoxifen with naturally abundant flavonol quercetin resulted in enhancement of $AUC_{0-\infty}$ and $C_{max}$ of the drug, with a considerable increase in oral bioavailability of tamoxifen in female rats. This combination treatment elevated also $AUC_{0-\infty}$ of 4-OH-TAM, but lowered significantly the metabolite-parent ratio, suggesting that quercetin promoted the intestinal absorption and inhibited the first-pass metabolism of tamoxifen [68]. Consistent with these results, coadministration of tamoxifen with flavanone glycoside naringin enhanced $AUC_{0-\infty}$ and $C_{max}$ of tamoxifen in female rats, leading to enhancement of oral bioavailability. Despite elevation of $AUC_{0-\infty}$ of 4-OH-TAM, the metabolite-parent ratio was still reduced in naringin-pretreated animals. Such alterations in pharmacokinetic profile of tamoxifen were presumably due to dual inhibition of CYP3A4 and P-gp by naringin [66]. Systemic exposure to orally administered tamoxifen was substantially enhanced also by the presence of flavonolignan silibinin that similarly to the other tested flavonoids elevated $AUC_{0-\infty}$ and $C_{max}$ of tamoxifen in experimental rats. Besides increasing $AUC_{0-\infty}$ also for 4-OH-TAM, silibinin considerably affected the formation of this active metabolite, as the metabolite-parent ratio was significantly reduced. Altered pharmacokinetics and improved oral bioavailability of tamoxifen were probably achieved via promotion of intestinal absorption and reduction of first-pass metabolism by silibinin [59]. In short, the substantial increase in oral bioavailability of tamoxifen in the presence of specific naturally occurring flavonoids (EGCG, baicalein, kaempferol, morin, myricetin, quercetin, naringin, silibinin) should be taken into consideration when tamoxifen and these phytochemicals (or their dietary supplements) are concomitantly used for the treatment or prevention of ER+ breast tumors. Such combinations might lead to lowering the effective drug doses and minimizing adverse side effects. However, before giving recommendations for clinical practice, the respective interactions definitely need to be further evaluated in humans.

On the other hand, the presence of isoflavone biochanin A induced no significant changes in the pharmacokinetic parameters of tamoxifen and 4-OH-TAM at lower doses (5-20 mg/kg) [81], but remarkably reduced oral bioavailability of the drug at higher doses (100 mg/kg) in female rats [60]. Although the lower doses of biochanin A did not affect the production of 4-

OH-TAM, $C_{max}$ of 4-OH-TAM was still considerably reduced [81]. Coadministration of oral tamoxifen with higher concentrations of biochanin A (100 mg/kg) led to significant decrease in $AUC_{0-\infty}$ and $C_{max}$ of both tamoxifen and 4-OH-TAM, with no apparent alterations in the metabolite-parent ratio [60]. This surprising finding indicates that the presence of biochanin A can substantially suppress the oral absorption and bioavailability of tamoxifen, and thereby influence also its anticancer efficacy. Although the exact molecular mechanisms behind this negative effect are still unclear, it is better for women under tamoxifen therapy to avoid the exposure to biochanin A-containing dietary supplements.

*3.1.2.1.2. Effects of Flavonoids on Anticancer Potential of Tamoxifen*

As tamoxifen has no access to first-pass metabolism in cultured cancer cells, most *in vitro* studies on antitumor potential of tamoxifen are performed using its active metabolite, 4-OH-TAM, as a model compound [27]. The results obtained by treatment of various breast cancer cells with combination of tamoxifen and structurally diverse flavonoids are compiled in Table 3.2 and discussed more thoroughly in the current subsection.

Several reports have studied anticancer action of tamoxifen in combination with green tea catechins in molecularly different breast cancer cells. Although three major green tea flavanols, epicatechin 3-gallate (ECG), epigallocatechin (EGC) and epigallocatechin 3-gallate (EGCG), all at 25 μM doses, were shown to exert no effect on cytotoxicity of 4-OH-TAM in human ER+ breast cancer (luminal A) cell line MCF-7, ECG (but not other flavanols) still induced a small but significant decrease in the cytotoxic potential of 4-OH-TAM in another ER+ cell line T47D [82]. It is well accepted that besides classical antiestrogenic action of tamoxifen, this drug can impact cellular signaling also in ER-independent manner. While none of the tested flavanols affected 4-OH-TAM-evoked cytotoxicity in triple-negative breast cancer (TNBC) cells HS578T, combination of EGCG (25 μM) and 4-OH-TAM produced synergistic cytotoxic response with increased apoptotic death in TNBC cells MDA-MB-231, suggesting that this combination may provide a possible new strategy for the treatment of estrogen-insensitive breast tumors [82]. Numerous other studies have also demonstrated that EGCG, even at considerably lower doses, can augment the growth inhibitory effects of 4-OH-TAM (or tamoxifen) in both ER+ as well as ER- breast cancer cells. In more detail, the combination of tamoxifen and EGCG (at the doses as low as 0.01-1 μM) synergistically inhibited proliferation of MCF-7 cells [3]. The presence of EGCG (5 μM) potentiated the growth inhibitory action of tamoxifen in both intact MCF-7 cells as well as estradiol-stimulated cells through downregulation of oncogenic S-phase kinase protein 2 (Skp2), an important regulatory point of G1/S phase cell cycle transition. However, the decrease in Skp2 protein led to an increase in p27 expression only in estradiol-stimulated cells contributing to synergistic antiproliferative action, suggesting that downregulation of Skp2 can impact the cell growth in several ways [43]. Moreover, EGCG was shown to overcome also drug resistance in tamoxifen-resistant MCF-7 cells (MCF-7/TAM), by suppressing endogenous expression of nuclear factor erythroid 2-related factor 2 (Nrf2) and its downstream target genes, such as heme oxygenase-1 (HO-1) and NAD(P)H:quinone oxidoreductase 1 (NQO1) [45]. Inhibition of proliferation was augmented when tamoxifen was combined with EGCG also in HER2-transfected MCF-7 cells (MCF-7/HER2/neu), representing luminal type B breast tumor. The potentiated antiproliferative action was accompanied by suppression of tyrosine kinase activity and occurred likewise in combination of tamoxifen with black tea polyphenols, theaflavin (TF)-1, TF-2 and TF-3 [30]. This finding is especially important as expression of HER2 has been found to be a critical factor behind resistance of ER+ breast tumors to tamoxifen treatment. In another HER2-positive breast cancer cell line with no expression of ERs or PRs, i.e., AU565 cells, combination of EGCG and tamoxifen synergistically enhanced growth inhibition through downregulation of Skp2 protein [43]. In TNBC cells, MDA-MB-231, coadministration of 4-OH-TAM and EGCG (25 μM) considerably enhanced cytotoxicity, resulting from apoptosis earlier and to a greater degree [44]. Moreover, when athymic nude mice implanted with MDA-MB-231 cells were treated with oral tamoxifen concomitantly with intraperitoneal injection of EGCG, tumor volume and weight were significantly reduced as compared to tamoxifen-treated mice. This superior antitumor effect was accompanied by significant decrease in epidermal growth factor receptor (EGFR), phosphorylated EGFR (pEGFR), mammalian target of rapamycin (mTOR) and CYP1B1 levels, probably representing important mechanisms for inhibition of tumor growth. Thus, tamoxifen can suppress the growth of ER- breast tumors when combined with EGCG, whereas the combination therapy was well tolerated and non-toxic to the mice [63]. Although the above-described promising results clearly indicate that EGCG could be applied as an adjuvant agent for tamoxifen, more studies with animal models as well as in human clinical trials are necessary to prove the efficacy of this combination therapy for the use in breast cancer treatment and prevention in the future. Further confirmation for beneficial role of combination therapy of tamoxifen and flavanols was obtained from the experiments with green tea extract (GTE), showing that GTE enhanced the inhibitory effects of tamoxifen on proliferation of ER+ human breast cancer cells MCF-7, T47D and ZR75, inducing a marked increase in apoptosis. In addition, MCF-7 xenografts were the smallest in mice treated with both GTE and tamoxifen, revealing also the highest levels of apoptosis and the lowest levels of angiogenesis and blood vessel density in tumor tissues, as compared to the animals given either agent alone. The growth inhibitory action of dual treatment was accompanied by suppression of ERα expression in malignant tissue, and blocking of ER-dependent transcription and E2-induced activation of mitogen-activated protein kinase (MAPK). No toxicity was observed with such combination therapy [40]. Moreover, in female C3H/OuJ mice (carrying the C3H mammary tumor virus type S and typically showing a high incidence of mammary tumors by 11 months of age), cotreatment with GTE in drinking water and subcutaneously inoculated tamoxifen resulted in a complete attenuation of spontaneous tumor formation and incidence, highlighting the potential of this combination therapy for breast cancer chemoprevention [3].

Among flavones, apigenin was shown to exert no significant impact on antiproliferative action of 4-OH-TAM in ER+ positive breast cancer cells MCF-7 and T47D, although apigenin could downregulate ERα expression in MCF-7 cells. In ER- MDA-MB435 cells, this combination did not exhibit any growth inhibitory effects [83]. However, cotreatment of MDA-MB-435 cells with apigenin and tamoxifen (in 1:1 combinations) led to an enhancement of antiproliferative activities. Similar effects were observed also when tamoxifen was combined with polymethoxylated flavones nobiletin and tangeretin [41]. The presence of another naturally abundant flavone, luteolin (even at low micromolar doses), sensitized tamoxifen-resistant MCF-7 cells to 4-OH-TAM-induced cytotoxic effects, by inhibiting cyclin E2 (CCNE2) protein expression and impeding G1/S phase cell cycle transition. While overexpression of CCNE2 might substantially contribute to E2-induced cell proliferation and act against antiestrogen-induced cell death, its high levels are considered as predictors of poor outcomes in breast cancer patients, particularly in women with luminal type A tumors. Therefore, luteolin might be an important adjuvant agent for tamoxifen therapy, targeting CCNE2 expression and overcoming drug resistance [22]. Somewhat unexpected results have been reported for cotreatment of MCF-7/6 cells with tamoxifen and citrus flavonoid tangeretin. While this combination therapy resulted in amplified inhibition of cell growth *in vitro* conditions, coadministration of these two agents in drinking water to tumor-bearing nude mice *in vivo* displayed a complete neutralization of tamoxifen-induced growth inhibition of subcutaneously inoculated MCF-7/6 tumors. Moreover, the median survival time of tumor-bearing mice cotreated with tamoxifen and tangeretin was significantly shortened as compared to mice treated with tamoxifen alone, i.e., 14 vs 56 weeks. This unfavorable action of tangeretin was explained by its suppression of the cytolytic activity of murine natural killer cells on MCF-7/6 cells *in vitro* [84]. These findings clearly demonstrate that dietary compounds can interfere with the oral tamoxifen and lead to decrease in therapeutic efficacy, suggesting that excessive consumption of tangeretin-added products and nutritional supplements should be avoided by breast cancer patients during tamoxifen treatment [84-86].

Despite abundant occurrence in the dietary plants, only one flavonol-type compound, i.e., quercetin, has been studied regarding to its potential impact on antitumor action of tamoxifen in breast cancer models. These studies revealed exciting results showing that while quercetin at high doses (100 μM) synergistically augmented tamoxifen-induced cell growth inhibition and apoptosis in ER+ MCF-7 cells, the presence of low concentrations (5 μM) of this flavonol significantly suppressed drug-elicited antiproliferative and apoptotic effects. Also, at low doses, quercetin counteracted tamoxifen-restricted metastatic ability, whereas combined treatment of cells with tamoxifen and high concentrations of quercetin synergistically inhibited metastatic processes. For such a dual role, quercetin regulated expression of diverse molecules involved in cell cycle progression (cyclin D1, cyclin E), apoptosis (p21, p53, Bax, caspases-3 and -9) and metastasis (MMP-2, MMP-9), in different directions dependent on its doses, through the ER pathways. Combined treatment with tamoxifen and quercetin indeed significantly affected the gene expression levels of several ER subtypes. At high doses, quercetin substantially promoted tamoxifen-induced decrease in the expression of both nuclear ERs (ERα66, ERβ) and membrane ERs (ERα36, GPR30). On the contrary, low concentrations of quercetin partially offset tamoxifen-mediated reduction of the expression of membrane ERs (ERα36, GPR30). In previous studies, these two membrane ERs have been considered to be relevant to poor prognosis, correlating with migratory and invasive abilities of malignant cells. Therefore, exposure to low micromolar doses of quercetin during tamoxifen treatment can modulate the relative ratios of ER subtypes, leading to changes in therapeutic efficacy and treatment outcomes [23]. In another study with MCF-7 cells, combination of tamoxifen and quercetin (in 1:2 weight ratio) led to an enhancement of drug-induced cytotoxicity, regardless of administering these agents as a free mixture or coencapsulated into poly (lactic-co-glycolic acid) (PLGA) nanoparticles [67]. In addition, quercetin (at 25 and 50 μM) could increase also sensitivity of tamoxifen resistant MCF-7 cells (MCF-7Ca/TAM-R) to 4-OH-TAM treatment, by upregulating ERα and downregulating Her-2 levels, and promoting apoptotic death. This chemosensitization effect was independent of whether quercetin and tamoxifen were administered simultaneously or sequentially with a 12-hour interval. However, as the physiological mechanisms of tamoxifen resistance in patients are obviously much more complex, interfering with the therapeutic efficacy of tamoxifen and its metabolites by quercetin definitely needs further comprehensive studies [34]. These *in vitro* results were confirmed using an *in vivo* model of ER+ mammary cancer, i.e., DMBA-induced breast tumors in female rats [18], where orally given nanoencapsulated formulation of dual agents, tamoxifen and quercetin, significantly enhanced tamoxifen-induced suppression of tumor growth, normalizing also the plasma levels of matrix metalloproteinase (MMP)-2 and MMP-9. No signs of hepatotoxicity or oxidative stress were detected, suggesting safety of this treatment. Also, no mortality was recorded among the animals treated with dual agents-loaded nanoparticles, whereas the death rate in tamoxifen-treated animals was about 50%. However, administration of free mixture of tamoxifen and quercetin led to no significant changes in tumor growth inhibition as well as mortality rate when compared to tamoxifen-alone treated rats. Therefore, increased *in vivo* antitumor efficacy of nanoencapsulated combination of tamoxifen and quercetin could be due to higher tumor accumulation of both drugs as a result of their improved oral bioavailabilities and sustained pharmacokinetics, rather than interfering with tamoxifen-induced antitumor mechanisms by quercetin [67]. In addition, the presence of quercetin has been shown to augment antiproliferative activity of tamoxifen also in ER-breast cancer models, as combination treatment of quercetin and tamoxifen induced more efficient growth inhibition in TNBC cells MDA-MB-435 than either agent alone [41]. Codelivery of quercetin and N-desmethyltamoxifen in multiwalled carbon nanotubes (MWCNTs)-based nanoconstructs to MDA-MB-231 cells also resulted in about sevenfold increase in cytotoxic responses of this tamoxifen metabolite. Considering that quercetin is a well-known P-gp efflux inhibitor, fast release of this flavonol from the nanoconjugate might contribute to higher intracellular accumulation of the drug, leading to substantially improved outcomes [87]. Moreover, coadministration of tamoxifen and quercetin, as a free mixture or entrapped to polyester nanosponge particles, to 4T1 murine mammary cancer cells (a well-known rodent model of TNBC) likewise increased tamoxifen-induced cytotoxic responses, although there were no significant differences in inhibition of cell viability between free mixture of dual agents and their nanoformulation [88]. These findings convincingly demonstrate that besides modulating the relative ratios of ER subtypes in ER+ breast cancer cells, the presence of quercetin can improve the therapeutic activity of tamoxifen also by intervening in hormone-independent pathways in TNBC cells.

Representatives of flavanones have also been combined with tamoxifen to evaluate their possible interactions and impacts on therapeutic efficacy in breast cancer models. Glycosidic form of citrus flavanone hesperetin, hesperetin 7-rutinoside or hesperidin, at doses over 20 μM, synergistically potentiated tamoxifen-induced inhibitory effects on the growth of ER+ breast cancer cells MCF-7 and T47D. Treatment of T47D cells with this combination promoted the arrest of cell cycle progression at G0/G1 phase and led to a significant increase in apoptosis, manifested as an increase in the ratio of pro- and antiapoptotic markers (Bax: Bcl-2), as well as reduced levels of ERα and EGFR expression. These results suggest that hesperidin could be used as an adjuvant agent to tamoxifen in the treatment of breast tumors, if further *in vivo* investigations will confirm the safety and efficacy of this combination [4]. The aglycone form of hesperidin, hesperetin, increased antiproliferative action of tamoxifen in TNBC cells MDA-MB-435, similarly to another flavanone aglycone, naringenin [41]. The presence of high doses of naringenin enhanced antitumor efficacy of tamoxifen also in ER+ MCF-7 cells, impairing cellular proliferation and viability [26, 27]. Combined treatment with tamoxifen and naringenin (200 μM) blocked the cell cycle progression at S and G2/M phases, suppressed migration and invasion of malignant cells, and promoted apoptotic death by stimulating the production of ROS and regulating the expression of mitochondrial apoptotic proteins. These activities were implemented via modulation of the expression of four different ER subtypes. While addition of naringenin elevated the levels of tamoxifen-suppressed ERβ and ERα36, it further reduced the transcription of ERα66 and GPR30 [27]. The intracellular signaling network triggered by cotreatment of MCF-7 cells with tamoxifen and naringenin (250 μM) was probably complex, involving reduction of overall levels of protein kinase B (AKT) and extracellular signal-regulated kinases 1 and 2 (ERK1/2), ultimately leading to induction of apoptosis to a greater extent than either agent alone [26]. Therefore, naringenin can potentially serve as an adjuvant therapy for tamoxifen in the treatment of ER+ breast tumors; however, the doses of this flavanone needed for potentiating the drug effectiveness are very high. Further enhancement of tamoxifen-induced cytotoxic responses was achieved by co-loading tamoxifen and naringenin into self-nanoemulsifying drug delivery system (SNEDDS), displaying a significant decrease in cellular viability and increase in apoptotic death of MCF-7 cells with respect to the use of tamoxifen-alone loaded nanocarriers or free suspensions. Combined treatment with nanoencapsulated tamoxifen and naringenin resulted in a superior inhibition of tumor growth and burden also in DMBA-treated female rats, being related to improved pharmacokinetics and oral bioavailability of the drug. Moreover, no animals receiving this dual-agent nanoformulation died during 60 days period, in contrast to 40% mortality rate among the rats who were administered tamoxifen-alone containing nanoparticles [89].

Probably the most exciting, but also controversial topic concerning the interactions between plant-derived flavonoids and tamoxifen is the role of isoflavones on the therapeutic efficacy of tamoxifen. The major soy isoflavones include genistein and daidzein, and these compounds are known for their weak estrogenic activities functioning through interaction with ERs. As phytoestrogens could have potentially adverse mitogenic effects on hormone-dependent tumor cells, intake of soy isoflavones concomitantly with antiestrogens has created confusion among breast cancer patients concerning possible unfavorable interactions with tamoxifen, which is why medical practitioners have discouraged women under tamoxifen therapy from consuming soy products or taking soy isoflavone supplements [39, 61, 90]. In addition, the precise molecular mechanisms of action of phytoestrogens have still remained ambiguous and diverse, whereas acting through ERs is apparently by no means their only mode of action [11, 39]. Moreover, effects of phytoestrogens at their physiological concentrations (less than 10 μM) seems to be dependent also on the estrogenic milieu, i.e., pre- or postmenopausal conditions [39]. Based on the current experimental knowledge, daidzein at low micromolar doses abrogated the growth inhibitory effects of 4-OH-TAM in ER+ (tamoxifen-sensitive) MCF-7 cells. However, in tamoxifen-resistant MCF-7 cells, MCF-7$^{MMU2}$, no effect on cell proliferation was observed after cotreatment with 4-OH-TAM and daidzein [39]. Also, coadministration of tamoxifen and daidzein exerted no effects on tumor growth *in vivo* in mice inoculated with ER+ T47D:A18 cells, while this combination therapy induced stimulation of malignant growth and produced tumors of greater size in the mice harboring protein kinase C (PKC)α-overexpressing and tamoxifen-resistant T47D:A18/PKCα tumors [50]. Therefore, simultaneous consumption of daidzein with tamoxifen treatment may not be safe, being possibly even harmful for patients with hormone-dependent breast cancers. On the contrary, dietary daidzein substantially improved tamoxifen-induced protection against mammary carcinogenesis in DMBA-treated female rats, reducing tumor multiplicity, tumor incidence and tumor burden and increasing tumor latency as compared to tamoxifen-alone treated animals. Coadministration of tamoxifen and daidzein led to a marked lowering in both DMBA-evoked as well as endogenous oxidative DNA damage in rat mammary glands, measured by decrease in 8-oxo-deoxyguanosine (8-oxo-dG) levels [61]. Considering that dietary intervention with tamoxifen and daidzein started a week before DMBA treatment, these results suggest that combined therapy with tamoxifen and daidzein might be beneficial for chemoprevention against mammary carcinogenesis, but not treatment of established breast tumors [50]. It is also possible that doses of isoflavones may play a determining role, as high concentrations of equol (100 μM), the main product of intestinal bacterial metabolism of daidzein, were shown to additively enhance 4-OH-TAM-induced inhibition of cell viability and promotion of apoptosis in ER+ MCF-7 cells. This proapoptotic action was related to decrease in Bcl-2 expression, promotion of cytochrome c release from the mitochondria to the cytosol, activation of caspases-9 and -7, and cleavage of poly (ADP-ribose) polymerase (PARP) and α-fodrin by combined treatment, more efficiently than either agent alone [19]. However, at lower doses (around 20 μM), the presence of equol contrarily antagonized the antitumor action of 4-OH-TAM in several ER+ breast cancer lines, MCF-7, T-47D and ZR-75-1, downregulating the expression of ER and PR in MCF-7 and ZR-75-1 cells [46]. As there are no human intervention studies performed to evaluate the effects of daidzein (or its metabolite equol) on therapeutic efficacy of tamoxifen against breast cancer, it is impossible to conclude whether the above-described data obtained from cultured cells and animal models are relevant also to humans.

**Table 3.2.** Effects of flavonoids on anticancer action of tamoxifen (TAM) and its major active metabolite 4-hydroxytamoxifen (4-OH-TAM) in breast tumor models (highlighted rows indicate undesired negative effects on anticancer efficacy)

| Flavonoid and its dosage | Tamoxifen and its dosage | Biological system | Assay method and time | Effect | Mechanisms | Ref. |
|---|---|---|---|---|---|---|
| FLAVANOLS | | | | | | |
| ECG; 25 µM | 4-OH-TAM; 0.01 µM | MCF-7 human breast cancer cells, ERα+ | SRB; 7 days | No effect on 4-OH-TAM-induced cytotoxicity | | [82] |
| ECG; 25 µM | 4-OH-TAM; 0.01 µM | T47D human breast cancer cells, ERα+ | SRB; 7 days | Decrease in cytotoxic potential of 4-OH-TAM | | [82] |
| ECG; 25 µM | 4-OH-TAM; 1 µM | MDA-MB-231 human breast cancer cells, ERα- | SRB; 7 days | No effect on 4-OH-TAM-induced cytotoxicity | | [82] |
| ECG; 25 µM | 4-OH-TAM; 0.1 µM | HS578T human breast cancer cells, ERα- | SRB; 7 days | No effect on 4-OH-TAM-induced cytotoxicity | | [82] |
| EGC; 25 µM | 4-OH-TAM; 0.01 µM | MCF-7 human breast cancer cells, ERα+ | SRB; 7 days | No effect on 4-OH-TAM-induced cytotoxicity | | [82] |
| EGC; 25 µM | 4-OH-TAM; 0.01 µM | T47D human breast cancer cells, ERα+ | SRB; 7 days | No effect on 4-OH-TAM-induced cytotoxicity | | [82] |
| EGC; 25 µM | 4-OH-TAM; 1 µM | MDA-MB-231 human breast cancer cells, ERα- | SRB; 7 days | No effect on 4-OH-TAM-induced cytotoxicity | | [82] |

| Flavonoid and its dosage | Tamoxifen and its dosage | Biological system | Assay method and time | Effect | Mechanisms | Ref. |
|---|---|---|---|---|---|---|
| EGC; 25 µM | 4-OH-TAM; 0.1 µM | HS578T human breast cancer cells, ERα- | SRB; 7 days | Increase in cytotoxic potential of 4-OH-TAM (not greater than that produced by EGC alone) | | [82] |
| EGCG; 25 µM | 4-OH-TAM; 0.01 µM | MCF-7 human breast cancer cells, ERα+ | SRB; 7 days | No effect on 4-OH-TAM-induced cytotoxicity | | [82] |
| EGCG; 0.01, 0.1, 1 µM | TAM; 0.001, 0.01, 0.1 µM | MCF-7 human breast cancer cells, ER+ | Counting colonies; 14 days | Synergistic inhibition of proliferation (CI<1) | | [3] |
| EGCG; 5 µM | TAM; 50-200 nM | MCF-7 human breast cancer cells | MTT; 24h | Synergistic increase in growth inhibition | Downregulation of Skp2 protein | [43] |
| EGCG; 5 µM | TAM; 100 nM | MCF-7 human breast cancer cells, stimulated with 100 nM E2 | MTT; 24h | Increase in growth inhibition | Decrease in Skp2, accumulation of p27 protein | [43] |
| EGCG; 10, 50, 100 µM | TAM; 0-10 µM | MCF-7/TAM human breast adenocarcinoma cells, TAM-resistant | MTT; 24h | 1.24-2.12-fold increase in sensitivity to TAM | Reduction of Nrf2 expression and signaling | [45] |
| EGCG; 40 µM | TAM; 1 µM | MCF-7/HER2/neu human breast cancer cells, estrogen-dependent, transfected with HER2/neu | MTT; 72h | Increase in antiproliferative effects of TAM | Suppression of tyrosine kinase activity | [30] |
| EGCG; 25 µM | 4-OH-TAM; 0.01 µM | T47D human breast cancer cells, ERα+ | SRB; 7 days | No effect on 4-OH-TAM-induced cytotoxicity | | [82] |
| EGCG; 5 µM | TAM; 100-400 nM | AU565 human breast cancer cells, overexpressing HER2 | MTT; 24h | Synergistic increase in growth inhibition | Downregulation of Skp2 protein | [43] |

**Table 3.2.** (Continued)

| Flavonoid and its dosage | Tamoxifen and its dosage | Biological system | Assay method and time | Effect | Mechanisms | Ref. |
|---|---|---|---|---|---|---|
| EGCG; 25 μM | 4-OH-TAM; 1 μM | MDA-MB-231 human breast cancer cells, ERα- | SRB; 7 days | Synergistic cytotoxicity | Increase in apoptosis | [82] |
| EGCG; 25 μM | 4-OH-TAM; 1 μM | MDA-MB-231 human breast cancer cells, ER- | SRB; 24, 36, 48h | Increase in cytotoxicity | Induction of apoptosis earlier and to a greater degree | [44] |
| EGCG; 25 mg/kg/day, i.p. | TAM; 75 μg/kg/day, p.o. | MDA-MB-231 cells inoculated into the right flank of 5-6 w-old female CD1 athymic nude mice | 10 weeks | Superior inhibition of tumor growth, decrease in tumor volume and weight | Suppression of EGFR, pEGFR and mTOR levels; decrease in CYP1B1 expression | [63] |
| EGCG; 25 μM | 4-OH-TAM; 0.1 μM | HS578T human breast cancer cells, ERα- | SRB; 7 days | No effect on 4-OH-TAM-induced cytotoxicity | | [82] |
| TF-1; 40 μM | TAM; 1 μM | MCF-7/HER2/neu human breast cancer cells, estrogen-dependent, transfected with HER2/neu | MTT; 72h | Increase in antiproliferative effects of TAM | Suppression of tyrosine kinase activity | [30] |
| TF-2; 40 μM | TAM; 1 μM | MCF-7/HER2/neu human breast cancer cells, estrogen-dependent, transfected with HER2/neu | MTT; 72h | Increase in antiproliferative effects of TAM | Suppression of tyrosine kinase activity | [30] |
| TF-3; 40 μM | TAM; 1 μM | MCF-7/HER2/neu human breast cancer cells, estrogen-dependent, transfected with HER2/neu | MTT; 72h | Increase in antiproliferative effects of TAM | Suppression of tyrosine kinase activity | [30] |

| Flavonoid and its dosage | Tamoxifen and its dosage | Biological system | Assay method and time | Effect | Mechanisms | Ref. |
|---|---|---|---|---|---|---|
| FLAVONES | | | | | | |
| Apigenin; 10 nM-10 μM | 4-OH-TAM; 0.1 μM | MCF-7 human breast cancer cells, ERα+ | MTS (CellTiter 96 Aqueous One Solution); 8 days | No significant effect on 4-OH-TAM-induced antiproliferation | Downregulation of ERα expression at mRNA and protein levels | [83] |
| Apigenin; 10 nM-10 μM | 4-OH-TAM; 0.1 μM | T47D human breast cancer cells, ERα+ | MTS (CellTiter 96 Aqueous One Solution); 9 days | Only a moderate insignificant blocking effect on 4-OH-TAM-induced antiproliferation | | [83] |
| Apigenin; 10 nM-10 μM | 4-OH-TAM; 0.1 μM | MDA-MB-435 human breast cancer cells, ERα- | MTS (CellTiter 96 Aqueous One Solution); 12 days | No antiproliferative effect | | [83] |
| Apigenin; 1:1 combination with TAM | TAM; 1:1 combination with apigenin | MDA-MB-435 human breast cancer cells, ER- | [$^3$H] Thymidine incorporation; 48h | Increase in antiproliferative action of TAM | | [41] |
| Luteolin; 5, 10 μM | 4-OH-TAM; 100 nM | TAM-R MCF-7 human mammary gland adenocarcinoma cells, TAM-resistant, luminal type A cells (ER+/PR+/Her2-) | MTT; 24h | Sensitization to 4-OH-TAM-induced cytotoxicity | Decrease in CCNE2 expression, inhibition of cell cycle entry into the S phase | [22] |
| Nobiletin; 1:1 combination with TAM | TAM; 1:1 combination with nobiletin | MDA-MB-435 human breast cancer cells, ER- | [$^3$H] Thymidine incorporation; 48h | Increase in antiproliferative action of TAM | | [41] |
| Tangeretin; 100 μM | TAM; 1 μM | MCF-7/6 human breast adenocarcinoma cells, ER+ | SRB; 5 days | Amplification of growth inhibition | | [84] |

**Table 3.2.** (Continued)

| Flavonoid and its dosage | Tamoxifen and its dosage | Biological system | Assay method and time | Effect | Mechanisms | Ref. |
|---|---|---|---|---|---|---|
| Tangeretin; 100 μM, in drinking water | TAM; 30 μM, in drinking water | MCF-7/6 cells inoculated into the mammary fat pad of female nude (Swiss nu/nu) mice | 16 weeks | Complete neutralization of inhibitory effect of TAM. Decrease in median survival time of mice (14 vs 56 weeks with TAM alone) | Inhibition of cytolytic effect of murine natural killer cells on MCF-7/6 cells | [84] |
| Tangeretin; 1:1 combination with TAM | TAM; 1:1 combination with tangeretin | MDA-MB-435 human breast cancer cells, ER- | [$^3$H] Thymidine incorporation; 48h | Increase in antiproliferative action of TAM | | [41] |
| FLAVONOLS | | | | | | |
| Quercetin; 5 μM | TAM; 5 μM | MCF-7 human breast carcinoma cells, ER+ | CCK-8; 24, 48, 72h. Real-time cellular impedance | Inhibition of TAM-induced antiproliferation, increase in cell viability. Partial prevention of TAM-induced cytotoxicity | Partial counteraction of TAM-inhibited migration and invasion (increase in MMP-2 and MMP-9); increase in S and G2/M phase cell populations (increase in cyclin D1 and cyclin E); attenuation of TAM-induced apoptosis (decrease in LDH, increase in GSH; | [23] |

| Flavonoid and its dosage | Tamoxifen and its dosage | Biological system | Assay method and time | Effect | Mechanisms | Ref. |
|---|---|---|---|---|---|---|
| | | | | | partial repression of TAM-induced caspases-3 and -9 activation and cyt c release; downregulation of p21 and p53; blocking of TAM-induced decline of ΔΨm; suppression of TAM-induced ROS generation). Regulation of ERs gene expression (partial offset of TAM-suppressed ERα36 and GPR30); increase in pS2 expression | |
| Quercetin; 100 μM | TAM; 5 μM | MCF-7 human breast carcinoma cells, ER+ | CCK-8; 24, 48, 72h. Real-time cellular impedance | Synergistic inhibition of cell proliferation | Suppression of migration and invasion (decrease in MMP-2 and MMP-9); increase in S phase cell population (decrease in cyclin D1 and cyclin E); promotion of TAM-induced apoptosis (increase in LDH, decrease in GSH; stimulation of TAM-induced caspases-3 and -9 activation and | [23] |

**Table 3.2.** (Continued)

| Flavonoid and its dosage | Tamoxifen and its dosage | Biological system | Assay method and time | Effect | Mechanisms | Ref. |
|---|---|---|---|---|---|---|
| | | | | | cyt c release; upregulation of Bax, p21 and p53; boosting of TAM-repressed ΔΨm; promotion of TAM-induced ROS generation). Strengthening of TAM-induced repression of nuclear ERs (ERα66, ERβ) and membrane ERs (ERα36, GPR30); suppression of pS2 expression | |
| Quercetin; 0.02-20 μg/ml; as free mixture or co-loaded with TAM to PLGA-NPs | TAM; 0.01-10 μg/ml; as free mixture or co-loaded with quercetin to PLGA-NPs | MCF-7 human breast adenocarcinoma cells | MTT; 24, 48, 72h | Increase in cytotoxicity compared to free TAM | | [67] |
| Quercetin; 25, 50 μM | 4-OH-TAM; 1 μM | MCF-7Ca/TAM-R human breast cancer cells, ER+, TAM-resistant | MTT; 48, 72h (simultaneously) or induction with quercetin for 12h followed by 4-OH-TAM | Decrease in cell survival rate, increase in sensitivity to 4-OH-TAM. No difference whether treated simultaneously or sequentially | Increase in apoptosis. Upregulation of ERα, downregulation of Her-2 | [34] |

| Flavonoid and its dosage | Tamoxifen and its dosage | Biological system | Assay method and time | Effect | Mechanisms | Ref. |
|---|---|---|---|---|---|---|
| Quercetin; 6 mg/kg, by oral gavage, once in 3 days for 30 days; as free mixture or co-loaded with TAM to PLGA-NPs | TAM; 3 mg/kg, by oral gavage, once in 3 days for 30 days; as free mixture or co-loaded with quercetin to PLGA-NPs | DMBA-induced breast cancer model in female SD rats, ER+ | 30 days | Increase in TAM-induced tumor suppression when quercetin was co-loaded with TAM to PLGA-NPs. Insignificant effect with free mixture. No mortality with NPs (after 60 days) | Normalization of plasma levels of MMP-2 and MMP-9 with TAM-quercetin-PLGA-NPs. No significant effect with free mixture | [67] |
| Quercetin; co-loaded with N-desmethyl TAM to TEG-MWCNT (1:3 w/w) | N-Desmethyl TAM; 0-500 mg/ml, co-loaded with quercetin to TEG-MWCNT | MDA-MB-231 human breast cancer cells, drug-resistant | MTT; 24h | Increase in N-desmethyl TAM-induced cytotoxicity | | [87] |
| Quercetin; 1:1 combination with TAM | TAM; 1:1 combination with quercetin | MDA-MB-435 human breast cancer cells, ER- | [$^3$H] Thymidine incorporation; 48h | Increase in antiproliferative action of TAM | | [41] |
| Quercetin; as free mixture or co-loaded with TAM to polyester nanosponge particles (1:1 w/w) | TAM; 0.01-10 µg/ml, as free mixture or co-loaded with quercetin to polyester nanosponge particles | 4T1 mouse mammalian breast cancer cells | MTT; 24, 48, 72h | Increase in cytotoxicity compared to free TAM | | [88] |
| FLAVANONES | | | | | | |
| Hesperetin; 1:1 combination with TAM | TAM; 1:1 combination with hesperetin | MDA-MB-435 human breast cancer cells, ER- | [$^3$H] Thymidine incorporation; 48h | Increase in antiproliferative action of TAM | | [41] |

**Table 3.2.** (Continued)

| Flavonoid and its dosage | Tamoxifen and its dosage | Biological system | Assay method and time | Effect | Mechanisms | Ref. |
|---|---|---|---|---|---|---|
| Hesperidin; 12.26-49.03 μg/ml | TAM; 7.71-30.83 μg/ml | MCF7 human breast adenocarcinoma cells, ER+ | MTT; 24h | Increase in antiproliferative effect of TAM | | [4] |
| Hesperidin; 17-68.01 μg/ml | TAM; 4.18-16.7 μg/ml | T47D human breast ductal carcinoma cells, ER+ | MTT; 24h | Synergistic increase in antiproliferative effect of TAM (CI<1) | Arresting cells at G0/G1 phase, increase in apoptosis (upregulation of Bax, downregulation of Bcl2); decrease in EGFR and ERα mRNA levels | [4] |
| Naringenin; 200 μM | TAM; 5 μM | MCF-7 human breast adenocarcinoma cells, ER+, expressing also ERα36 and GPR30 | Real-time cellular impedance; every 5 min to 96h | Additive inhibition of cell proliferation | Suppression of cell migration and invasion (downregulation of MMP-2 and MMP-9); blocking cell cycle at S and G2/M phases (increase in p53 and p21 mRNA expression, decrease in cyclin D and cyclin E expression); promotion of apoptosis (decrease in Bcl-2/Bax ratio, stimulation of ROS production); regulation of nuclear ERs (ERα, ERβ) and membrane ERs (ERα36, GPR30) | [27] |

| Flavonoid and its dosage | Tamoxifen and its dosage | Biological system | Assay method and time | Effect | Mechanisms | Ref. |
|---|---|---|---|---|---|---|
| Naringenin; 250 µM | TAM; 100 nM | MCF-7 human breast cancer cells | Guava easy-Cyte$^{TM}$ Flow Cytometry; 7 days | Increase in cytostatic and cytotoxic activities of TAM | Increase in apoptosis (activation of caspases-7 and -9, cleavage of PARP). Decrease in ERK1/2 and AKT expression | [26] |
| Naringenin; co-loaded with TAM into SNEDDS | TAM; 3.12-100 µM, co-loaded with naringenin into SNEDDS | MCF-7 human breast adenocarcinoma cells | MTT; 24h | Improving cytotoxicity with respect to TAM-SNEDDS, TAM-naringenin suspension and TAM suspension | Increase in apoptosis | [89] |
| Naringenin; co-loaded with TAM into SNEDDS, oral administration | TAM; 45 mg/kg, co-loaded with naringenin into SNEDDS, oral administration for 3 consecutive weeks at weekly interval | DMBA-induced female Wistar rat breast cancer model, ER+ | 30 days | Superior decrease in tumor growth and tumor burden. Complete survival of animals (vs 40% mortality in TAM-SNEDDS group) | | [89] |
| Naringenin; 1:1 combination with TAM | TAM; 1:1 combination with naringenin | MDA-MB-435 human breast cancer cells, ER- | [$^3$H] Thymidine incorporation; 48h | Increase in antiproliferative action of TAM | | [41] |
| ISOFLAVONES | | | | | | |
| Daidzein; 1, 10 µM | 4-OH-TAM; 100 nM | MCF-7 human breast cancer cells, TAM-sensitive | MTT; 72h | Abrogation of growth inhibitory effect of 4-OH-TAM | | [39] |
| Daidzein; 1, 10 µM | 4-OH-TAM; 100 nM | MCF-7$^{MMU2}$ human breast cancer cells, TAM-resistant | MTT; 72h | No effect, no increase in cell proliferation | | [39] |

**Table 3.2.** (Continued)

| Flavonoid and its dosage | Tamoxifen and its dosage | Biological system | Assay method and time | Effect | Mechanisms | Ref. |
|---|---|---|---|---|---|---|
| Daidzein; 0.144 g/kg diet | TAM; 1.5 mg/animal, p.o. daily for 5 days | T47D:A18 hormone-dependent human breast cancer cells injected s.c. into the axillary mammary fat pads of ovariectomized BALB/c athymic mice | 22 weeks | No effect on tumor growth | | [50] |
| Daidzein; 0.144 g/kg diet | TAM; 1.5 mg/animal, p.o. daily for 5 days | T47D:A18/PKCα human breast cancer cells (TAM-resistant) injected s.c. into the axillary mammary fat pads of ovariectomized BALB/c athymic mice | 11 weeks | Stimulation of tumor growth; producing tumor of greater size than TAM alone | | [50] |
| Daidzein; 105 mg/kg diet | TAM; 0.125 mg/kg diet | DMBA-induced mammary tumors in female Sprague-Dawley rats, ER+ | 114 days | Increase in TAM-induced protection against mammary carcinogenesis. Improving the suppressive effect of TAM on tumor incidence, multiplicity and burden | Synergistic protection against oxidative DNA damage (decrease in 8-oxo-dG levels) | [61] |
| Equol; 100 μM | 4-OH-TAM; 10 μM | MCF-7 human breast cancer cells, estrogen-dependent | MTT; 72h | Additive increase in antiproliferative effect of 4-OH-TAM | Additive increase in apoptosis (decrease in Bcl-2 expression, promotion of cyt c release to the cytosol, increase in caspases-9 and -7 activation, cleavage of PARP and α-fodrin) | [19] |

| Flavonoid and its dosage | Tamoxifen and its dosage | Biological system | Assay method and time | Effect | Mechanisms | Ref. |
|---|---|---|---|---|---|---|
| Equol; 22.3 μM (=$IC_{50}$) | 4-OH-TAM; molar ratio with equol of 1:2 | MCF-7 human breast cancer cells, hormone receptor+ | MTS; 72h | Antagonistic effect against 4-OH-TAM (CI>1) | Decrease in ER and PR expression; downregulation of cyclin D1 | [46] |
| Equol; 18.3 μM(=$IC_{50}$) | 4-OH-TAM; molar ratio with equol of 1:2 | ZR-75-1 human breast cancer cells, hormone receptor+ | MTS; 72h | Antagonistic effect against 4-OH-TAM (CI>1) | Decrease in ER and PR expression | [46] |
| Equol; 16.2 μM (=$IC_{50}$) | 4-OH-TAM; molar ratio with equol of 1:4 | T-47D human breast cancer cells, hormone receptor+ | MTS; 72h | Antagonistic effect against 4-OH-TAM (CI>1) | | [46] |
| Genistein; 1-10 μg/ml (3.7-37 μM) | TAM; 100 nM, 1 μM | MCF-10$A_1$ human mammary dysplastic cells, ER+, devoid of metastatic potential | Methylene blue staining; 72h | Synergistic antiproliferative effect | | [91] |
| Genistein; 1-10 μg/ml (3.7-37 μM) | TAM; 100 nM, 1 μM | MCF-ANeoT human mammary dysplastic cells, ER+, devoid of metastatic potential | Methylene blue staining; 72h | Synergistic antiproliferative effect | | [91] |
| Genistein; 1-10 μg/ml (3.7-37 μM) | TAM; 100 nM, 1 μM | MCF-$T_6$3B human mammary dysplastic cells, ER+, devoid of metastatic potential | Methylene blue staining; 72h | Synergistic antiproliferative effect | | [91] |
| Genistein; 1-10 μg/ml (3.7-37 μM) | TAM; 100 nM, 1 μM | MCF-7 human breast cancer cells, ER+, with the least metastatic potential | Methylene blue staining; 72h | Additive growth inhibition | | [91] |
| Genistein; 25, 50 μM | TAM; 3, 6 μM | MCF-7 human breast cancer cells, estrogen-dependent | Counting; 72h | Potentiation of cell growth inhibition (less than additive effect) | | [8] |

**Table 3.2.** (Continued)

| Flavonoid and its dosage | Tamoxifen and its dosage | Biological system | Assay method and time | Effect | Mechanisms | Ref. |
|---|---|---|---|---|---|---|
| Genistein; 0.069-150 μM | TAM; 0.14-100 μM | MCF-7 human breast cancer cells, ERα+, ERβ+, very low level of erbB2 | MTS (CellTiter 96 Aqueous One Solution); 72h | Reversal of growth inhibitory effect of TAM, stimulation of growth at lower doses (<30 μM genistein and <10 μM TAM). Growth inhibition at higher doses | | [11] |
| Genistein; 1 μM | Tamoxifen; 10 μM | MCF-7 human breast cancer cells, high ERα/ERβ ratio | Crystal Violet; 48h | Decrease in TAM efficacy, increase in cell viability | Decrease in TAM-induced ROS production, autophagy and apoptosis; increase in CAT protein, increase in S phase cell cycle arrest | [17] |
| Genistein; 1 μM | Tamoxifen; 10 μM | MCF7+ERβ, ERβ-overexpressing MCF-7 human breast cancer cells | Crystal Violet; 48h | Slight decrease in TAM-induced inhibition of cell viability (milder than in parent MCF-7 cells) | Decrease in TAM-induced ROS production (milder than in parent MCF-7 cells). No significant changes in autophagy and apoptosis | [17] |
| Genistein; 2, 10 μM | TAM; 0.4 μM | MCF-7/Neo human breast cancer cells, ER+, erbB2 normal | MTT; 6 days | Abrogation of TAM-induced inhibitory effect; increase in cell proliferation and TAM resistance | Increase in ER activity | [32] |

| Flavonoid and its dosage | Tamoxifen and its dosage | Biological system | Assay method and time | Effect | Mechanisms | Ref. |
|---|---|---|---|---|---|---|
| Genistein; 2, 10 μM | TAM; 0.4 μM | MCF-7/erbB-2 human breast cancer cells, ER+, transfected with human erbB2 (luminal type B cells) | MTT; 6 days | Abrogation of TAM-induced inhibitory effect; increase in cell proliferation and TAM resistance | Increase in ER activity; activation of ER-erbB2 crosstalk | [32] |
| Genistein; 1, 10 μM | 4-OH-TAM; 100 nM | MCF-7 human breast cancer cells, TAM-sensitive | MTT; 72h | Abrogation of growth inhibitory effect of 4-OH-TAM; stimulation of cell growth | | [39] |
| Genistein; 10 μM | 4-OH-TAM; 0.1 μM | MCF-7 human breast cancer cells, ERα+ | MTS (CellTiter 96 Aqueous One Solution); 8 days | Blocking antiproliferative effect of 4-OH-TAM | Downregulation of ERα expression at mRNA and protein levels | [83] |
| Genistein; 1, 10 μM | 4-OH-TAM; 100 nM | MCF-7$^{MMU2}$ human breast cancer cells, TAM-resistant | MTT; 72h | No effect, no increase in cell proliferation | | [39] |
| Genistein; 1 μM-10 μM | 4-OH-TAM; 0.1 μM | MCF-7 human breast cancer cells and H295R human adrenocortico-carcinoma cells co-culture (at 5:1 ratio) | MTT; 9 days | Overcoming 4-OH-TAM-induced growth inhibition, induction of cell proliferation | | [37] |
| Genistein; 1000 ppm, with diet | TAM; 2.5 or 5 mg, as implants placed in i.p. region of mice | MCF-7 cells injected into two sites on the flank of ovariectomized athymic BALB/c nude mice; implanted with E2 (0.25 mg) in i.p. region of mice | 32 weeks | Negation of TAM inhibitory effect on tumor growth, increase in tumor sizes | Reversal of TAM-induced inhibition of cyclin D1, pS2 and PR expression. Lowering plasma levels of E2 | [9] |

**Table 3.2.** (Continued)

| Flavonoid and its dosage | Tamoxifen and its dosage | Biological system | Assay method and time | Effect | Mechanisms | Ref. |
|---|---|---|---|---|---|---|
| Genistein; 250, 500, 1000 ppm, as dietary supplement | TAM; 3 mg, as implant | MCF-7 cells injected s.c. into four sites on the flank of female ovariectomized athymic nude mice; implanted with estrogen (0.08 mg) | 35 weeks | Negation of TAM inhibitory effect on tumor growth and prevalence (at 250 and 500 ppm; no effect at 1000 ppm) | Abrogation of TAM inhibitory effect on cell proliferation and inducing effect on cell apoptosis (at 250 and 500 ppm; synergistic effect on apoptosis at 1000 ppm). Abrogation of TAM inhibitory effect on cyclin D1 gene expression (at 250 and 500 ppm; no effect at 1000 ppm). Counteraction of TAM inhibitory effect on PR gene expression (at all doses) | [10] |
| Genistein; 0.07%, added to diet | TAM; 25 mg, implanted s.c., 90-day release | MCF-7 cells implanted orthotopically into a mammary fat pad of female SCID mice; implanted s.c. with E2 pellets (0.72 mg, 90-day release) | ~12 weeks | Synergistic effect on delaying tumor growth | Increase in apoptotic index. Reduction of serum E2 level. Decrease in pS2 and EGFR expression | [8] |

| Flavonoid and its dosage | Tamoxifen and its dosage | Biological system | Assay method and time | Effect | Mechanisms | Ref. |
|---|---|---|---|---|---|---|
| Genistein; 1 μM | Tamoxifen; 10 μM | T47D human breast cancer cells, low ERα/ERβ ratio | Crystal Violet; 48h | Increase in TAM-induced inhibition of cell viability | Decrease in ROS production; increase in TAM-induced autophagy and apoptosis (rise in PARP cleavage) | [17] |
| Genistein; 1.0 μM | TAM; 1.0 μM | T47-D human ductal breast cancer cells, ER+ | MTS (CellTiter 96 Aqueous One Solution); 48h | Reversal of TAM-induced cell growth inhibition | Reversal of TAM-induced G1 phase cell cycle arrest | [51] |
| Genistein; 10 nM-10 μM | 4-OH-TAM; 0.1 μM | T47D human breast cancer cells, ERα+ | MTS (CellTiter 96 Aqueous One Solution); 9 days | Blocking antiproliferative effect of 4-OH-TAM | | [83] |
| Genistein; 0.206 g/kg diet | TAM; 1.5 mg/animal, p.o. daily for 5 days | T47D:A18 hormone-dependent human breast cancer cells injected s.c. into the axillary mammary fat pads of ovariectomized BALB/c athymic mice | 22 weeks | No effect on tumor growth | | [50] |
| Genistein; 0.206 g/kg diet | TAM; 1.5 mg/animal, p.o. daily for 5 days | T47D:A18/PKCα human breast cancer cells (TAM-resistant) injected s.c. into the axillary mammary fat pads of ovariectomized BALB/c athymic mice | 11 weeks | Stimulation of tumor growth; producing tumor of greater size than TAM alone | | [50] |

**Table 3.2.** (Continued)

| Flavonoid and its dosage | Tamoxifen and its dosage | Biological system | Assay method and time | Effect | Mechanisms | Ref. |
|---|---|---|---|---|---|---|
| Genistein, 3.125-25 μM | TAM; 0.625-5 μM | BT-474 human breast cancer cells, ER+, HER2-overexpressing | Counting; 72h | Synergistic inhibition of cell growth | Potentiation of G1 phase cell cycle arrest, synergistic increase in apoptosis (decrease in survivin expression). Downregulation of EGFR, HER2 and ERα levels | [36] |
| Genistein; 0.1-20 μM | TAM; 1 μM | 78717, 78617, 85815, 85819 mammary tumor cell lines derived from MMTV-wt-erbB2/neu transgenic mice, ERα-, ERβ+, high levels of erbB2 | MTS (CellTiter 96 Aqueous One Solution); 72h | Reversal of growth inhibitory effect of TAM, stimulation of growth at low doses (0.1-0.3 μM). Synergistic growth inhibition at higher doses | | [11] |
| Genistein; 500 ppm, from postnatal day 15 onward (lifetime exposure), with diet | TAM; 15 mg/kg, with diet (when the first tumor reached 1.4 cm in diameter) | Female Sprague-Dawley rats with DMBA-induced ER+ mammary tumors | 30 weeks | Improving response to TAM therapy; decrease in de novo resistance to TAM, lowering the risk of tumor recurrence | Downregulation of UPR and autophagy-related genes (GRP78, IRE1α, ATF4, Beclin-1) and genes linked to immunosuppression (TGFβ, Foxp3); upregulation of cytotoxic T-cell marker CD8α in the tumors | [18] |

| Flavonoid and its dosage | Tamoxifen and its dosage | Biological system | Assay method and time | Effect | Mechanisms | Ref. |
|---|---|---|---|---|---|---|
| Genistein; 500 ppm, after DMBA (adult exposure), with diet | TAM; 15 mg/kg, with diet (when the first tumor reached 1.4 cm in diameter) | Female Sprague-Dawley rats with DMBA-induced ER+ mammary tumors | 30 weeks | Lowering the risk of tumor recurrence; no effect on de novo resistance to TAM | | [18] |
| Genistein; 500 ppm, after TAM addition (post-diagnosis exposure), with diet | TAM; 15 mg/kg, with diet (when the first tumor reached 1.4 cm in diameter) | Female Sprague-Dawley rats with DMBA-induced ER+ mammary tumors | 30 weeks | Increase in de novo resistance to TAM | | [18] |
| Genistein; 140 mg/kg diet | TAM; 0.125 mg/kg diet | DMBA-induced mammary tumors in female Sprague-Dawley rats, ER+ | 114 days | Decrease in TAM-induced protection against mammary carcinogenesis. Weakening the suppressive effect of TAM on tumor incidence and multiplicity | No effect on DMBA-induced oxidative DNA damage (measured by 8-oxo-dG levels) | [61] |
| Genistein; 25 μM | TAM; 1 μM | MDA-MB-157 human breast cancer cells, ERα- | MTT; 3 days | Re-sensitization of cells to TAM-induced anticancer action | Restoring ERα expression | [20] |
| Genistein; 1-10 μg/ml (3.7-37 μM) | TAM; 100 nM, 1 μM | MDA-231 human breast cancer cells, ER-, with moderate metastatic potential | Methylene blue staining; 72h | Additive growth inhibition | | [91] |

**Table 3.2.** (Continued)

| Flavonoid and its dosage | Tamoxifen and its dosage | Biological system | Assay method and time | Effect | Mechanisms | Ref. |
|---|---|---|---|---|---|---|
| Genistein; 25 μM | TAM; 1 μM | MDA-MB-231 human breast cancer cells, ERα- | MTT; 3 days | Re-sensitization of cells to TAM-induced anticancer action | Restoring ERα expression through epigenetic pathways (by reducing HDAC and DNMT activities) | [20] |
| Genistein; 250 mg/kg, daily diet (from 2 weeks pre-injection) | TAM; 25 mg/pellet with 21 days release, implanted s.c. under the neck area (2 weeks post-injection) | MDA-MB-231 cells injected orthotopically into the mammary fat pad of female immunodeficient Nu/Nu nude mice (Crl:NU-Foxn1nu) | 4 weeks | Increase in therapeutic sensitivity to TAM; increase in tumor growth inhibitory rate | Decrease in the percentage of proliferating cells. Epigenetic reactivation of ERα, decrease in HDAC and DNMT activities | [20] |
| Genistein; 10 nM-10 μM | 4-OH-TAM; 0.1 μM | MDA-MB-435 human breast cancer cells, ERα- | MTS (CellTiter 96 Aqueous One Solution); 12 days | No antiproliferative effect | | [83] |
| Genistein; 1-10 μg/ml (3.7-37 μM) | TAM; 100 nM, 1 μM | MDA-435 human breast cancer cells, ER-, expressing the highest metastatic potential | Methylene blue staining; 72h | Additive growth inhibition | | [91] |
| Genistein; 5, 10, 15 μM | TAM; 5, 10, 15 μM | MDA-MB-435 human breast carcinoma cells, ER- | Counting; 3 days | Synergism in growth inhibition (CI<1) | Synergistic reduction of $IP_3$ concentration | [64] |
| Genistein; 2, 5, 10 μM | TAM; 0.25, 0.50, 0.75 μM | MDA-MB-435 human breast carcinoma cells, ER- | Counting colonies; 7 days | Synergism in cytotoxicity (CI<1) | Synergistic reduction of $IP_3$ concentration | [64] |

| Flavonoid and its dosage | Tamoxifen and its dosage | Biological system | Assay method and time | Effect | Mechanisms | Ref. |
|---|---|---|---|---|---|---|
| Genistein; 1:1 combination with TAM | TAM; 1:1 combination with genistein | MDA-MB-435 human breast cancer cells, ER- | [$^3$H] Thymidine incorporation; 48h | Increase in antiproliferative action of TAM | | [41] |
| Genistein; 250 mg/kg, daily diet | TAM; 25 mg tablet, implanted s.c. for 3 weeks (when tumor size reaches ~400 mm$^3$) | C3(1)-SV40 Tag transgenic mice (spontaneous breast cancer model developing hormone-independent tumors) | 5 weeks | Increase in therapeutic sensitivity to TAM; increase in tumor growth inhibitory rate | Decrease in the percentage of proliferating cells. Epigenetic reactivation of ERα, decrease in HDAC and DNMT activities | [20] |
| Glabridin; 1 µM | Tamoxifen; 10 µM | MCF-7 human breast adenocarcinoma cells | MTT; 72h | Enhancement of antiproliferative effect of TAM | No effect on TAM-induced expression of ESR1 and bcl-2 genes | [14] |
| SYNTHETIC FLAVONOIDS | | | | | | |
| Aminoflavone; 100 nM | 4-OH-TAM; 0.5 or 1 µM | TamR MCF-7 human luminal A breast cancer cells, TAM-resistant | Alamar Blue; 72h | Restoring sensitivity to 4-OH-TAM, blocking of 4-OH-TAM-stimulated proliferation | Decrease in α6-integrin/Src/Akt signaling | [74] |
| Aminoflavone; 2 µM | 4-OH-TAM; 1 or 10 µM | BT-474 human luminal B breast cancer cells, TAM-resistant | Alamar Blue; 120h | Restoring sensitivity to 4-OH-TAM, blocking of 4-OH-TAM-stimulated proliferation | Decrease in α6-integrin expression | [74] |

Much more experiments have been conducted combining tamoxifen with the major soy isoflavone, genistein, in molecularly different breast cancer models, both ER+ and ER- tumors. Combination of tamoxifen and genistein (3.7-37 μM) exerted synergistic antiproliferative activities in several breast dysplastic cell lines, positive to ERs but still missing malignant characteristics (metastatic potential), MCF-10$A_1$, MCF-ANeoT and MCF-$T_6$3B. However, in ER+ breast cancer cells MCF-7, the combined effect on growth inhibition was less prominent and additive in its nature. These results suggest that genistein, similarly to daidzein, could be therapeutically more important at the beginning of carcinogenesis, i.e., in the cases of mammary dysplasia, calling for *in vivo* animal studies for testing this combination as a chemopreventive mean to reduce breast cancer risk [91]. Although potentiation of tamoxifen-induced growth inhibition of MCF-7 cells in the presence of higher doses of genistein (25, 50 μM) has been confirmed also in other reports (being still less than the theoretic additive effect) [8, 11], combination of tamoxifen with low micromolar concentrations of genistein led to contrary results promoting cell proliferation. In fact, genistein at less than 30 μM doses reversed growth inhibitory effects of tamoxifen in MCF-7 cells [11]. At 1 μM concentration, genistein decreased antitumor efficacy of tamoxifen and raised cellular viability in both the parent MCF-7 cells with a high ERα/ERβ ratio as well as ERβ-overexpressing MCF-7 cells, although the antagonistic effect was considerably greater in the parent cells. This action was accompanied by increase in the protein levels of antioxidant enzymes (catalase), reducing production of tamoxifen-induced ROS, besides decrease in autophagy and apoptosis in intact MCF-7 cells, but still not in ERβ-overexpressing cells. These results demonstrate that the ERα/ERβ ratio can be another important factor determining the effect of combination treatment of tamoxifen and isoflavones in breast cancer cells [17]. In addition, the presence of genistein (2, 10 μM) abrogated tamoxifen-induced growth inhibition and induced enhanced cell proliferation and tamoxifen resistance in not only MCF-7 cells, but particularly HER2-transfected MCF-7 cells (MCF-7/erbB-2, representing luminal type B cancer), by increasing ER activity and stimulating crosstalk between ER and HER2 pathways [32]. Similar results have been observed also by combining genistein at its lower doses (1, 10 μM) with tamoxifen active metabolite, 4-OH-TAM, showing that cotreatment of MCF-7 cells with this combination resulted in blocking of 4-OH-TAM-induced antiproliferative effects and instead promoted cellular growth, through downregulation of ERα expression [39, 83]. However, no effects on cell growth were detected in tamoxifen-resistant

MCF-7 cells [39]. Abrogation of 4-OH-TAM-evoked antitumor activities by physiologically achievable genistein doses (1-10 μM) was described also in a co-culture model of MCF-7 cells and human adrenocortical carcinoma cells H295R. Similar to cancer-associated fibroblasts, H295R cells can secrete and respond to several cytokines, such as TNFα and IL-8, thereby mimicking more closely the real surrounding where breast tumors develop [37]. In accordance with these *in vitro* results, addition of genistein (1000 ppm) negated tamoxifen-induced inhibition of estradiol-mediated growth of MCF-7 xenografts in ovariectomized athymic mice, leading to tumors of greater size. The presence of dietary genistein significantly lowered the plasma estradiol levels that were produced by estradiol implants (0.25 mg), and reversed tamoxifen-evoked decrease in the expression of estradiol-responsive genes, including cyclin D1, pS2 and PR [9]. Genistein at low oral doses (250 and 500 ppm) similarly antagonized the inhibitory effects of tamoxifen on MCF-7 tumor growth and prevalence in estradiol (0.08 mg)-implanted ovariectomized mice, by abrogating antiproliferative and apoptotic effects of tamoxifen, at least in part, via regulation of cyclin D1 and PR gene expression and lowering circulating estradiol concentrations. However, in this preclinical model, 1000 ppm genistein diet did not interfere with the inhibitory action of tamoxifen on tumor growth, but rather exerted a synergistic effect on apoptotic death [10]. As opposed to the previous results, the presence of genistein (0.07%) or soy phytochemical concentrate (0.2%) in the diet was shown to synergistically enhance the preventive effects of tamoxifen on development of MCF-7 tumors, delaying the growth of xenografts in estradiol (0.72 mg)-implanted mice, and inducing tumors of smaller weight and volume. Combined treatment with tamoxifen and genistein (or soy phytochemical concentrate) led to a synergistic increase in apoptotic index, with downregulation of pS2 and EGFR expression and reduction of serum estradiol levels in MCF-7 cells-inoculated mice [8]. Such inconsistencies of *in vivo* results could be caused by the interaction of dietary genistein with different levels of implanted estradiol and tamoxifen; raising by all means the safety concerns of consuming dietary genistein supplements in patients with ER+ breast cancer under tamoxifen therapy [10].

Conflicting results have been published also for another ER+ breast cancer cell line, T47D, representing similarly to MCF-7 cells luminal type A tumors, but having differently from MCF-7 cells low ERα/ERβ ratio. Cotreatment of these cells with tamoxifen and genistein (1 μM) resulted in a slight increase in drug-induced inhibition of cell viability, due to an increment in autophagic and apoptotic deaths [17]. However, in another study with 1 μM genistein, its combination with tamoxifen led to abrogation of tamoxifen-induced cell growth inhibition, accompanied by reversal of drug-induced G1 phase cell cycle arrest [51]. Genistein (10 nM-10 μM) blocked antiproliferative effects and reduced therapeutic action also of 4-OH-TAM, promoting the growth of T47D cells [83]. Moreover, while coadministration of genistein and tamoxifen did not affect the tumor growth in T47D:A18 xenograft-bearing mice, this combination treatment stimulated tumor growth to a greater extent than either agent alone in the ovariectomized athymic mice implanted with tamoxifen-resistant T47D:A18/PKCα cells, suggesting once more that simultaneous consumption of isoflavone supplements with tamoxifen may not be safe [50]. In addition, genistein (3.125-25 μM) was found to synergistically augment tamoxifen-induced growth inhibition in ER+, HER2-overexpressing human breast cancer cells BT-474 (representing luminal type B tumors) via arresting the cell cycle progression at G1 phase, promoting apoptosis, and suppressing EGFR, HER2 and ERα expression [36]. Despite the synergistic growth inhibitory effects observed also by treatment of several ERβ+, HER2-overexpressing murine mammary tumor cells (78717, 78617, 85815, 85819) with tamoxifen in the presence of higher doses of genistein, at low concentrations (0.1-0.3 μM), this isoflavone still reversed the antitumor action of tamoxifen and unfavorably stimulated malignant progression [11]. Abrogation of tamoxifen-associated mammary tumor prevention was observed also in MMTV-wt-erbB-2/neu transgenic mice fed the low-dose (but not high-dose) isoflavone enriched diet, manifesting as higher rate of tumor development and shortened tumor latency [11]. Furthermore, experiments with DMBA-induced ER+ mammary tumors in rats have also displayed somewhat controversial results. The action of dietary genistein (500 ppm) has been associated with the timing when exposure to genistein started. In more detail, lifetime genistein exposure (from postnatal day 15 onward, mimicking the soy food intake of Asian women) improved responsiveness of tumors to tamoxifen therapy by reducing de novo drug resistance and the risk of recurrence. These beneficial effects were related to downregulation of genes involved in unfolded protein response and prosurvival autophagy, and upregulation of markers of antitumor immunity. Local mammary cancer recurrence was lowered also by addition of genistein immediately after the DMBA treatment, mimicking soy food intake among some Western women who start soy consumption during their adulthood. In all experimental animals, the treatment of tamoxifen was initiated when the first tumor reached 1.4 cm in diameter. However, among the subset of rats where genistein intake began during tamoxifen treatment, i.e., post diagnosis, de novo resistance to tamoxifen was oppositely significantly increased [18]. Although these results suggest that genistein might provide some additional protection to tamoxifen in the prevention and delay of breast carcinogenesis, being possibly harmful in the treatment of existing tumors, another study did still not confirm this implication. In fact, dietary intervention with genistein and tamoxifen, started one week before inducing tumors with DMBA, led to a decrease in tamoxifen-induced protection against carcinogenesis, reducing drug-induced suppression of tumor incidence and multiplicity in female rats [61]. Therefore, the reported *in vitro* and *in vivo* experimental results, still controversial and conflicting in many aspects, suggest that consumption of genistein-containing soy products and dietary supplements may be detrimental for patients with ER+ breast tumors (or women at high risk of developing breast cancer) while receiving tamoxifen, leading to decrease in the effectiveness of hormonal therapy, exhibiting soy as a potent risk factor. Further studies are needed to unravel the molecular mechanisms by which genistein overcomes the inhibitory effects of tamoxifen on estradiol-dependent tumor growth and promotes the malignant progression.

On the other hand, addition of genistein to tamoxifen treatment has been found to invariably augment the antitumor responses in different ER- breast cancer cell lines. It is well accepted that besides acting on ERs, tamoxifen can exert cytotoxic activities also by modulating different hormone-independent cellular signaling pathways. As these activities usually occur at considerably higher doses of tamoxifen [63, 64], the ability of genistein to potentiate antitumor responses could lead to lowering the therapeutically effective concentrations of tamoxifen in refractory hormone-independent breast tumor models. Indeed, at low micromolar doses, genistein interfered with anticancer action of tamoxifen in TNBC cells MDA-MB-435, resulting in synergism in both growth inhibition and cytotoxicity [64]. Enhanced antiproliferative effects by cotreating MDA-MB-435 cells with tamoxifen and genistein were demonstrated also in other studies [41, 91]. However, combination of genistein (up to 10 μM) with tamoxifen active metabolite, 4-OH-TAM, had no effect on the growth of MDA-MB-435 cells [83]. In addition, genistein (3.7-37 μM) interfered with tamoxifen-induced antitumor action also in TNBC cells MDA-MB-231, displaying additive antiproliferative effects [91]. Furthermore, in TNBC lines MDA-MB-231 and MDA-MB-157, genistein (25 μM) re-sensitized cells to tamoxifen-induced anticancer action by restoring the expression of ERα through modulation of epigenetic pathways involving histone modification and DNA methylation. The same mechanism was described also *in vivo* by pretreating MDA-MB-231 xenograft-bearing mice with dietary genistein, for two weeks before injection of tumor cells and continued throughout the study. Administration of tamoxifen to these mice led to a dramatic increase in tumor growth inhibition as compared to individual agents-treated animals, and these beneficial effects were due, at least in part, to epigenetic reactivation of ERα. Dietary genistein enhanced the antitumor properties of tamoxifen also in a spontaneous breast cancer model, C3(1)-SV40 Tag transgenic mice by re-sensitizing hormone-independent tumors to antihormone therapy [20]. Accordingly, combination of tamoxifen with genistein might be of strong therapeutic importance in treating refractory ER- breast tumors in the future. Further *in vivo* animal studies and subsequent human trials are needed to assess the safety and efficacy of this dual regimen for potential clinical application.

Despite conflicting results of experimental works about interactions between soy components and tamoxifen on breast cancer progression, current epidemiological evidence has rather suggested that soy foods do not counteract the benefits of tamoxifen therapy in breast cancer survivors. Serum levels of tamoxifen and its metabolites were unrelated to self-reported intake of soy or circulating concentrations of isoflavones among Asian American women with breast cancer who were users of tamoxifen [52]. In accordance, no association was found between dietary intake of soy isoflavones and the risk of recurrence among tamoxifen-treated Chinese women with a diagnosis of early or locally advanced hormone-dependent breast cancer [55]. Similarly, isoflavone intake was not related to the risk of a second breast cancer event in early-stage breast cancer survivors, irrespective of the use of tamoxifen, in the Women`s Healthy Eating and Living (WHEL) study. Although the interaction between soy intake and tamoxifen use on mortality was insignificant, the trend toward lower mortality with increasing soy intake was still stronger among women who had ever used tamoxifen [56]. Moreover, consumption of soy isoflavones two years after diagnosis at levels comparable to those in Asian populations seemed to reduce the risk of cancer recurrence among tamoxifen-treated female breast cancer survivors, mostly Caucasians, in the Life After Cancer Epidemiology (LACE) study [16]. In the Shanghai Breast Cancer Survival Study, postdiagnosis consumption of soy isoflavones was associated with reduced mortality and disease recurrence in Chinese women, regardless of the status of ERs in tumors or the use of tamoxifen. Tamoxifen was related to enhanced survival only in those women with ER+ tumors who had low or moderate levels of soy food intake and did not lead to further improvement of survival rates in women who had the highest level of soy food intake (more than 60 mg isoflavones per day) [21]. Intake of soy food was inversely associated with the risk of recurrence also among American and Chinese women with a diagnosis of invasive breast cancer in the After Breast Cancer Pooling Project (ABCPP), whereas this relation appeared to be slightly stronger in women with ER+ tumors who were tamoxifen users and consumed higher amount of isoflavones (more than 10 mg isoflavones per day) as compared to their counterparts who did not receive tamoxifen and consumed the lowest amount of isoflavones (less than 4 mg isoflavones per day) [54].

Last but not least, the potential effect of some synthetic flavonoids on therapeutic efficacy of tamoxifen has also been studied in several breast cancer models. Among them, aminoflavone was found to increase sensitivity to 4-OH-TAM in tamoxifen-resistant ER+ MCF-7 cells (TamR MCF-7) and luminal type B breast cancer cells BT-474. Moreover, aminoflavone prevented also 4-OH-TAM-stimulated increase in cell viability. This chemosensitization effect was achieved via decrease in α6-integrin expression and inhibition of downstream Src/Akt signaling pathway. Elevated α6-integrin levels in malignant tissue have been indeed associated with poor overall survival among breast cancer patients, conferring both cancer stemness as well as drug resistance [74].

#### *3.1.2.1.3. Effects of Flavonoids on Tamoxifen-Induced Toxicities*

With the widespread therapeutic and prophylactic use of tamoxifen, adverse side effects of this drug have become a major focus of concern, particularly its organ toxicity. Several studies have shown that tamoxifen can cause hepatotoxicity, including toxic hepatitis, massive hepatic steatosis or multifocal hepatic fatty infiltration, sub-massive hepatic necrosis and even cirrhosis in humans. Tamoxifen-induced fatty liver is observed in more than 30% of breast cancer patients who have received adjuvant tamoxifen treatment [92, 93]. Administration of tamoxifen leads to oxidative liver damage and it has been elucidated to be a potent hepatocarcinogen in rodents, resulting from oxygen radical overproduction during the drug metabolism. Generation of reactive oxygen intermediates that covalently bind to cellular macromolecules can induce genotoxic damage and initiate carcinogenesis. Thus, tamoxifen-evoked toxicity occurs primarily through oxidant mechanisms, and is not related to its ER-dependent activities [71-73, 92].

As oxidative stress has been demonstrated to underlie in the pathogenesis of tamoxifen-induced organ toxicity [92], natural antioxidants, especially flavonoids could scavenge free radicals and attenuate oxidative damage, providing protection to healthy tissues. Although the knowledge about possible role of phytochemicals on tamoxifen-induced toxicity is scarce, a few studies have shown important protective activities of specific flavonoids against tamoxifen-induced toxicity. These data are compiled and presented in Table 3.3. In fact, the presence of flavanol catechin could significantly reduce tamoxifen-induced lipid peroxidation, hydrogen peroxide generation and protein carbonyl contents in the liver and kidney tissues of the male mice, besides increasing the levels of tamoxifen-reduced cytochrome P450 (CYP) content. In addition, administration of catechin to tamoxifen-treated mice also normalized the levels of diverse non-enzymatic antioxidants and antioxidant enzymes, including restoration of glutathione redox status, thereby attenuating tamoxifen-induced hepato-renal toxicity [92, 93]. Such protective effects were demonstrated in both tissue homogenates of the liver and kidney [92], as well as liver mitochondrial preparation of mice [93]. Moreover, oral treatment of female rats with 1.5% green tea extract likewise led to alleviation of tamoxifen-induced liver injury, by suppressing drug-induced lipid peroxidation, elevating drug-reduced levels of antioxidant enzymes and decreasing drug-elicited activities of liver transaminases [71]. In addition, coadministration of tamoxifen with flavonol quercetin in the form of PLGA-nanoparticles abolished tamoxifen-induced hepatotoxicity in DMBA-treated female rats. Although such protective action was manifested as prevention of drug-evoked oxidative stress and normalization of liver histopathological appearance, it was still observed only with coencapsulated nanoparticles, and not using free mixture of tamoxifen and quercetin [67]. Codelivery of tamoxifen and naringenin on nanocarrier system resulted also in some protection against tamoxifen-induced hepatotoxicity in DMBA-treated rats, but this effect was again detected only with dual-loaded nanoparticles and not free mixture [89]. Further experimental studies with substantially expanded spectrum of flavonoids are highly needed to find out more effective combinations between tamoxifen and plant-derived flavonoids for prevention of drug-induced toxicity.

**Table 3.3.** Effects of flavonoids on tamoxifen (TAM)-induced toxicities

| Flavonoid and its dosage | Tamoxifen and its dosage | Biological system | Effects | Mechanisms | Ref. |
|---|---|---|---|---|---|
| FLAVANOLS | | | | | |
| Catechin; 40 mg/kg bw, by gavage for 10 consecutive days | TAM; 50 mg/kg bw, single i.p. dose on the 9$^{th}$ day with catechin | Swiss albino male mice | Prevention of TAM-induced hepato-renal toxicity | Decrease in TAM-induced LPO, $H_2O_2$ and PC levels; increase in TAM-reduced CYP content; restoring normalcy in non-enzymatic antioxidants (GSH, GSSG, T-SH, AsA) and antioxidant enzymes (GST, GPx, GR, G6-PD, CAT, SOD) in liver and kidney | [92] |
| Catechin; 40 mg/kg bw, p.o. for 10 consecutive days | TAM; 50 mg/kg bw, single i.p. dose on the 9$^{th}$ day with catechin | Swiss albino male mice | Protection against TAM-induced oxidative damage in liver mitochondria | Attenuation of TAM-increased oxidative stress parameters (LPO, PC, superoxide); restoring TAM-reduced non-enzymatic and enzymatic antioxidants of liver mitochondria (GSH, T-SH, MnSOD, GPx) | [93] |
| FLAVONOLS | | | | | |
| Quercetin; 6 mg/kg, by oral gavage, once in 3 days for 30 days; as free mixture or co-loaded with TAM to PLGA-NPs | TAM; 3 mg/kg, by oral gavage, once in 3 days for 30 days; as free mixture or co-loaded with quercetin to PLGA-NPs | DMBA-induced breast cancer model in female SD rats | Abolishing TAM-induced hepatotoxicity and oxidative stress, normalization of liver histopathological appearance with TAM-quercetin-PLGA-NPs. No effect with free mixture | | [67] |
| FLAVANONES | | | | | |
| Naringenin; co-loaded with TAM into SNEDDS | TAM; 45 mg/kg, co-loaded with naringenin into SNEDDS, for 3 consecutive weeks at weekly interval | DMBA-induced female Wistar rat breast cancer model | Protective effect against TAM hepatotoxicity | Decrease in ALT and AST levels in plasma, and TBARS in liver tissue; increase in GSH in liver homogenates | [89] |

Based on the above-described studies with rodents, supplementation of antioxidant flavonoids, especially flavanols, might be beneficial in abrogation of tamoxifen-induced organ toxicity. If this protective function will be confirmed in patients, flavonoids might be important adjuvant agents in hormonal cancer therapy. In fact, combination of tamoxifen with specific flavonoids cannot only augment drug-induced anticancer activities, allowing to lower the therapeutically effective doses of tamoxifen and thereby reduce adverse side effects, but can also directly avoid the toxic reactions caused by tamoxifen in the body, by preventing drug-evoked oxidative stress. Such dual benefits might be of strong therapeutic importance for enhancing clinical outcome and improving quality of life of breast cancer patients in the future.

#### *3.1.2.1.4. Effects of Flavonoid-Rich Natural Products on Anticancer Efficacy and Toxicity of Tamoxifen*

In addition to individual flavonoids, some flavonoid-rich natural products have also been investigated toward combinatory action with tamoxifen in different breast cancer models. These studies revealed both potentiating as well as attenuating effects on drug-induced anticancer activities and their results are compiled in Table 3.4. In more detail, coadministration of tamoxifen with purified cocoa polyphenolic extract resulted in synergistic cytotoxicity in both ER+ breast cancer cells MCF-7 as well as ER- cells SKBR3. This extract contains a wide spectrum of monomeric and oligomeric flavonoids naturally present in cocoa and its beneficial effects on therapeutic efficacy of tamoxifen definitely need further *in vivo* studies [28]. Also, the presence of Tualang honey that is rich in both flavonoids and phenolic acids promoted antitumor action of tamoxifen in breast cancer cells [25]. On the contrary, combination of tamoxifen with the extract of *Tamarindus indica* L. seeds led to a complete elimination of cytotoxic effects [75]. Also, the traditional Chinese formula Baihe Zhimu Tang, consisting of plant-derived extracts, significantly attenuated the effectiveness of tamoxifen in MCF-7 tumor-bearing mice, by reducing the concentrations of 4-OH-TAM and endoxifen in animals. Although this extract has been widely used to naturally alleviate symptoms of depression and anxiety, based on the current experimental data, its concomitant use with tamoxifen should be avoided [57].

**Table 3.4.** Effects of flavonoid-rich natural products on anticancer action and toxicity of tamoxifen (TAM) (highlighted rows indicate undesired negative effects on anticancer efficacy)

| Flavonoid-rich natural product | Tamoxifen and its dosage | Biological system | Effects | Mechanisms | Ref. |
|---|---|---|---|---|---|
| ANTICANCER ACTION | | | | | |
| Polyphenolic cocoa extract; 250 ng/μl | TAM; 1, 10 μM | MCF-7 human breast cancer cells, ER+ | Synergistic cytotoxicity, decrease in cell viability | Increase in apoptosis | [28] |
| Polyphenolic cocoa extract; 250 ng/μl | TAM; 1, 10 μM | SKBR3 human breast cancer cells, ER- | Synergistic cytotoxicity, decrease in cell viability | | [28] |
| Tualang honey, 1% | TAM; 2.5-15 μM | MCF-7 human breast cancer cells, ER+ | Promotion of TAM-induced anticancer activity | Increase in apoptosis (activation of caspases-3/7, -8 and -9; decrease in $\Delta\Psi m$) | [25] |
| Tualang honey, 1% | TAM; 2.5-15 μM | MDA-MB-231 human breast cancer cells, ER- | Promotion of TAM-induced anticancer activity | Increase in apoptosis (activation of caspases-3/7, -8 and -9; decrease in $\Delta\Psi m$) | [25] |
| Extract of *Tamarindus indica* L. seeds; 47.3 μg/ml | TAM; 0.8 μg/ml | MCF-7 human breast cancer cells, ER+ | Complete elimination of cytotoxicity | | [75] |
| Baihe Zhimu formula; 2 or 8 g/kg, intragastrically once-daily for 8 consecutive weeks | TAM; 4 mg/kg, intragastrically once-daily for 8 consecutive weeks | MCF-7 cells inoculated s.c. into female nude mice | Attenuation of TAM effectiveness, decrease in TAM-induced inhibition of tumor growth | Decrease in serum concentrations of 4-OH-TAM and endoxifen | [57] |
| TOXICITY | | | | | |
| Polyphenolic extract from *Ichnocarpus frutescence* (L.) R.Br. leaves; 200 mg/kg bw daily for 10 days before and 7 days after TAM (prophylactic) or simultaneously with TAM for 18 days (curative treatment) | TAM; 45 mg/kg/day, i.p. administration for 7 successive days | Wistar rats of either sex | Protection against TAM-induced hepatic damage, improvement of histological appearance of liver | Decrease in TAM-elevated AST, ALT, ALP and γ-GT levels, lowering of bilirubin concentration. Reduction of TAM-induced lipid peroxidation. Increase in TAM-reduced GSH levels | [73] |

**Table 3.4.** (Continued)

| Flavonoid-rich natural product | Tamoxifen and its dosage | Biological system | Effects | Mechanisms | Ref. |
|---|---|---|---|---|---|
| Polyphenolic fraction of *Desmostachya bipinnata* Stapf (L.); 100 or 200 mg/kg/day, oral administration for 21 days | TAM; 45 mg/kg/day, oral administration for 21 days | Female Sprague-Dawley rats | Inhibition of TAM-induced hepatic injury and oxidative stress, attenuation of hepatocellular necrosis | Decrease in TAM-induced SGOT, SGPT, ALP, TG, cholesterol, urea, uric acid, bilirubin and creatinine levels. Increase in antioxidant enzyme activities (GSH, GPx, SOD, CAT). Decrease in TAM-evoked lipid peroxidation in liver | [72] |

On the other hand, oral administration of polyphenolic extract from *Ichnocarpus frutescence* (L.) R.Br. leaves to tamoxifen-treated rats, either prophylactically or curatively, provided protection against drug-induced liver damage by regulating the levels of serum biochemical parameters and preventing elevated lipid peroxidation. At that, prophylactic treatment with polyphenolic extract led to somewhat stronger protection against hepatic damage caused by tamoxifen-induced oxidative stress [73]. Moreover, polyphenolic fraction of a perennial grass, *Desmostachya bipinnata* Stapf (L.), was also able to protect female rats against tamoxifen-induced hepatotoxicity, by normalizing liver functional parameters, improving antioxidant enzyme activities and inhibiting drug-induced oxidative stress. These activities were accompanied by restoration of normal hepatic architecture, reducing tamoxifen-induced centrilobular necrosis, feathery degeneration and fatty changes [72]. Further studies are required to purify and characterize the individual bioactive components (flavonoids) that are responsible for hepatoprotective activities of these extracts, and examine the potential use of these agents as adjuvants to tamoxifen treatment.

Taken together, although potentiation of tamoxifen activities by natural products may reduce the required effective doses of tamoxifen with a resultant decrease in adverse reactions of the drug, such combinations may also lead to undesired outcomes, by abrogating drug-induced antitumor effects. Therefore, utmost caution should be required when breast cancer patients on tamoxifen therapy decide to consume, for any purpose, supplemental herbal extracts.

#### *3.1.2.2. Raloxifene*

Raloxifene is another SERM-type antiestrogen that is structurally similar to tamoxifen [94, 95] (Figure 3.2). Raloxifene can produce ER antagonistic effects in the breast tissue and uterine endometrium, and behaves as ER agonist in bone and lipid metabolism, elevating bone mineral density and reducing total and low-density lipoprotein cholesterol levels [94, 95]. Due to its tissue selectivity, fewer side effects may be observed with the use of raloxifene as compared to the first generation SERMs [94]. Thus, unlike tamoxifen that is known to induce uterine cancer, raloxifene therapy is not related to adverse uterine effects [35, 95]. Accordingly, raloxifene has been approved by the US Food and Drug Administration (FDA) for the prevention of postmenopausal osteoporosis and breast cancer in high-risk patients [94].

Similarly to tamoxifen, also raloxifene undergoes extensive biotransformation in the body, but it does not appear to be metabolized by the cytochrome P450 (CYP) pathway [94]. The bioavailability of raloxifene has been estimated to be about 39% in rats, and only 2% in humans, due to its extensive first pass metabolism after oral administration [94, 96]. Raloxifene was shown to be largely conjugated in rat intestine and hepatic microsomes, whereas intestinal metabolism played a more important role than its presystemic metabolism in the liver [94]. Although metabolic pathways of raloxifene in rats and humans are rather similar, the major interspecies difference lies on the main metabolite, being raloxifene 6-β-glucuronide in rats and 4-β-glucuronide in humans [94, 96]. Thus, the total raloxifene that enters the systemic circulation includes both intact and conjugated drug [94]. In addition, raloxifene is also the substrate of efflux pumps, such as P-gp and MRP on enterocytes [94]. The most of raloxifene is eliminated in the feces directly or via bile and only negligible amounts, i.e., below 6%, appear in the urine [94]. Therefore, interactions between other agents that are eliminated by the Phase II metabolism are likely, affecting possibly the therapeutic efficacy of raloxifene.

Like tamoxifen, also raloxifene has been demonstrated to act not only through ERs, as besides ER+ breast tumors, cytotoxic responses of raloxifene were found also in some ER- breast cancer cells [95]. Thus, identification of adjuvant agents to increase the efficacy of raloxifene might be important for lowering the dose of the drug and reducing exposure burden to this antiestrogen. However, a concern has arisen about possible interactions of raloxifene and flavonoids-containing dietary supplements that can be used by breast cancer patients without the knowledge of their physicians.

#### *3.1.2.2.1. Effects of Flavonoids on Pharmacokinetics of Raloxifene*

Although both raloxifene as well as phytochemicals undergo an extensive intestinal and hepatic bioconversion before reaching the circulation, the current information about possible effects of plant-derived flavonoids on pharmacokinetic profile and oral bioavailability of raloxifene is still unacceptably scarce (Table 3.5). Studies with human intestinal microsomes have shown that two green tea flavanols, ECG and EGCG, can improve pharmacokinetic parameters (AUC) of raloxifene, behaving as intestinal UGT inhibitors and suppressing glucuronidation of the drug [96]. Also, the presence of flavone apigenin led to a significant increase in $AUC_{0-\infty}$ and $C_{max}$ values of intact raloxifene in rats, improving oral bioavailability of the drug through inhibition of glucuronidation and sulfation of raloxifene in the intestine [94]. These results suggest that concomitant oral administration of raloxifene with certain flavonoids might modulate systemic exposure to the drug and thereby impact also its therapeutic efficacy. Such interactions should not be disregarded, as elevated drug concentrations can possibly raise the risk of adverse side effects if their levels reach toxic threshold.

**Table 3.5.** Effects of flavonoids on pharmacokinetic parameters of raloxifene

| Flavonoid and its dosage | Raloxifene and its dosage | Biological system | Effects | Purported mechanism | Ref. |
|---|---|---|---|---|---|
| FLAVANOLS | | | | | |
| ECG; 0.5-8 μM | Raloxifene; 0.25-10 μM | Human intestinal microsomes | Increase in AUC | Inhibition of intestinal glucuronidation of raloxifene | [96] |
| EGCG; 1-16 μM | Raloxifene; 0.25-10 μM | Human intestinal microsomes | Increase in AUC | Inhibition of intestinal glucuronidation of raloxifene | [96] |
| FLAVONES | | | | | |
| Apigenin; 5 or 10 mg/kg, as single oral administration | Raloxifene; 10 mg/kg, as a single oral dose | Wistar rats | Increase in $AUC_{0-\infty}$ and $C_{max}$, enhancement of oral bioavailability of raloxifene | Inhibition of phase II metabolism and efflux transporter function | [94] |

*3.1.2.2.2. Effects of Flavonoids on Anticancer Potential of Raloxifene*

Besides influencing pharmacokinetics of raloxifene, green tea flavanol EGCG (25 μM) was demonstrated to augment also raloxifene-induced cytotoxic responses in TNBC cells MDA-MB-231. Cotreatment of these ER- cells with EGCG and raloxifene led to induction of an earlier and greater apoptosis than either agent alone, probably due to reduced phosphorylation of EGFR, AKT, mTOR and S6K proteins and elevated phosphorylation of p38 and JNK1/2 levels. Furthermore, these changes were accompanied by decrease in the nuclear localization of p65, a major subunit of NF-κB, suggesting that combination of raloxifene and EGCG can effectively suppress mitogenic and survival signaling in MDA-MB-231 cells [35, 95] (Table 3.6). Further studies are warranted to investigate this combination *in vivo* ER- breast cancer models; however, evaluation of interactions between raloxifene and EGCG in ER+ mammary tumors is also highly important, considering prescription of this drug to women at high risk of developing invasive breast cancer and widespread availability of EGCG-containing supplements on the market.

**Table 3.6.** Effects of flavonoids on anticancer action of raloxifene in breast tumor models

| Flavonoid and its dosage | Raloxifene and its dosage | Biological system | Assay method and time | Effect | Mechanisms | Ref. |
|---|---|---|---|---|---|---|
| FLAVANOLS | | | | | | |
| EGCG; 25 μM | Raloxifene; 1-5 μM | MDA-MB-231 human breast cancer cells, ER- | SRB; 48h, 7 days | Increase in cytotoxicity | Induction of apoptosis earlier and to a greater extent. Decrease in phosphorylation of EGFR and AKT | [95] |
| EGCG; 25 μM | Raloxifene 4 μM | MDA-MB-231 human breast cancer cells, ER-, erbB2/Her-2- | Western blotting; 12, 18h | | Decrease in phosphorylation of EGFR, AKT, mTOR and S6K; increase in phosphorylation of p38 and JNK1/2. Reduction of p65 nuclear translocation | [35] |

### *3.1.2.3. Centchroman*

Centchroman (also known as ormeloxifene) is a widely used non-steroidal oral contraceptive in India. This drug is categorized as SERM and resembles tamoxifen [5, 42, 97] (Figure 3.2). Considering several adverse reactions related to long-term use of tamoxifen, centchroman can be a promising agent for breast cancer, as this compound has been found to exhibit potent anticancer activities and have very few side effects [5, 42]. As a typical SERM, centchroman can exert ER antagonistic properties in breast, uterus and ovarian tissues, while behaving as an ER agonist in bone [5, 97].

#### *3.1.2.3.1. Effects of Flavonoids on Anticancer Potential of Centchroman*

Combined effects of centchroman and soy isoflavones (daidzein, genistein) have been tested in different breast cancer models, both ER+ and ER-, and these results are compiled in Table 3.7. Interactions between these agents in

ER- breast cancer cells clearly indicate that targeting ERs is by far not the only mechanism through which centchroman can act in malignant cells. Specifically, the presence of daidzein (at 25 and 50 μM) led to a synergistic augmentation of centchroman-induced cytotoxicity though increasing apoptotic death in both ER+ breast cancer cells MCF-7 as well as TNBC cells MDA-MB-231. This anticancer effect was mediated through production of intracellular ROS, disruption of mitochondrial membrane potential, alterations of pro- and antiapoptotic protein expression, activation of caspases -9 and -3/7, and cleavage of PARP; and these apoptotic events were triggered by downregulating PI3K/AKT signaling pathway. Moreover, as combination of centchroman and daidzein could not affect the viability of non-tumorigenic human mammary epithelial cells MCF-10A, the synergistic cell killing effect seemed to be specific for cancerous cells [42]. In similar manner, genistein supplementation (at 25 and 50 μM) also synergistically potentiated centchroman cytotoxicity in a variety of molecularly different breast cancer cells (ER+ cells MCF-7 and T-47D; ER- cells MDA-MB-231, MDA-MB-468 and 4T1), while exerting no effect in non-tumorigenic human mammary epithelial cells MCF-10A [5, 97]. The molecular mechanisms behind this augmented cell killing involved the arrest of cell cycle progression at G2/M phase and induction of ROS-dependent apoptosis. Combined treatment with centchroman and genistein caused dysregulation of apoptotic proteins Bax and Bcl-2 ratio leading to mitochondrial dysfunction, activation of caspases-9 and -3/7, and cleavage of PARP; mediated through significant suppression of PI3K/AKT/NF-κB cell survival signaling. In addition, the combination of centchroman and genistein resulted in markedly enhanced suppression of tumor growth in 4T1 syngeneic mouse model, manifesting as a significant decrease in tumor volume and weight with a considerable prolongation of animal survival as compared to the mice treated with either agent alone [97]. Hence, soy isoflavones (genistein and daidzein) may enhance centchroman-mediated suppression of mammary malignant growth, supporting the use of these flavonoids as potential adjuncts to centchroman therapy for management of breast cancer. Further studies on *in vivo* animal models with subsequent human trials are highly needed to elucidate possibilities for clinical application of these combinational treatments in the future.

**Table 3.7.** Effects of flavonoids on anticancer action of centchroman in breast tumor models

| Flavonoid and its dosage | Centchroman and its dosage | Biological system | Assay method and time | Effect | Mechanisms | Ref. |
|---|---|---|---|---|---|---|
| ISOFLAVONES | | | | | | |
| Daidzein; 25, 50 μM | Centchroman; 5, 10 μM | MCF-7 human breast cancer cells, ER+ | SRB; 48h | Synergistic cytotoxic effects (CI<1) | Increase in apoptosis (generation of ROS; disruption of ΔΨm; increase in Bax, upregulation of caspases-9 and -7; cleavage of PARP). Inhibition of PI3K/AKT/mTOR pathway | [42] |
| Daidzein; 25, 50 μM | Centchroman; 5, 10 μM | MDA-MB-231 human breast cancer cells, ER- | SRB; 48h | Synergistic cytotoxic effects (CI<1) | Increase in apoptosis (generation of ROS; disruption of ΔΨm; decrease in Bcl-xL, increase in Bax, upregulation of caspases-9 and -3; cleavage of PARP). Inhibition of PI3K/AKT pathway | [42] |
| Genistein; 25, 50 μM | Centchroman; 5, 10 μM | MCF-7 human breast cancer cells, ER+ | SRB; 48h | Synergistic cytotoxic effect | | [5] |
| Genistein; 50 μM | Centchroman; 10 μM | MCF-7 human breast cancer cells, ER+ | SRB; 48h | Synergistic cytotoxic effect | Arresting cells at G2/M phase (downregulation of cyclin B1, upregulation of phospho-cdc2); increase in apoptosis (generation of ROS, disruption of ΔΨm, increase in cytosolic cyt c, upregulation of Bax, downregulation of Bcl-2 and Bcl-xL, activation of caspases-9 and -7, cleavage of PARP). Inhibition of PI3K/Akt/mTOR/NF-κB signaling | [97] |

| Flavonoid and its dosage | Centchroman and its dosage | Biological system | Assay method and time | Effect | Mechanisms | Ref. |
|---|---|---|---|---|---|---|
| Genistein; 25, 50 μM | Centchroman; 5, 10 μM | T-47D human breast cancer cells; ER+ | SRB; 48h | Synergistic cytotoxic effect | | [5] |
| Genistein; 25, 50 μM | Centchroman; 5, 10 μM | MDA-MB-231 human breast cancer cells, ER- | SRB; 48h | Synergistic cytotoxic effect | | [5] |
| Genistein; 50 μM | Centchroman; 10 μM | MDA-MB-231 human breast cancer cells, ER- | SRB; 48h | Synergistic cytotoxic effect | Arresting cells at G2/M phase (downregulation of cyclin B1, upregulation of phospho-cdc2); increase in apoptosis (generation of ROS, disruption of $\Delta\Psi m$, increase in cytosolic cyt c, upregulation of Bax, downregulation of Bcl-2 and Bcl-xL, activation of caspases-9 and -3, cleavage of PARP). Inhibition of PI3K/Akt/NF-κB signaling | [97] |
| Genistein; 25, 50 μM | Centchroman; 5, 10 μM | MDA-MB-468 human breast cancer cells, ER- | SRB; 48h | Synergistic cytotoxic effect (except 10 μM drug + 25 μM genistein) | | [5] |
| Genistein; 50 μM | Centchroman; 10 μM | 4T1 murine breast cancer cells | SRB; 48h | Synergistic cytotoxic effect | | [97] |
| Genistein; 200 mg/kg, p.o., thrice a week for 3 weeks | Centchroman; 10 mg/kg, p.o., thrice a week for 3 weeks | 4T1 cells injected onto the left mammary fat pad of adult female BALB/c mice | 21 days | Enhanced suppression of tumor growth, decrease in tumor volume and weight. Prolongation of mice survival | | [97] |

### *3.1.2.4. Fulvestrant*

Fulvestrant (ICI 182 780) is a selective estrogen receptor downregulator (SERD) that, unlike tamoxifen and other SERMs, does not exhibit any ER agonistic activities [7, 53] (Figure 3.2). This drug is sold under the brand name Faslodex and results in degradation of ERs, thereby completely eliminating the effects of estrogens on the cells. Due to this action, fulvestrant lacks cross resistance with other hormonal cancer therapies [7, 53]. This ER antagonist is approved in both the United States and Europe for the treatment of ER+ metastatic breast cancer or locally advanced unresectable disease in postmenopausal women, whereas hot flashes represent the most commonly occurring adverse side effects noticed during administration of fulvestrant [53].

#### *3.1.2.4.1. Effects of Flavonoids on Anticancer Potential of Fulvestrant*

As presented in Table 3.8, the data about possible effects of plant-derived flavonoids on anticancer potential of fulvestrant are very scarce. It has been shown that equol, a bacterial metabolite of soy isoflavone daidzein, affected antiproliferative activity of fulvestrant in a manner dependent on both its concentration as well as cell line used. While equol, at its 50% and 75% effective doses, showed synergistic effects with fulvestrant in ER+ breast cancer cells MCF-7, these interactions were antagonistic in another ER+ cell line ZR-75-1, and either synergistic or antagonistic in ER+ cells T-47D. However, equol augmented fulvestrant-induced ER downregulation in all three cell lines [46]. As different effects were observed in diverse ER+ breast cancer cells, it is probable that interactions between equol and fulvestrant involved, at least in part, modulation of ER-independent cellular pathways. Although further preclinical research is needed to unravel the underlying molecular mechanisms, these results still indicate that the use of equol (daidzein) during the treatment of breast cancer with fulvestrant requires caution. Dose-dependent effects were observed also when MCF-7 xenograft-bearing ovariectomized athymic mice (implanted with estradiol pellets) were concomitantly treated with phytoestrogen-containing soy extract and fulvestrant. While at 50 mg/kg/day, this extract slightly potentiated the growth inhibitory action of the drug leading to tumors of smaller weight, at 100 mg/kg/day, it partially negated anticancer activity of fulvestrant. At lower dose, the soy extract enhanced the effect of fulvestrant on reducing the expression of estradiol target genes (cyclin D1, PR, TSP-1, KLK6); as opposed to suppression of antiestrogenic action of the drug at higher dose, resulting in reversion of the drug-induced downregulation of these genes.

**Table 3.8.** Effects of flavonoids on anticancer action of fulvestrant (ICI 182 780) in breast tumor models (highlighted rows indicate undesired negative effects on anticancer efficacy)

| Flavonoid and its dosage | Fulvestrant and its dosage | Biological system | Assay method and time | Effect | Mechanisms | Ref. |
|---|---|---|---|---|---|---|
| ISOFLAVONES | | | | | | |
| Equol; 22.3 μM (=$IC_{50}$) | Fulvestrant; molar ratio with equol of 1:1 | MCF-7 human breast cancer cells, hormone receptor-positive | MTS; 72h | Synergistic effect (CI<1) | Increase in fulvestrant-induced downregulation of ER expression | [46] |
| Equol; 16.2 μM (=$IC_{50}$) | Fulvestrant; molar ratio with equol of 1:4 | T-47D human breast cancer cells, hormone receptor-positive | MTS; 72h | Synergistic effect at 50% effective doses (CI<1); antagonistic effect at 75% effective doses) (CI>1) | Increase in fulvestrant-induced downregulation of ER expression | [46] |
| Equol; 18.3 μM (=$IC_{50}$) | Fulvestrant; molar ratio with equol of 1:1 | ZR-75-1 human breast cancer cells, hormone receptor-positive | MTS; 72h | Antagonistic effect against fulvestrant (CI>1) | Increase in fulvestrant-induced downregulation of ER expression | [46] |
| SYNTHETIC FLAVONOIDS | | | | | | |
| Aminoflavone; various | Fulvestrant (Faslodex); 100 nM | MCF-7 human breast cancer cells, ER+ | MTT | Synergistic cytotoxicity | | [98] |

This study again raises concerns about the consumption of isoflavone supplements concomitantly with fulvestrant therapy in postmenopausal women with ER+ breast cancer [53].

In addition, influence of a synthetic flavonoid, aminoflavone, was also studied on anticancer potential of fulvestrant, showing a synergistic growth inhibition of MCF-7 cells [98].

### 3.1.3. Influence of Flavonoids on Therapeutic Action of Aromatase Inhibitors

Aromatase (cytochrome P450 19, CYP19) is a key enzyme in estrogen biosynthesis [15, 29]. Estrogen can be produced from cholesterol, and aromatase catalyzes the last and rate-limiting aromatization steps converting androstenedione and testosterone to estrone (E1) and estradiol (E2), respectively [15, 29, 47, 99]. While the highest levels of aromatase activity are present in the ovaries of premenopausal women, extraovarian organs (mainly adipose tissue and skin) are the predominant tissue sources of estrogens in postmenopausal women [15]. In addition, elevated levels of aromatase expression and activity are found in and around the cancerous breast tissue, with estrogen concentrations many times higher in malignant neoplasm than in the systemic circulation [6, 15, 29, 99]. Such locally produced estrogen can be responsible for stimulating the growth and proliferation of mammary tumors [6, 29].

In recent years, aromatase inhibitors (AIs), such as exemestane, anastrozole and letrozole, have been developed for adjuvant treatment of ER+ breast cancer in postmenopausal women, either as initial therapy or after a course of tamoxifen [15, 29, 47]. AIs, which can be both steroidal and nonsteroidal compounds, suppress aromatase enzyme activity leading to decrease in circulating levels of estrogens to nearly undetectable levels, thereby controlling the growth of estrogen-responsive breast tumors [47, 69]. Studies have shown that AIs can be even more effective than tamoxifen in treating advanced breast cancer, reducing the risk of recurrence and improving the survival rate of patients [6, 15, 29, 69]. However, since AIs suppress estrogen synthesis in the whole body, patients treated with these drugs are threatened by conditions typically associated with estrogen deficiency, such as reduced bone mineral density and musculoskeletal complications as well as unfavorable blood lipid profile and increased coronary heart disease risk [29, 47, 69]. The presence of flavonoids-containing natural products might be helpful in increasing breast selective responses of AIs and reducing systemic toxicity of the currently approved drugs; moreover, certain flavonoids can themselves exert some aromatase inhibitory activity [47, 69, 100]. Nevertheless, very little is still known about the possible impact of plant-derived flavonoids on anticancer efficacy of clinically used AIs, and this is unfortunate considering that AIs are increasingly being prescribed to women with ER+ breast cancer.

#### *3.1.3.1. Exemestane*

Exemestane is one of the most effective and widely used AIs [6] (Figure 3.2). This steroidal agent is a third-generation AI that binds irreversibly to the active site of the enzyme and induces long-term decrease in estrogen levels [6, 69]. However, as side effects, exemestane can cause bone loss putting patients at elevated risk of osteoporosis and bone fractures [6]. Moreover, acquired resistance to this drug is another major clinical concern, leading to relapse of the disease in postmenopausal patients with ER+ breast cancer [38, 100].

##### *3.1.3.1.1. Effects of Flavonoids on Anticancer Potential of Exemestane*

Regarding to severe bone detrimental effects accompanying the use of exemestane, combination therapies with natural agents that can enhance sensitivity of malignant cells to this AI and thereby reduce toxicity to normal tissues would be of great importance. The current knowledge about co-effects of plant-derived flavonoids and exemestane on breast cancer models is summarized in Table 3.9. It has been found that combination of exemestane with flavone luteolin, either as free mixture or being coloaded into different zein nanosphere systems, resulted in an enhanced cytotoxicity as compared to the drug alone in both ER+ breast cancer cells MCF-7 as well as murine TNBC cells 4T1. Co-delivery of exemestane and luteolin in tumor-targeted zein nanospheres created the possibility to overcome limited aqueous solubility and high lipophilicity of exemestane, thereby increasing the drug bioavailability [38]. However, as enhanced cytotoxicity of dual treatment was observed in both ER+ as well as ER- mammary tumor cells, molecular mechanisms under such action involved, at least in part, also ER-independent events. In similar manner, combination of exemestane and flavanone hesperetin, either as free mixture or different dual-loaded nanoformulations, led to a significant increase in cytotoxic responses in MCF-7 cells, as compared to either drug alone. Moreover, the presence of hesperetin potentiated exemestane-induced tumor growth inhibition also in

Ehrlich ascites tumor-bearing mice leading to neoplasms of smaller volume, by significantly reducing proliferation inside the malignancy and promoting necrosis. At that, coencapsulation of exemestane and hesperetin into the tumor-targeted protein-lipid nanohybrid system (boronic-targeted albumin-shell oily-core nanocapsules) led to the strongest inhibition of tumor growth in experimental mice [6]. Therefore, combined treatment of breast tumors with exemestane and specific flavonoids might serve as a promising novel strategy for improvement of therapeutic outcome, allowing reduction of the effective drug doses and side effects, and lessening also the development of drug resistance. The spectrum of test flavonoids with possible ability to augment exemestane anticancer activities definitely needs to be expanded in the future *in vitro* and *in vivo* studies, with the aim to allow exemestane-taking patients to make more informed choices on food products and supplements.

#### *3.1.3.2. Anastrozole*

Anastrozole, sold under the brand name Arimidex, is a third-generation nonsteroidal AI that has been approved for the treatment of ER+ breast cancer in postmenopausal women, to prevent disease recurrence and improve clinical outcome [47, 48, 55] (Figure 3.2). Studies have suggested that this AI can be superior to tamoxifen providing some disease-free survival advantage [47]. Anastrozole has been used also to prevent breast cancer in postmenopausal women at high risk for the disease [48]. However, since its aromatase inhibiting activity is not tissue-specific, anastrozole-induced estrogen deficiency can cause bone demineralization, markedly elevating the risk of osteoporosis [47, 48]. Therefore, to potentiate the antiestrogenic activities of anastrozole in malignant tissue and concurrently reduce its toxicity in healthy organs, combinations with plant-derived flavonoids might be of great clinical importance. However, no such experimental studies have been reported yet.

The only indication for a potentially beneficial effect of soy isoflavones comes from an epidemiological study, showing an inverse association between the intake of soy isoflavones and the risk of recurrence among postmenopausal ER+ breast cancer patients receiving adjuvant anastrozole therapy after surgical resection. In fact, the recurrence rate for postmenopausal patients under anastrozole treatment was 18.7% lower among patients in the highest quartile of soy intake (>42.3 mg/day) than those in the lowest quartile (<15.2 mg/day) [55]. Although it is possible that

**Table 3.9.** Effects of flavonoids on anticancer action of exemestane in breast tumor models

| Flavonoid and its dosage | Exemestane and its dosage | Biological system | Assay method and time | Effect | Mechanisms | Ref. |
|---|---|---|---|---|---|---|
| FLAVONES | | | | | | |
| Luteolin; 5-100 μg/ml, as free mixture, or co-loaded with exemestane to zein NSs, lactoferrin-targeted zein NSs or PEGylated zein NSs | Exemestane; 5-100 μg/ml, as free mixture, or co-loaded with luteolin to zein NSs, lactoferrin-targeted zein NSs or PEGylated zein NSs | MCF-7 human breast adenocarcinoma cells | MTT; 24h | Increase in cytotoxicity compared to free exemestane | | [38] |
| Luteolin; 5-100 μg/ml, as free mixture, or co-loaded with exemestane to zein NSs, lactoferrin-targeted zein NSs or PEGylated zein NSs | Exemestane; 5-100 μg/ml, as free mixture, or co-loaded with luteolin to zein NSs, lactoferrin-targeted zein NSs or PEGylated zein NSs | 4T1 murine breast cancer cells | MTT; 24h | Increase in cytotoxicity compared to free exemestane | | [38] |
| FLAVANONES | | | | | | |
| Hesperetin; 0-30 μM, as free mixture, or co-loaded with exemestane to albumin-shell oily-core NCs or boronic-targeted albumin-shell oily-core NCs | Exemestane; 0-30 μM, as free mixture, or co-loaded with hesperetin to albumin-shell oily-core NCs or boronic-targeted albumin-shell oily-core NCs | MCF-7 human breast cancer cells | MTT; 24h | Increase in cytotoxicity compared to free exemestane | | [6] |
| Hesperetin; 0-30 μM, as free mixture, or co-loaded with exemestane to oil-in-water nanoemulsion | Exemestane; 0-30 μM, as free mixture, or co-loaded with hesperetin to oil-in-water nanoemulsion | MCF-7 human breast cancer cells | MTT; 24h | Increase in cytotoxicity compared to free exemestane | | [6] |
| Hesperetin; 7.5 mg/kg, i.v. injection, biweekly for 3 weeks, as free mixture, or co-loaded with exemestane to albumin-shell oily-core NCs or boronic-targeted albumin-shell oily-core NCs | Exemestane; 30 mg/kg, i.v. injection, biweekly for 3 weeks, as free mixture, or co-loaded with hesperetin to albumin-shell oily-core NCs or boronic-targeted albumin-shell oily-core NCs | Ehrlich ascites tumor (EAT) cells injected into the left side of the mammary fat pad of female BALB/C mice | 21 days | Increase in inhibition of tumor volume compared to exemestane alone | Induction of necrosis, decrease in expression of Ki-67 | [6] |

concomitant treatment with anastrozole and soy isoflavones might exert synergistic inhibitory effects on estrogen synthesis, further preclinical studies are highly needed to identify bioactive soy component(s) interacting with anastrozole therapy as well as molecular mechanisms underlying their combinational action.

*3.1.3.2.1. Effects of Flavonoids on Anastrozole-Induced Toxicities*

A few in vivo studies with female ovariectomized rats have shown that the presence of biochanin A can be beneficial for reducing anastrozole-induced toxic side effects (Table 3.10). Intraperitoneal injection of this isoflavone ameliorated anastrozole-induced adverse effects on bone health by decreasing drug-induced serum levels of bone turnover biomarkers (bone alkaline phosphatase, osteocalcin, parathyroid hormone, tartrate-resistant acid phosphatase), and increasing drug-reduced calcium and phosphate levels in serum and bone. The rise of serum levels of TNFα, total cholesterol and triglycerides observed after treatment with anastrozole, was also declined by combined treatment with anastrozole and biochanin A. Moreover, while anastrozole caused marked degenerative changes and severe decrease in the bone density of ovariectomized rats, the presence of biochanin A led to a significant increase in the bone mineral density and radiopacity of tibias and lumbar vertebrae, besides regaining also the normal matrix architecture of femur neck regions [47]. It is well known that a significant decline in estrogen contributes to an elevated rate of bone remodeling and creates an imbalance between bone formation and bone resorption, causing bone loss and fractures. If further studies confirm alleviating role of biochanin A on anastrozole-induced detrimental effects on bone health also in humans, this natural compound could be an important adjuvant to anastrozole therapy improving the quality of life of patients with ER+ breast cancer. Furthermore, biochanin A was shown to exert beneficial activities also in renal and cutaneous tissues of anastrozole-treated ovariectomized rats. Coadministration of anastrozole with biochanin A led to a significant decrease in the drug-elevated levels of kidney injury biomarkers (urea, creatinine, uric acid), and a marked increase in the drug-reduced serum levels of GSH, catalase and total antioxidant capacity, thereby guarding against oxidative stress. In addition, the presence of biochanin A evoked a significant increase in anastrozole-reduced levels of IL-4 and GATA3 in the skin of experimental rats. Combined treatment with biochanin A and anastrozole reversed also drug-induced upregulation of renal TNFα and iNOS expression and downregulation of cutaneous TGFβ levels. In accordance with these molecular changes, biochanin A was able to moderately reduce anastrozole-induced vascular, degenerative and necrotic lesions in the renal tissue, and ameliorate morphological alterations in skin of rats [48]. Therefore, biochanin A might be an important supplement for breast cancer patients under anastrozole therapy, providing protection to different healthy organs against detrimental changes that are caused by drug-induced estrogen deprivation in the whole body. Further studies are highly needed to investigate interactions between anastrozole and biochanin A more closely, exploring also potential co-effects on anticancer activities, before any implications for clinical practice can be drawn.

#### *3.1.3.3. Letrozole*

Letrozole, sold under the brand name Femara, is a third-generation non-steroidal AI [15, 101] (Figure 3.2). This imidazole derivative suppresses aromatase enzyme activity and total-body aromatization by more than 99% [15, 99-101]. Letrozole is approved as a first-line therapy for the treatment of local or metastatic ER+ breast cancer in postmenopausal women [69, 99, 101]. Moreover, it is used also for management of hormone-sensitive male breast cancer [101]. Because of the tissue-nonspecific action, side effects of letrozole result from prolonged estrogen deprivation, including increased bone turnover and a more atherogenic blood lipid profile [69].

##### *3.1.3.3.1. Effects of Flavonoids on Anticancer Potential of Letrozole*

Several plant-derived flavonoids have been investigated concerning their potential impact on letrozole-induced anticancer effects in ER+ breast cancer model MCF-7. The results of these studies are compiled in Table 3.11 and they clearly indicate that the presence of specific flavonoids might be both beneficial but also detrimental on therapeutic efficacy of letrozole. In fact, while flavone luteolin had no significant effect on letrozole-induced suppression of xenograft growth in aromatase-expressing MCF-7 tumor-bearing ovariectomized mice, without affecting also the drug-reduced plasma estradiol levels [69], polymethoxylated flavone nobiletin as well as flavanone hesperetin, both at low micromolar doses, markedly compromised aromatase inhibitory activity of letrozole in testosterone-treated MCF-7 cells *in vitro* [99, 100]. However, in ovariectomized female mice injected with aromatase-overexpressing MCF-7 cells (MCF-7aro) and treated with androstenedione, oral administration of citrus flavanone hesperetin did still not counteract letrozole-induced suppression of tumor growth, nor affected also the plasma estradiol levels [29].

**Table 3.10.** Effects of flavonoids on anastrozole-induced toxicities

| Flavonoid and its dosage | Anastrozole and its dosage | Biological system | Effects | Mechanisms | Ref. |
|---|---|---|---|---|---|
| ISOFLAVONES | | | | | |
| Biochanin A; 5 mg/kg bw, i.p. injection | Anastrozole; 0.5 mg/kg bw, p.o. as tablets | Female Sprague-Dawley rats, bilaterally ovariectomized | Alleviation of anastrozole-induced bone health decrements | Decrease in anastrozole-induced bone turnover biomarkers in serum (BALP, OC, PTH, TRAP, TNFα). Increase in anastrozole-reduced serum and bone calcium and phosphate levels. Increase in anastrozole-reduced bone density and radiopacity of tibias and vertebrae; regaining normal cortical bone architecture of femur neck region | [47] |
| Biochanin A; 5 mg/kg bw, daily, i.p. | Anastrozole; 0.5 mg/kg bw, daily, p.o. | Female Wistar rats, ovariectomized | Improvement of side effects of anastrozole. Amelioration of biochemical, molecular and ultrastructural changes of renal and cutaneous tissue | Decrease in serum levels of urea, creatinine, uric acid and MDA. Increase in serum CAT, GSH and TAC; and cutaneous IL-4 and GATA3 levels. Downregulation of renal TNFα and iNOS expression, upregulation of cutaneous TGFβ expression | [48] |

Although the metabolite of daidzein, equol, was found to exert synergistic action with letrozole in aromatase-overexpressing MCF-7 cells (E10arom) [46], dietary administration of soy isoflavone genistein negated tumor growth inhibitory effects of letrozole in athymic ovariectomized mice harboring aromatase-expressing MCF-7 xenografts and treated with androstenedione. This unfavorable action of genistein was accompanied by reversal of letrozole-suppressed plasma estradiol levels and pS2 expression in tumors. Also, while letrozole significantly decreased the expression of cellular proliferation marker in tumors, the presence of genistein attenuated this effect [15]. In addition, combined treatment of letrozole and genistein overcome letrozole-induced growth inhibitory effects also in a co-culture model of MCF-7 cells and human adrenocortical carcinoma cells H295 that, in several aspects, resemble cancer-associated fibroblasts. As breast tumor surrounding fibroblasts can express aromatase enzyme after their stimulation by tumor cells-secreted cytokines, providing in turn estradiol to epithelial cancer cells, this co-culture model could better mimic the complex *in vivo* conditions [37]. Moreover, genistein (at 1 μM) antagonized the efficacy also of a combination therapy with letrozole and palbociclib, a cyclin-dependent kinase inhibitor, in ER+ breast cancer cells MCF-7 and T47D, by reversing the drug combination-induced antiproliferative action through interfering with mTOR signaling [13]. Further preclinical studies are definitely needed to unravel molecular mechanisms underlying interactions between letrozole and genistein in aromatase-expressing ER+ breast cancer cells. Nevertheless, as dietary genistein can adversely impact breast cancer therapy, caution is warranted for the use of isoflavones-containing supplements by post-menopausal women taking letrozole treatment.

*3.1.3.3.2. Effects of Flavonoids on Letrozole-Induced Toxicities*

Although flavone luteolin was shown to not impact letrozole therapeutic efficacy in aromatase-overexpressing MCF-7 tumor-bearing ovariectomized mice, this flavonoid still exerted beneficial effects in alleviating drug-induced toxicity. In fact, the presence of luteolin produced favorable changes in the blood lipid profile by increasing plasma high-density lipoprotein (HDL) concentrations and reducing letrozole-elevated LDL/HDL ratio in mice. However, no improvement in the bone status of animals was observed after cotreatment with letrozole and luteolin [69] (Table 3.12). Nevertheless, dietary administration of flavanone hesperetin prevented letrozole-induced bone deterioration in the same breast cancer mouse model, by reversing drug-induced bone loss [29]. In clinical practice, bisphosphonates are usually administered for counteracting bone deterioration caused by chronic AI therapy. As bisphosphonates themselves have several undesirable side effects, including esophagitis, ulcers, renal dysfunction and atrial fibrillation, safer alternatives are highly needed to alleviate undesirable effects of AIs [29]. In this context, specific flavonoids might be important adjuvants to letrozole therapy, reducing drug-induced toxicity and thereby improving the quality of life of breast cancer patients. Moreover, as letrozole has been used also for the treatment of hormone-sensitive male breast cancer, studies with male rats have shown that the presence of flavonol quercetin can induce a protective effect against drug-induced injury on testicular tissue. Oral administration of quercetin for 10 days after 3-months long letrozole treatment helped to restore the plasma hormone levels (testosterone, luteinizing hormone, follicle-stimulating hormone) to near normal and reduce drug-elevated lipid peroxidation, besides reversing letrozole-induced abnormalities and damage of seminiferous tubules of the testes. The appearance of testicular tissue after combined treatment with letrozole and quercetin was revealed to be rather normal [101].

### 3.1.4. Conclusions from Preclinical Knowledge with Dietary Recommendations to Breast Cancer Patients

Although the results obtained *in vitro* and *in vivo* cancer models need to be confirmed in clinical trials before any specific recommendations can be created for patients undergoing hormonal breast cancer treatment, it is inconceivable and also unethical that human trials will be undertaken with those drug-flavonoid combinations that have revealed detrimental effects in preclinical studies. However, the knowledge about these interactions is even more valuable, potentially leading to decrease in therapeutic efficacy and increase in the risk of recurrence, thereby impairing clinical outcome. On the other hand, the *in vitro* and *in vivo* experimental studies on possible impact of plant-derived flavonoids on therapeutic efficacy and toxicity of hormonal breast cancer therapies, i.e., antiestrogens and aromatase inhibitors, must be expanded and intensified in the future, as these interactions may be extensive and concern more and more women diagnosed with breast cancer worldwide.

**Table 3.11.** Effects of flavonoids on anticancer action of letrozole in breast tumor models (highlighted rows indicate undesired negative effects on anticancer efficacy)

| Flavonoid and its dosage | Letrozole and its dosage | Biological system | Assay method and time | Effect | Mechanisms | Ref. |
|---|---|---|---|---|---|---|
| FLAVONES | | | | | | |
| Luteolin; 20 mg/kg bw/ day, with diet | Letrozole; 2 µg/day, s.c. injection | MCF-7 cells transfected with human CYP19 (MCF-7aro) injected into the two flanks of ovariectomized female athymic mice; injected s.c. with androstenedione (0.1 mg/day) | 84 days | No effect on letrozole-induced suppression of xenograft growth, tumor weight, plasma E2 concentration and uterine wet weight | No effect on letrozole-induced changes in cell cycle and apoptotic markers | [69] |
| Nobiletin; 1 µM | Letrozole;1 µM | MCF-7 human breast cancer cells; treated with 100 nM testosterone | Aromatase activity; 48h | Compromising letrozole-induced aromatase inhibition | No effect on aromatase (CYP19) gene expression | [100] |
| FLAVANONES | | | | | | |
| Hesperetin; 1, 5, 25 µM | Letrozole; 0.1, 1, 10 µM | MCF-7 human breast cancer cells, ER+; treated with 100 nM testosterone | Aromatase activity; 48h | Attenuating letrozole-induced inhibition of aromatase activity | No effect on aromatase (CYP19) gene expression | [99] |
| Hesperetin; 5 µM | Letrozole;1 µM | MCF-7 human breast cancer cells; treated with 100 nM testosterone | Aromatase activity; 48h | Compromising letrozole-induced aromatase inhibition | No effect on aromatase (CYP19) gene expression | [100] |

**Table 3.11.** (Continued)

| Flavonoid and its dosage | Letrozole and its dosage | Biological system | Assay method and time | Effect | Mechanisms | Ref. |
|---|---|---|---|---|---|---|
| Hesperetin; 5000 ppm, with diet | Letrozole; 2 μg/day, s.c. injection | MCF-7 cells transfected with human CYP19 (MCF-7aro) injected into the two flanks of ovariectomized female athymic mice; injected s.c. with androstenedione (0.1 mg/day) | 84 days | No effect on letrozole-induced suppression of xenograft growth, tumor weight, plasma estrogen concentration, pS2 mRNA level and uterine wet weight | | [29] |
| ISOFLAVONES | | | | | | |
| Equol; molar ratio with letrozole of 1:1 | Letrozole; molar ratio with equol of 1:1 | E10arom, MCF-7 human breast cancer cells, hormone receptor-positive, overexpressing aromatase | MTS; 72h | Synergistic effect (CI<1) | | [46] |
| Genistein; 250, 500, 1000 ppm, with diet | Letrozole; 1 mg, implanted s.c. on the backs of mice | MCF-7Ca cells (transfected with human aromatase gene) injected into two sites on the backs of athymic ovariectomized Balb/c nude mice; androstenedione (5 mg) implanted s.c. on the backs of mice | 31 weeks | Dose-dependent negation of inhibitory effect of letrozole on tumor growth | Overwhelming of inhibitory effects of letrozole on cellular proliferation in tumors, plasma E2 levels, expression of pS2 mRNA and protein in tumors, and uterine wet weight | [15] |
| Genistein; 100 nM-10 μM | Letrozole; 0.1 μM | MCF-7 human breast cancer cells and H295R human adrenocortico-carcinoma cells co-culture (at 5:1 ratio) | MTT; 9 days | Overcoming letrozole-induced growth inhibition, induction of cell proliferation | | [37] |

**Table 3.12.** Effects of flavonoids on letrozole-induced toxicities

| Flavonoid and its dosage | Letrozole and its dosage | Biological system | Effects | Mechanisms | Ref. |
|---|---|---|---|---|---|
| FLAVONES | | | | | |
| Luteolin; 20 mg/kg bw/day, with diet | Letrozole; 2 μg/day, s.c. injection | MCF-7 cells transfected with human CYP19 (MCF-7aro) injected into the two flanks of ovariectomized female athymic mice; injected s.c. with androstenedione (0.1 mg/day) | Favorable change of plasma lipid profile, decrease in letrozole-elevated LDL/HDL ratio. No improvement of bone status | | [69] |
| FLAVONOLS | | | | | |
| Quercetin; 50 mg/kg bw, by gavage for 10 consecutive days after letrozole dosing | Letrozole; 0.04 mg/kg bw, for 3 months | Sexually mature male Wistar rats | Protection against letrozole-induced injury on testicular tissue | Increase in letrozole-reduced plasma levels of testosterone, LH, FSH and serum E2. | [101] |
| | | | | Increase in letrozole-reduced body and testis weights. Reversal of letrozole-induced elevation of lipid peroxidation (decrease in MDA and NO levels, increase in GSH-Px in blood). Reduction of letrozole-induced abnormalities and damage of seminiferous tubules, restoration of normal appearance of testicular tissue | |
| FLAVANONES | | | | | |
| Hesperetin; 5000 ppm, with diet | Letrozole; 2 μg/day, s.c. injection | MCF-7 cells transfected with human CYP19 (MCF-7aro) injected into the two flanks of ovariectomized female athymic mice; injected s.c. with androstenedione (0.1 mg/day) | Protection against letrozole-induced bone deterioration; reversal of letrozole-induced bone loss | | [29] |

The most important findings that can be highlighted on the basis of our current knowledge are the following:

- Some flavonoids (such as EGCG, baicalein, kaempferol, morin, myricetin, quercetin, naringin and silibinin) can considerably affect the pharmacokinetic fate of TAMOXIFEN when administered concomitantly with this antiestrogen. Promotion of intestinal absorption of tamoxifen through reduction of the P-gp-mediated efflux and inhibition of CYP3A4-catalyzed drug metabolism in the small intestine and liver in the presence of these flavonoids can lead to enhanced oral bioavailability, and increase the anticancer effect of tamoxifen. If these results, currently experimentally proven in rats, will be confirmed also in clinical studies with humans, these combination therapies might lead to lowering the effective doses of tamoxifen, thereby minimizing also its adverse side effects. However, the presence of isoflavone biochanin A is shown to exert contrary effects, i.e., reduce oral bioavailability of tamoxifen. Therefore, no generalization about the beneficial role of flavonoids on pharmacokinetic profile of tamoxifen can be made, and further experimental studies in rat models as well as clinical trials with humans are highly needed. Until more data will be available, it is recommended to women under long-term tamoxifen therapy not to consume dietary supplements with high doses of biochanin A content.
- Numerous *in vitro* cell culture studies and *in vivo* animal works have demonstrated both beneficial (potentiating) as well as detrimental (inhibiting) effects of plant-derived flavonoids on antitumor potential of TAMOXIFEN in molecularly different breast tumors. Therefore, women taking tamoxifen should be careful in consuming any concomitant dietary supplements, not to decrease the therapeutic efficacy and inflict damage on themselves. As natural supplements usually contain a mixture of several compounds, the action of each individual component in combination with tamoxifen might not be known. For this reason, intake of a specific flavonoid rather than their mixtures or plant extracts should be preferred, if at all. Based on the current experimental studies, solely beneficial effects (with no contraindications) have been described for combination of tamoxifen with EGCG, luteolin, hesperidin or naringenin. Development of combination regimens with these

natural agents might lead to lowering the therapeutically efficient doses of tamoxifen and reduce its adverse side effects in the future. However, as the current studies are performed with cultured cells or animal models only, their results should be first confirmed in clinical trials with humans, before any evidence-based recommendations can be given for clinical practice. A special caution must be exercised with exposure to soy isoflavones, known also as phytoestrogens possessing weak estrogenic activity, while receiving tamoxifen treatment. Although genistein can be beneficial in suppressing menopausal symptoms, such as hot flashes, genistein-containing dietary supplements can antagonize the antiproliferative effects of tamoxifen and stimulate the growth of breast tumors. Also, daidzein can abrogate the therapeutic effects of tamoxifen in ER+ breast cancer cells. Therefore, intake of soy isoflavones should better be avoided by women who have been prescribed tamoxifen for either treatment or prevention of breast cancer. In addition, patients should minimize also the consumption of tangeretin-added products and dietary supplements, as tangeretin might be able to abrogate the growth inhibitory effects of tamoxifen *in vivo* breast cancer models, due to suppression of the host`s immune defense against the tumor. Such tangeretin-added products can involve various beverages and food items that are enriched with tangerine peel oil [84].

- Women on the long-term TAMOXIFEN therapy are threatened by the drug-induced toxicity, mainly by oxidative damage to the liver, as the majority of tamoxifen metabolism occurs in the hepatic tissue. Based on a few experiments with rodents, specific flavonoids (especially catechins) can scavenge free radicals and normalize redox status in the liver, thereby providing protection against tamoxifen-induced hepatotoxicity. If this function will be confirmed in patients, carefully selected flavonoids might be important adjuvants for long-term tamoxifen therapy in the future.
- Based on experimental studies, green tea flavanol EGCG might be an important adjuvant for RALOXIFENE therapy. The presence of EGCG can improve oral bioavailability of the drug by inhibiting its metabolic conversion in the intestine and potentiate raloxifene-induced cytotoxic activities in breast cancer cells. If further *in vivo* studies and clinical trials will confirm these results, EGCG could be recommended as an auxiliary agent to postmenopausal women who

are prescribed raloxifene for preventing breast cancer and/or osteoporosis, allowing lowering of the effective drug doses.

- Laboratorial studies have shown that concomitant use of CENTCHROMAN and soy isoflavones (genistein, daidzein) might lead to synergistic potentiation of drug-induced anticancer effects. If clinical trials with humans will confirm these experimental results, the doses of centchroman must be appropriately adjusted (lowered) when used concurrently with dietary isoflavone supplements. Women who take centchroman for the treatment of advanced breast cancer should be aware of these possible interactions.
- It would be reasonable to recommend that postmenopausal women under FULVESTRANT therapy avoid the consumption of soy isoflavone supplements, as based on *in vitro* and *in vivo* experimental studies it is possible that ingredients of soy extracts (or the bacterial metabolite of daidzein, equol) can negate antiestrogenic and anticancer activities of the drug. Further preclinical and clinical research is needed to unravel these possibilities and allow breast cancer patients to make informed decisions on the intake of soy-containing dietary supplements during the treatment with fulvestrant.
- Postmenopausal breast cancer patients receiving aromatase inhibitor therapy are threatened by severe detrimental effects on the bone health with elevated risk for osteoporosis and bone fractures, due to drug-induced suppression of estrogen synthesis in the whole body. For the same reason, a more atherogenic blood lipid profile and increased coronary heart disease risk are often observed in women under long-term adjuvant therapy with aromatase inhibitors. Experimental studies with rodents have found that the presence of biochanin A can be beneficial in alleviating ANASTROZOLE-induced bone health decrements, while luteolin mitigated LETROZOLE-evoked adverse effects on blood lipid profile. If these results will be further confirmed in human trials, supplements of specific flavonoids might be helpful to ameliorate toxicity of aromatase inhibitors and thereby improve the quality of life of breast cancer patients. However, as the presence of soy isoflavone genistein is found to be able to attenuate LETROZOLE-induced anticancer effects both *in vitro* as well as *in vivo* models of ER+ breast cancer, great caution is required when consuming isoflavone-containing dietary supplements during letrozole therapy.

- Many women under hormonal cancer therapy decide to consume different flavonoid-rich herbal products to mitigate drug-induced side effects or manage possible depression and anxiety resulting from both diagnosis as well as cancer treatment. As the ingredients of these herbal products are largely unexplored and may counteract antitumor action of the drugs, it is better to avoid the use of any herbal supplements during treatment course, not to inflict damage on themselves.

## 3.2. Interfering of Flavonoids with Hormonal Prostate Cancer Therapies

### 3.2.1. Prostate Cancer as a Hormone-Dependent Tumor

Prostate cancer is the second most common cancer type diagnosed in men, being the fifth leading cause of cancer-related death among males. In 2020, there were more than 1.41 million new prostate cancer cases with over 375,000 deaths worldwide [2]. The incidence rate of prostate cancer elevates with age [102]. Other risk factors include environmental impacts, such as dietary habits and lifestyle, whereas a genetic component can also play a definite role in prostate tumorigenesis [102, 103]. As the development of prostate cancer is initially androgen-dependent, primary treatment modalities include regulation of the synthesis of androgens or blocking the androgen receptors, i.e., androgen deprivation therapy or surgical castration [103-106]. At later stages, prostate cancer becomes androgen-independent, and its growth and survival do not depend anymore on body androgens [104]. Progression from a hormone-sensitive phase to a hormone-independent phase occurs through multiple steps; however, once castration-resistant prostate cancer is developed, it is highly lethal due to metastasis and acquiring of resistance to available therapies [103]. Although chemotherapy has remained an option for the treatment of castration-resistant prostate cancer, it is still a major clinical problem with a great need for more effective therapeutic strategies [103, 107].

In comparison with breast cancer hormonal treatment, considerably less studies have been performed about possible impact of phytochemicals on the efficacy of prostate cancer hormonal therapies, as interactions with only three antiandrogenic drugs, i.e., bicalutamide, flutamide and enzalutamide (Figure 3.4), have been investigated. On the other hand, prostate cancer patients as well as men at high risk of developing prostate cancer frequently consume one or more dietary supplements, including herbal extracts [105]. Moreover, long-term androgen deprivation therapy has been associated with a variety of adverse side effects, including hypertension, unfavorable blood lipid profile with a high predisposition to cardiovascular diseases, diabetes, degeneration of muscles and bone, as well as low libido [106], whereas many patients receiving antiandrogens may seek alleviation to these conditions from the use of flavonoids-containing dietary supplements. The current knowledge about interactions between antiandrogens and plant-derived flavonoids, although very limited, is discussed in the subsection 3.2.2.

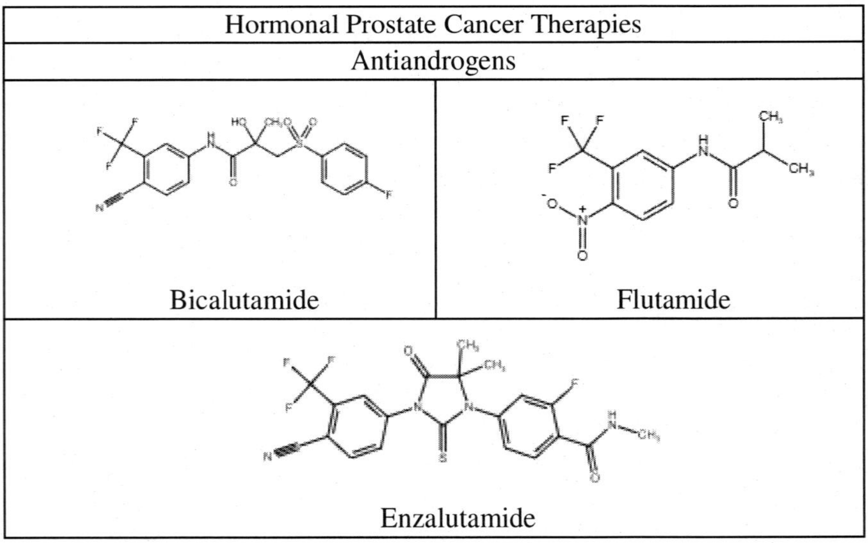


**Figure 3.4.** Structural formulas of hormonal prostate cancer therapies studied in combination with flavonoids.

### 3.2.2. Influence of Flavonoids on Therapeutic Action of Antiandrogens

#### *3.2.2.1. Bicalutamide*

Bicalutamide, sold under the brand name Casodex, is a first-generation non-steroidal antiandrogen medication approved for the treatment of androgen-dependent prostate cancer [102, 104, 108] (Figure 3.4). This drug is typically used in combination with a gonadotropin-releasing hormone analog or surgical removal of the testicles, resulting in a complete androgen blockade and death of androgen-dependent cells [102, 109]. Bicalutamide suppresses production of testicular androgens but blocks also androgen receptors (ARs) present on prostate tissue, besides being responsible for ARs degradation. Efficacy of bicalutamide therapy is assessed by decrease in prostate specific antigen (PSA) and testosterone levels [104]. However, administration of bicalutamide causes drug accumulation and toxicities. Its major side effects include hot flashes, sexual dysfunction, gynecomastia and breast tenderness, anemia, liver problems, nephrotoxicity, lung damage, constipation and back pain [104, 108, 109]. Furthermore, long-term treatment with bicalutamide can cause ARs to be mutated, starting to act as a receptor agonist and leading to failure of antiandrogen therapy. As a result, prostate cancer grows even in the environment of low-level androgens [108]. Taking into account numerous beneficial properties of plant-derived flavonoids, their combination with bicalutamide therapy might be helpful in combating drug-induced toxicities and delaying the development of drug resistance. However, the research in this field is still very scarce today, as well as the information about possibly detrimental coeffects is completely lacking.

*3.2.2.1.1. Effects of Flavonoids on Anticancer Potential of Bicalutamide*

Recent studies have shown that cotreatment of prostate cancer cells with bicalutamide and a few specific flavonoids might be important in augmenting drug-induced anticancer potential (Table 3.13). The presence of green tea flavanol EGCG (at 30 and 40 μM) resulted in a significant potentiation of bicalutamide-induced cytotoxic responses in both AR+ (NRP-152) as well as AR- cells (NRP-154) derived from dorsolateral prostate of N-methyl-N-nitrosourea-treated rats, whereas this effect was even stronger in AR-non-expressing cells. Enhancement of anticancer efficacy in AR- prostate cells suggests that some other mechanisms rather than AR-dependent signaling must be involved in the action of this combination; however, the precise cellular events are currently unknown [102]. In similar manner, combination treatment of bicalutamide with citrus flavanone hesperetin, either as free mixture or coloaded into nanoparticles, increased drug-induced cytotoxicity in AR- human prostate cancer cells PC-3. This superior activity was accompanied by induction of apoptosis with enhanced mitochondrial disruption and modulation of the progression of cell cycle. In addition, co-encapsulation of both agents into nanoparticles revealed higher accumulation of drug inside the tumor cells, in turn leading to stronger anticancer activities [108]. Further studies are highly needed to unravel molecular mechanisms behind cytotoxic responses observed by treatment of AR- prostate cancer cells with combination of bicalutamide and flavonoids, to determine the possibilities for using EGCG or hesperetin as adjuvants for bicalutamide therapy in clinical practice. It is well accepted that human prostate cancer tissue is heterogenous containing both AR+ as well as AR- cells [110]; therefore, finding a combinational strategy for simultaneous targeting of both androgen-dependent and androgen-independent cells is highly attractive. Bicalutamide, being a drug of choice for androgen-sensitive prostate cancer, can be therapeutically effective also against androgen-insensitive tumor cells, when combined with specific flavonoids.

*3.2.2.1.2. Effects of Flavonoids on Bicalutamide-Induced Toxicities*

Besides enhancing therapeutic efficacy of bicalutamide in prostate cancer cells, flavanone hesperetin has been shown to provide also protective effects against drug-related nephrotoxicity in male rats. In fact, combined treatment with bicalutamide and hesperetin, co-delivered as nanoemulsifying system, led to a significant decrease in the levels of biochemical markers of nephrotoxicity (serum urea and creatinine), suggesting the protective role against renal toxicity. Moreover, the presence of hesperetin could also restore the normal architecture of kidney that was distorted by bicalutamide treatment [109] (Table 3.14). Therefore, codelivery of bicalutamide with hesperetin may represent a useful novel approach for management of prostate cancer in the future.

### *3.2.2.2. Flutamide*

Flutamide is another first-generation non-steroidal antiandrogen medication that is widely prescribed for the treatment of both benign prostatic hyperplasia as well as prostate cancer [106] (Figure 3.4). This drug acts as an androgen receptor antagonist and thereby prevents androgen-dependent growth of prostate cancer cells [111]. The major side effects of flutamide therapy include breast enlargement and tenderness, feminization, sexual dysfunction and hot flashes, besides leading also to elevated serum levels of total cholesterol, LDL and triglycerides, rendering patients at higher risk to cardiovascular diseases [106].

**Table 3.13.** Effects of flavonoids on anticancer action of bicalutamide in prostate tumor models

| Flavonoid and its dosage | Bicalutamide and its dosage | Biological system | Assay method and time | Effect | Mechanisms | Ref. |
|---|---|---|---|---|---|---|
| FLAVANOLS | | | | | | |
| EGCG; 30, 40 μM | Bicalutamide; 10 μM | NRP-152 non-tumorigenic cells derived from dorsolateral prostate of Lobund-Wistar rats treated with MNU, cytokeratin 14+ and AR+; basal epithelial cells | CV; 72h | Potentiation of bicalutamide-induced cell number decrease | Non-significant increase in bicalutamide-induced apoptotic events | [102] |
| EGCG; 30, 40 μM | Bicalutamide; 10 μM | NRP-154 tumorigenic cells derived from dorsolateral prostate of Lobund-Wistar rats treated with MNU, cytokeratin 18+ and AR-; secretory epithelial cells | CV; 72h | Potentiation of bicalutamide-induced cell number decrease | Increase in bicalutamide-induced apoptotic events | [102] |
| FLAVANONES | | | | | | |
| Hesperetin; 12.5-200 μM, as free mixture or co-loaded with bicalutamide to PCL-CS NPs | Bicalutamide; 12.5-200 μM, as free mixture or co-loaded with hesperetin to PCL-CS NPs | PC-3 human prostate cancer cells, androgen-independent | MTT; 24, 48h | Increase in cytotoxicity compared to free bicalutamide | Increase in apoptosis (enhancement of $\Delta\Psi m$). Increase in G1-S phase cell cycle arrest (for NPs only) | [108] |

**Table 3.14.** Effects of flavonoids on bicalutamide-induced toxicities

| Flavonoid and its dosage | Bicalutamide and its dosage | Biological system | Effects | Mechanisms | Ref. |
|---|---|---|---|---|---|
| FLAVANONES | | | | | |
| Hesperetin; 20 mg/kg, oral delivery, co-loaded with bicalutamide to SNEDDS | Bicalutamide; 20 mg/kg, oral delivery, co-loaded with hesperetin to SNEDDS | Male Sprague-Dawley rats | Protective effect against nephrotoxicity. Restoration of normal architecture of kidney. Overcoming of tissue toxicity | Decrease in the levels of nephrotoxicity biochemical markers (creatinine and serum urea) | [109] |

#### *3.2.2.2.1. Effects of Flavonoids on Flutamide-Induced Toxicities*

Although there are no reports available about potential effects of plant-derived flavonoids on anticancer efficacy of flutamide in prostate cancer models, in a few studies, the role of flavonoids on flutamide-related toxicities have been explored (Table 3.15). As a result, it was found that flavonol morin could suppress flutamide-induced markers of lipid peroxidation in blood samples of male rabbits, preventing oxidative damage to cell membranes, lipoproteins and other lipid-containing cellular structures. In addition, the presence of morin exerted also a protective effect against flutamide-induced changes in cholesterol profile, by lowering total cholesterol levels and elevating HDL content, suggesting that morin can reduce toxic potential of flutamide [111]. Another flavonoid with similar beneficial properties on flutamide-related toxicities was found to be soy isoflavone daidzein. Subchronic treatment of male rats with flutamide in the presence of orally administered daidzein significantly alleviated drug-induced changes in blood lipid profile, redox balance, expression of matrix degrading genes, and prostate architecture. Daidzein was able to decrease flutamide-induced levels of total cholesterol, LDL and triglycerides, while increasing HDL content and endogenous antioxidant levels. Moreover, daidzein could restore also flutamide-suppressed AR expression in ventral prostate of rats [106]. Beneficial roles of these two flavonoids, morin and daidzein, in minimizing drug-related adverse effects are definitely worth of further studies to elucidate possibilities for the use of these dietary supplements as adjuvants for prostate cancer patients under flutamide therapy, retarding their susceptibility to cardiovascular diseases.

### *3.2.2.3. Enzalutamide*

Enzalutamide is a second-generation non-steroidal antiandrogen medication that is used for the treatment of prostate cancer [105] (Figure 3.4). This drug acts as an AR antagonist; however, like earlier androgen deprivation therapies, enzalutamide has a short duration of efficacy due to primary or acquired resistance [105]. Moreover, the use of enzalutamide is associated with several adverse side effects, including fatigue, gynecomastia, sexual dysfunction, hot flashes, headache, diarrhea and back pain.

**Table 3.15.** Effects of flavonoids on flutamide-induced toxicities

| Flavonoid and its dosage | Flutamide and its dosage | Biological system | Effects | Mechanisms | Ref. |
|---|---|---|---|---|---|
| FLAVANOLS | | | | | |
| Morin; 50 mg/kg bw, p.o. | Flutamide; 12.5 mg/kg bw, p.o. | Male white New Zeeland rabbits | Protective effect against flutamide-induced toxicity | Antiperoxidative action on flutamide-induced lipid peroxidation (decrease in MDA and 4-HNE, increase in GSH and NO levels). Protective effect on flutamide-induced changes in cholesterol profile (decrease in total cholesterol, increase in HDL content) | [111] |
| ISOFLAVONES | | | | | |
| Daidzein; 20 or 60 mg/kg bw, 3h after flutamide, for 60 days, p.o. | Flutamide; 30 mg/kg bw, for 60 days | Male Wistar rats | Protective effect against flutamide-induced toxicity | Decrease in flutamide-induced levels of total cholesterol, LDL and TG; increase in HDL. Restoration of AR expression; decrease in uPAR and MMP-9 levels. Restoration of activity of antioxidant enzymes (GSH, GPx, GR and CAT); decrease in TBARS and NO; increase in SOD levels. Restoration of prostate architecture disrupted by flutamide | [106] |

*3.2.2.3.1. Effects of Flavonoids on Anticancer Potential of Enzalutamide*

Based on the recent innovative studies, prostate cancer can remain dependent on androgen receptor signaling even after castration, being mediated by different cellular mechanisms [103, 105]. Although enzalutamide is approved for the treatment of castration-resistant prostate cancer, its efficacy is limited due to not only mutation and amplification of AR, but also the generation of splice variants of AR protein, such as AR splice variant 7 (AR-V7) that is constitutively active and lacks a functional ligand-binding domain, evading binding of antiandrogens. Therefore, AR-V7 can represent a potential key target for novel strategies of prostate cancer therapy [103, 105]. Recent studies have shown that specific plant-derived flavonoids can suppress this protein leading to synergistic anticancer activities, when combined with enzalutamide treatment (Table 3.16). In fact, flavone luteolin enhanced therapeutic efficacy of enzalutamide in human castration-resistant prostate cancer cells 22Rv1 by reducing the expression of both AR as well as AR-V7. In 22Rv1 tumor-bearing castrated nude mice, this effect was mediated by induction of microRNA 8080 (miR-8080) levels by oral luteolin, leading to reduction of AR-V7 expression and suppression of xenograft growth [103]. Similarly, the presence of flavonol quercetin (at 5 or 10 μM) downregulated splicing factor hnRNPA1, reduced the expression of AR-V7, and antagonized sustained and ligand-independent AR signaling in human prostate cancer cells 22Rv1 and C4-2B, resulting in synergistic decrease in cellular viability and clonogenic ability when administered concomitantly with enzalutamide. Also, quercetin re-sensitized enzalutamide-resistant prostate cancer cells 22Rv1-Enza-R and C4-2B-Enza-R to enzalutamide, through suppression of full-length AR and AR-V7 levels and downregulation of AR signaling. Moreover, cotreatment of 22Rv1 xenograft-bearing mice with enzalutamide and quercetin led to a synergistic inhibition of malignant growth with almost complete abolishment of tumors [105]. Therefore, certain plant-derived flavonoids (luteolin, quercetin) can improve therapeutic resistance to enzalutamide and augment efficacy of hormonal prostate cancer therapy, by suppressing the alternative splicing of AR.

**Table 3.16.** Effects of flavonoids on anticancer action of enzalutamide in prostate tumor models

| Flavonoid and its dosage | Enzalutamide and its dosage | Biological system | Assay method and time | Effect | Mechanisms | Ref. |
|---|---|---|---|---|---|---|
| FLAVONES | | | | | | |
| Luteolin; 10, 25, 50 μM | Enzalutamide; 10 μM | 22Rv1 human prostate cancer cells, castration-resistant prostate cancer | WST-1; 48h | Increase in therapeutic efficacy of enzalutamide. Induction of cell growth inhibition (no effect by drug alone) | Decrease in AR and AR-V7 | [103] |
| Luteolin; 100 ppm, daily, from diet | Enzalutamide; 10 mg/kg/day, i.p. injection, 5 times weekly | 22Rv1 cells implanted s.c. into castrated nude mice | 12 days | Increase in therapeutic efficacy of enzalutamide. Suppression of tumor growth (no effect by drug alone) | Induction of miR-8080 level; reduction of AR-V7 expression | [103] |
| FLAVONOLS | | | | | | |
| Quercetin; 5, 10 μM | Enzalutamide; 20 μM | C4-2B human prostate cancer cells | Counting; 48h | Synergistic decrease in cell survival. Reduction of clonogenic ability | Synergistic decrease in mRNA and protein levels of hnRNPA1, AR and AR-V7; downregulation of AR signaling | [105] |
| Quercetin; 5, 10 μM | Enzalutamide; 20 μM | C4-2B-Enza-R human prostate cancer cells, enzalutamide-resistant | Counting; 48h | Synergistic decrease in cell survival; re-sensitization to enzalutamide. Reduction of clonogenic ability | Synergistic decrease in mRNA and protein levels of hnRNPA1, AR and AR-V7; downregulation of AR signaling | [105] |
| Quercetin; 5, 10 μM | Enzalutamide; 20 μM | 22Rv1 human prostate cancer cells | Counting; 48h | Synergistic decrease in cell survival. Reduction of clonogenic ability | Synergistic decrease in mRNA and protein levels of hnRNPA1, AR and AR-V7; downregulation of AR signaling | [105] |

| Flavonoid and its dosage | Enzalutamide and its dosage | Biological system | Assay method and time | Effect | Mechanisms | Ref. |
|---|---|---|---|---|---|---|
| Quercetin; 5, 10 μM | Enzalutamide; 20 μM | 22Rv1-Enza-R human prostate cancer cells, enzalutamide-resistant | Counting; 48h | Synergistic decrease in cell survival; re-sensitization to enzalutamide. Reduction of clonogenic ability | Synergistic decrease in mRNA and protein levels of hnRNPA1, AR and AR-V7; downregulation of AR signaling | [105] |
| Quercetin; 20 mg/kg, i.p. daily for 5 days/week | Enzalutamide; 25 mg/kg, via oral gavage, for 5 days/week | 22Rv1 cells injected s.c. into the flanks of male SCID mice | 3 weeks | Synergistic suppression of xenograft growth. Re-sensitization of enzalutamide-resistant xenografts to enzalutamide; complete abolishment of tumors | Downregulation of hnRNPA1, AR and AR-V7 mRNA and protein levels in tumor tissues; suppression of Ki-67 | [105] |

### 3.2.3. Conclusions from Preclinical Knowledge with Dietary Recommendations to Prostate Cancer Patients

According to the current experimental knowledge, no counteractive effects of plant-derived flavonoids have been reported so far on anticancer action of antiandrogens (bicalutamide, flutamide, enzalutamide) in different prostate cancer models. However, the amount of these studies is still very limited, and further *in vitro* and *in vivo* preclinical research is highly needed. The conclusions from the present information can be summed as following:

- Based on *in vitro* and *in vivo* experimental studies, citrus flavanone hesperetin can be a favorable adjunct to BICALUTAMIDE therapy by increasing drug-induced cytotoxic responses in prostate cancer cells, and reducing drug-related toxicity to renal functions and kidney morphology. If these results will be further confirmed in human trials, prostate cancer patients receiving bicalutamide therapy might obtain some important benefits from the intake of hesperetin-containing supplements in improving their clinical outcome and quality of life.
- Laboratorial studies with experimental animals have revealed a significant protective action of few flavonoids (morin, daidzein) against FLUTAMIDE-induced oxidative damage and unfavorable blood lipid profile. If human trials will confirm these findings, supplements of specific flavonoids might become important adjuvants to flutamide therapy for improvement of patient condition and prevention of cardiovascular diseases associated with the chronic use of antiandrogens.
- Investigation into prostate cancer cell cultures as well as experimental mice have shown that certain flavonoids (luteolin, quercetin) can prevent the resistance to ENZALUTAMIDE therapy by suppressing the expression of aberrant variants of AR. Although further human studies are highly needed, it is expected that supplemental intake of these plant-derived agents could be beneficial in retarding the development of resistance and prolonging the effectiveness of antiandrogen treatment. Future clinical trials should evaluate this possibility in prostate cancer patients receiving enzalutamide therapy to improve their clinical outcome.

## References

[1] Baum M. Historical and cultural determinants in the evolution of adjuvant endocrine therapy: a tale of two hemispheres, separated by a common language. *Oncology* 2012; 26: 559, 562, 567.

[2] Sung H, Ferlay J, Siegel RL, Laversanne M, Soerjomataram I, Jemal A, Bray F. Global Cancer Statistics 2020: GLOBOCAN estimates of incidence and mortality worldwide for 36 cancers in 185 countries. *CA Cancer J Clin* 2021; 71: 209-49.

[3] Sakata M, Ikeda T, Imoto S, Jinno H, Kitagawa Y. Prevention of mammary carcinogenesis in C3H/OuJ mice by green tea and tamoxifen. *Asian Pac J Cancer Prev* 2011; 12: 567-71.

[4] Khamis AA, Ali EM, El-Moneim MA, Abd-Alhaseeb MM, El-Magd MA, Salim EI. Hesperidin, piperine and bee venom synergistically potentiate the anticancer effect of tamoxifen against breast cancer cells. *Biomed Pharmacother* 2018; 105: 1335-43.

[5] Kaushik S, Shyam H, Sharma R, Balapure AK. Genistein synergizes centchroman action in human breast cancer cells. *Indian J Pharmacol* 2016; 48: 637-42.

[6] Gaber M, Hany M, Mokhtar S, Helmy MW, Elkodairy KA, Elzoghby AO. Boronic-targeted albumin-shell oily-core nanocapsules for synergistic aromatase inhibitor/herbal breast cancer therapy. *Mater Sci Eng C Mater Biol Appl* 2019; 105: 110099.

[7] Boszkiewicz K, Sawicka E, Piwowar A. The impact of xenoestrogens on effectiveness of treatment for hormone-dependent breast cancer – current state of knowledge and perspectives for research. *Ann Agric Environ Med* 2020; 27: 526-34.

[8] Mai Z, Balckburn GL, Zhou JR. Soy phytochemicals synergistically enhance the preventive effect of tamoxifen on the growth of estrogen-dependent human breast carcinoma in mice. *Carcinogenesis* 2007; 28: 1217-23.

[9] Ju YH, Doerge DR, Allred KF, Allred CD, Helferich WG. Dietary genistein negates the inhibitory effect of tamoxifen on growth of estrogen-dependent human breast cancer (MCF-7) cells implanted in athymic mice. *Cancer Res* 2002; 62: 2474-7.

[10] Du M, Yang X, Hartman JA, Cooke PS, Doerge DR, Ju YH, Helferich WG. Low-dose dietary genistein negates the therapeutic effect of tamoxifen in athymic nude mice. *Carcinogenesis* 2012; 33: 895-901.

[11] Liu B, Edgerton S, Yang X, Kim A, Ordonez-Ercan D, Mason T, Alvarez K, McKimmey C, Liu N, Thor A. Low-dose dietary phytoestrogen

abrogates tamoxifen-associated mammary tumor prevention. *Cancer Res* 2005; 65: 879-86.

[12] Messina MJ, Wood CE. Soy isoflavones, estrogen therapy, and breast cancer risk: analysis and commentary. *Nutr J* 2008; 7: 17.

[13] Warth B, Raffeiner P, Granados A, Huan T, Fang M, Forsberg EM, Benton HP, Goetz L, Johnson CH, Siuzdak G. Metabolomics reveals that dietary xenoestrogens alter cellular metabolism induced by palbociclib/letrozole combination cancer therapy. *Cell Chem Biol* 2018; 25: 291-300.

[14] Jen SH, Wei MP, Yin AC. The combinatory effects of glabridin and tamoxifen on Ishikawa and MCF-7 cell lines. *Nat Prod Commun* 2015; 10: 1573-6.

[15] Ju YH, Doerge DR, Woodling KA, Hartman JA, Kwak J, Helferich WG. Dietary genistein negates the inhibitory effect of letrozole on the growth of aromatase-expressing estrogen-dependent human breast cancer cells (MCF-7Ca) in vivo. *Carcinogenesis* 2008; 29: 2162-8.

[16] Guha N, Kwan ML, Quesenberry Jr CP, Weltzien EK, Castillo AL, Caan BJ. Soy isoflavones and risk of cancer recurrence in a cohort of breast cancer survivors: the Life After Cancer Epidemiology study. *Breast Cancer Res Treat* 2009; 118: 395-405.

[17] Pons DG, Nadal-Serrano M, Torrens-Mas M, Oliver J, Roca P. The phytoestrogen genistein affects breast cancer cells treatment depending on the ERα/ERβ ratio. *J Cell Biochem* 2016; 117: 218-29.

[18] Zhang X, Cook KL, Warri A, Cruz IM, Rosim M, Riskin J, Helferich W, Doerge D, Clarke R, Hilakivi-Clarke L. Lifetime genistein intake increases the response of mammary tumors to tamoxifen in rats. *Clin Cancer Res* 2017; 23: 814-24.

[19] Charalambous C, Pitta CA, Constantinou AI. Equol enhances tamoxifen`s anti-tumor activity by induction of caspase-mediated apoptosis in MCF-7 breast cancer cells. *BMC Cancer* 2013; 13: 238.

[20] Li Y, Meeran SM, Patel SN, Chen H, Hardy TM, Tollefsbol TO. Epigenetic reactivation of estrogen receptor-alpha (ERalpha) by genistein enhances hormonal therapy sensitivity in ERalpha-negative breast cancer. *Mol Cancer* 2013; 12: 9.

[21] Shu XO, Zheng Y, Cai H, Gu K, Chen Z, Zheng W, Lu W. Soy food intake and breast cancer survival. *JAMA* 2009; 302: 2437-43.

[22] Tu SH, Ho CT, Liu MF, Huang CS, Chang HW, Chang CH, Wu CH, Ho YS. Luteolin sensitises drug-resistant human breast cancer cells to tamoxifen via the inhibition of cyclin E2 expression. *Food Chem* 2013; 141: 1553-61.

[23] Xu Z, Zhao D, Zheng X, Huang B, Xia X, Pan X. Quercetin exerts bidirectional regulation effects on the efficacy of tamoxifen in estrogen receptor-positive breast cancer therapy: An in vitro study. *Environ Toxicol* 2020; 35: 1179-93.

[24] Memariani Z, Abbas SQ, Ul Hassan SS, Ahmadi A, Chabra A. Naringin and naringenin as anticancer agents and adjuvants in cancer combination therapy: Efficacy and molecular mechanisms of action, a comprehensive narrative review. *Pharmacol Res* 2021; 171: 105264.

[25] Yaacob NS, Nengsih A, Norazmi MN. Tualang honey promotes apoptotic cell death induced by tamoxifen in breast cancer cell lines. *Evid Based Complement Alternat Med* 2013; 2013: 989841.

[26] Hatkevich T, Ramos J, Santos-Sanchez I, Patel YM. A naringenin-tamoxifen combination impairs cell proliferation and survival of MCF-7 breast cancer cells. *Exp Cell Res* 2014; 327: 331-9.

[27] Xu Z, Huang B, Liu J, Wu X, Luo N, Wang X, Zheng X, Pan X. Combinatorial anti-proliferative effects of tamoxifen and naringenin: The role of four estrogen receptor subtypes. *Toxicology* 2018; 410: 231-46.

[28] Oleaga C, Garcia M, Sole A, Ciudad CJ, Izquierdo-Pulido M, Noe V. CYP1A1 is overexpressed upon incubation of breast cancer cells with a polyphenolic cocoa extract. *Eur J Nutr* 2012; 51: 465-76.

[29] Li F, Chow S, Cheung WH, Chan FL, Chen S, Leung LK. The citrus flavonone hesperetin prevents letrozole-induced bone loss in a mouse model of breast cancer. *J Nutr Biochem* 2013; 24: 1112-6.

[30] Way TD, Lee HH, Kao MC, Lin JK. Black tea polyphenol theaflavins inhibit aromatase activity and attenuate tamoxifen resistance in HER2/neu-transfected human breast cancer cells through tyrosine kinase suppression. *Eur J Cancer* 2004; 40: 2165-74.

[31] Li Y, Meeran SM, Tollefsbol TO. Combinatorial bioactive botanicals re-sensitize tamoxifen treatment in ER-negative breast cancer via epigenetic reactivation of ERα expression. *Sci Rep* 2017; 7: 9345.

[32] Yang X, Yang S, McKimmey C, Liu B, Edgerton SM, Bales W, Archer LT, Thor AD. Genistein induces enhanced growth promotion in ER-positive/erbB-2-overexpressing breast cancers by ER-erbB-2 cross talk and p27/kip1 downregulation. *Carcinogenesis* 2010; 31: 695-702.

[33] Waks AG, Winer EP. Breast cancer treatment: A review. *JAMA* 2019; 321: 288-300.

[34] Wang H, Tao L, Qi K, Zhang H, Feng D, Wei W, Kong H, Chen T, Lin Q. Quercetin reverses tamoxifen resistance in breast cancer cells. *J BUON* 2015; 20: 707-13.

[35] Stuart EC, Jarvis RM, Rosengren RJ. In vitro mechanism of action for the cytotoxicity elicited by the combination of epigallocatechin gallate and raloxifene in MDA-MB-231 cells. *Oncol Rep* 2010; 24: 779-85.

[36] Mai Z, Blackburn GL, Zhou JR. Genistein sensitizes inhibitory effect of tamoxifen on the growth of estrogen receptor-positive and HER2-overexpressing human breast cancer cells. *Mol Carcinog* 2007; 46: 534-42.

[37] van Duursen MB, Smeets EE, Rijk JC, Nijmeijer SM, van den Berg M. Phytoestrogens in menopausal supplements induce ER-dependent cell proliferation and overcome breast cancer treatment in an in vitro breast cancer model. *Toxicol Appl Pharmacol* 2013; 269: 132-40.

[38] El-Lakany SA, Elgindy NA, Helmy MW, Abu-Serie MM, Elzoghby AO. Lactoferrin-decorated vs PEGylated zein nanospheres for combined aromatase inhibitor and herbal therapy of breast cancer. *Expert Opin Drug Deliv* 2018; 15: 835-50.

[39] Limer JL, Parkes AT, Speirs V. Differential response to phytoestrogens in endocrine sensitive and resistant breast cancer cells in vitro. *Int J Cancer* 2006; 119: 515-21.

[40] Sartippour MR, Pietras R, Marquez-Garban DC, Chen HW, Heber D, Henning SM, Sartippour G, Zhang L, Lu M, Weinberg O, Rao JY, Brooks MN. The combination of green tea and tamoxifen is effective against breast cancer. *Carcinogenesis* 2006; 27: 2424-33.

[41] Guthrie N, Gapor A, Chambers AF, Carroll KK. Palm oil tocotrienols and plant flavonoids act synergistically with each other and with tamoxifen in inhibiting proliferation and growth of estrogen receptor-negative MDA-MB-435 and -positive MCF-7 human breast cancer cells in culture. *Asia Pac J Clin Nutr* 1997; 6: 41-5.

[42] Kaushik S, Shyam H, Sharma R, Balapure AK. Dietary isoflavone daidzein synergizes centchroman action via induction of apoptosis and inhibition of PI3K/Akt pathway in MCF-7/MDA MB-231 human breast cancer cells. *Phytomedicine* 2018; 40: 116-24.

[43] Huang HC, Way TD, Lin CL, Lin JK. EGCG stabilizes p27kip1 in E2-stimulated MCF-7 cells through down-regulation of the Skp2 protein. *Endocrinology* 2008; 149: 5972-83.

[44] Stuart EC, Larsen L, Rosengren RJ. Potential mechanisms for the synergistic cytotoxicity elicited by 4-hydroxytamoxifen and epigallocatechin gallate in MDA-MB-231 cells. *Int J Oncol* 2007; 30: 1407-12.

[45] Esmaeili MA. Combination of siRNA-directed gene silencing with epigallocatechin-3-gallate (EGCG) reverses drug resistance in human breast cancer cells. *J Chem Biol* 2015; 9: 41-52.

[46] Hatono M, Ikeda H, Suzuki Y, Kajiwara Y, Kawada K, Tsukioki T, Kochi M, Suzawa K, Iwamoto T, Yamamoto H, Shien T, Yamane M, Taira N, Doihara H, Toyooka S. Effect of isoflavones on breast cancer cell development and their impact on breast cancer treatments. *Breast Cancer Res Treat* 2021; 185: 307-16.

[47] Mohamed AA, Ahmed MM, Gomaa M, Ebraheim LL. Bone health consequence of adjuvant anastrozole in monotherapy or associated with biochanin-A in ovariectomized rat model. *Life Sci* 2018; 212: 159-67.

[48] Galal AA, Mohamed AA, Khater SI, Metwally MM. Beneficial role of biochanin A on cutaneous and renal tissues of ovariectomized rats treated with anastrozole. *Life Sci* 2018; 201: 9-16.

[49] Quella SK, Loprinzi CL, Barton DL, Knost JA, Sloan JA, LaVasseur BI, Swan D, Krupp KR, Miller KD, Novotny PJ. Evaluation of soy phytoestrogens for the treatment of hot flashes in breast cancer survivors: A North Central Cancer Treatment Group Trial. *J Clin Oncol* 2000; 18: 1068-74.

[50] Tonetti DA, Zhang Y, Zhao H, Lim SB, Constantinou AI. The effect of the phytoestrogens genistein, daidzein, and equol on the growth of tamoxifen-resistant T47D/PKC alpha. *Nutr Cancer* 2007; 58: 222-9.

[51] Jones JL, Daley BJ, Enderson BL, Zhou JR, Karlstad MD. Genistein inhibits tamoxifen effects on cell proliferation and cell cycle arrest in T47D breast cancer cells. *Am Surg* 2002; 68: 575-8.

[52] Wu AH, Pike MC, Williams LD, Spicer D, Tseng CC, Churchwell MI, Doerge DR. Tamoxifen, soy, and lifestyle factors in Asian American women with breast cancer. *J Clin Oncol* 2007; 25: 3024-30.

[53] Gallo D, Mantuano E, Fabrizi M, Ferlini C, Mozzetti S, De Stefano I, Scambia G. Effects of a phytoestrogen-containing soy extract on the growth-inhibitory activity of ICI 182 780 in an experimental model of estrogen-dependent breast cancer. *Endocr Relat Cancer* 2007; 14: 317-24.

[54] Nechuta SJ, Caan BJ, Chen WY, Lu W, Chen Z, Kwan ML, Flatt SW, Zheng Y, Zheng W, Pierce JP, Shu XO. Soy food intake after diagnosis of breast cancer and survival: an in-depth analysis of combined evidence from cohort studies of US and Chinese women. *Am J Clin Nutr* 2012; 96: 123-32.

[55] Kang X, Zhang Q, Wang S, Huang X, Jin S. Effect of soy isoflavones on breast cancer recurrence and death for patients receiving adjuvant endocrine therapy. *CMAJ* 2010; 182: 1857-62.

[56] Caan BJ, Natarajan L, Parker B, Gold EB, Thomson C, Newman V, Rock CL, Pu M, Al-Delaimy W, Pierce JP. Soy food consumption and breast cancer prognosis. *Cancer Epidemiol Biomarkers Prev* 2011; 20: 854-8.

[57] Li H, Wu C, Liu Y, Zhang S, Gao X. Baihe Zhimu formula attenuates the efficacy of tamoxifen against breast cancer in mice through modulation of CYP450 enzymes. *BMC Complement Altern Med* 2019; 19: 240.

[58] Li C, Lim SC, Kim J, Choi JS. Effects of myricetin, an anticancer compound, on the bioavailability and pharmacokinetics of tamoxifen and its main metabolite, 4-hydroxytamoxifen, in rats. *Eur J Drug Metab Pharmacokinet* 2011; 36: 175-82.

[59] Kim CS, Choi SJ, Park CY, Li C, Choi JS. Effects of silybinin on the pharmacokinetics of tamoxifen and its active metabolite, 4-hydroxytamoxifen in rats. *Anticancer Res* 2010; 30: 79-85.

[60] Singh SP, Wahajuddin, Raju KS, Ali MM, Kohli K, Jain GK. Reduced bioavailability of tamoxifen and its metabolite 4-hydroxytamoxifen after oral administration with biochanin A (an isoflavone) in rats. *Phytother Res* 2012; 26: 303-7.

[61] Constantinou AI, White BE, Tonetti D, Yang Y, Liang W, Li W, van Breemen RB. The soy isoflavone daidzein improves the capacity of tamoxifen to prevent mammary tumours. *Eur J Cancer* 2005; 41: 647-54.

[62] Suganuma M, Sueoka E, Sueoka N, Okabe S, Fujiki H. Mechanisms of cancer prevention by tea polyphenols based on inhibition of TNF-alpha expression. *Biofactors* 2000; 13:67-72.

[63] Scandlyn MJ, Stuart EC, Somers-Edgar TJ, Menzies AR, Rosengren RJ. A new role for tamoxifen in oestrogen receptor-negative breast cancer when it is combined with epigallocatechin gallate. *Br J Cancer* 2008; 99: 1056-63.

[64] Shen F, Xue X, Weber G. Tamoxifen and genistein synergistically down-regulate signal transduction and proliferation in estrogen receptor-negative human breast carcinoma MDA-MB-435 cells. *Anticancer Res* 1999; 19: 1657-62.

[65] Shin SC, Piao YJ, Choi JS. Effects of morin on the bioavailability of tamoxifen and its main metabolite, 4-hydroxytamoxifen, in rats. *In Vivo* 2008; 22: 391-5.

[66] Choi JS, Kang KW. Enhanced tamoxifen bioavailability after oral administration of tamoxifen in rats pretreated with naringin. *Arch Pharm Res* 2008; 31: 1631-6.

[67] Jain AK, Thanki K, Jain S. Co-encapsulation of tamoxifen and quercetin in polymeric nanoparticles: implications on oral bioavailability, antitumor efficacy, and drug-induced toxicity. *Mol Pharm* 2013; 10: 3459-74.

[68] Shin SC, Choi JS, Li X. Enhanced bioavailability of tamoxifen after oral administration of tamoxifen with quercetin in rats. *Int J Pharm* 2006; 313: 144-9.

[69] Li F, Wong TY, Lin SM, Chow S, Cheung WH, Chan FL, Chen S, Leung LK. Coadministrating luteolin minimizes the side effects of the aromatase inhibitor letrozole. *J Pharmacol Exp Ther* 2014; 351: 270-7.

[70] Chen J, Halls SC, Alfaro JF, Zhou Z, Hu M. Potential beneficial metabolic interactions between tamoxifen and isoflavones via cytochrome P450-mediated pathways in female rat liver microsomes. *Pharm Res* 2004; 21: 2095-104.

[71] El-Beshbishy HA. Hepatoprotective effect of green tea (Camellia sinensis) extract against tamoxifen-induced liver injury in rats. *J Biochem Mol Biol* 2005; 38: 563-70.

[72] Rahate KP, Rajasekaran A. Hepatoprotection by active fractions from Desmostachya bipinnata stapf (L.) against tamoxifen-induced hepatotoxicity. *Indian J Pharmacol* 2015; 47: 311-5.

[73] Kumarappan C, Vijayakumar M, Thilagam E, Balamurugan M, Thiagarajan M, Senthil S, Das SC, Mandal SC. Protective and curative effects of polyphenolic extracts from Ichnocarpus frutescense leaves on experimental hepatotoxicity by carbon tretrachloride and tamoxifen. *Ann Hepatol* 2011; 10: 63-72.

[74] Campbell PS, Mavingire N, Khan S, Rowland LK, Wooten JV, Opoku-Agyeman A, Guevara A, Soto U, Cavalli F, Loaiza-Perez AI, Nagaraj G, Denham LJ, Adeoye O, Jenkins BD, Davis MB, Schiff R, Brantley EJ. AhR ligand aminoflavone suppresses α6-integrin-Src-Akt signaling to attenuate tamoxifen resistance in breast cancer cells. *J Cell Physiol* 2018; 234: 108-21.

[75] Guneidy RA, Gad AM, Zaki ER, Ibrahim FM, Shokeer A. Antioxidant or pro-oxidant and glutathione transferase P1-1 inhibiting activities for Tamarindus indica seeds and their cytotoxic effect on MCF-7 cancer cell line. *J Genet Eng Biotechnol* 2020; 18: 74.

[76] Srinivas NR. Recent trends in preclinical drug-drug interaction studies of flavonoids – Review of case studies, issues and perspectives. *Phytother Res* 2015; 29: 1679-91.

[77] Albassam AA, Markowitz JS. An appraisal of drug-drug interactions with green tea (Camellia sinensis). *Planta Med* 2017; 83: 496-508.

[78] Shin SC, Choi JS. Effects of epigallocatechin gallate on the oral bioavailability and pharmacokinetics of tamoxifen and its main metabolite, 4-hydroxytamoxifen, in rats. *Anticancer Drugs* 2009; 20: 584-8.

[79] Li C, Kim M, Choi H, Choi J. Effects of baicalein on the pharmacokinetics of tamoxifen and its main metabolite, 4-hydroxytamoxifen, in rats: possible role of cytochrome P450 3A4 and P-glycoprotein inhibition by baicalein. *Arch Pharm Res* 2011; 34: 1965-72.

[80] Piao Y, Shin SC, Choi JS. Effects of oral kaempferol on the pharmacokinetics of tamoxifen and one of its metabolites, 4-hydroxytamoxifen, after oral administration of tamoxifen to rats. *Biopharm Drug Dispos* 2008; 29: 245-9.

[81] Singh SP, Wahajuddin, Ali MM, Kohli K, Jain GK. Liquid chromatography-mass spectrometry method for the quantification of tamoxifen and its metabolite 4-hydroxytamoxifen in rat plasma: application to interaction study with biochanin A (an isoflavone). *J Chromatogr B Analyt Technol Biomed Life Sci* 2011; 879: 2845-51.

[82] Chisholm K, Bray BJ, Rosengren RJ. Tamoxifen and epigallocatechin gallate are synergistically cytotoxic to MDA-MB-231 human breast cancer cells. *Anticancer Drugs* 2004; 15: 889-97.

[83] Seo HS, DeNardo DG, Jacquot Y, Laios I, Vidal DS, Zambrana CR, Leclercq G, Brown PH. Stimulatory effect of genistein and apigenin on the growth of breast cancer cells correlates with their ability to activate ER alpha. *Breast Cancer Res Treat* 2006; 99: 121-34.

[84] Bracke ME, Depypere HT, Boterberg T, Van Marck VL, Vennekens KM, Vanluchene E, Nuytinck M, Serreyn R, Mareel MM. Influence of tangeretin on tamoxifen`s therapeutic benefit in mammary cancer. *J Natl Cancer Inst* 1999; 91: 354-9.

[85] Bracke ME, Boterberg T, Depypere HT, Stove C, Leclercq G, Mareel MM. The citrus methoxyflavone tangeretin affects human cell-cell interactions. *Adv Exp Med Biol* 2002; 505: 135-9.

[86] Depypere HT, Bracke ME, Boterberg T, Mareel MM, Nuytinck M, Vennekens K, Serreyn R. Inhibition of tamoxifen`s therapeutic benefit by tangeretin in mammary cancer. *Eur J Cancer* 2000; 36Suppl4: S73.

[87] Kumar M, Sharma G, Misra C, Kumar R, Singh B, Katare OP, Raza K. N-desmethyl tamoxifen and quercetin-loaded multiwalled CNTs: A synergistic approach to overcome MDR in cancer cells. *Mater Sci Eng C Mater Biol Appl* 2018; 89: 274-82.

[88] Lockhart JN, Stevens DM, Beezer DB, Kravitz A, Harth E. Dual drug delivery of tamoxifen and quercetin: Regulated metabolism for anticancer treatment with nanosponges. *J Control Release* 2015; 220: 751-7.

[89] Sandhu PS, Kumar R, Beg S, Jain S, Kushwah V, Katare OP, Singh B. Natural lipids enriched self-nano-emulsifying systems for effective co-delivery of tamoxifen and naringenin: Systematic approach for improved breast cancer therapeutics. *Nanomedicine* 2017; 13: 1703-13.

[90] This P, Magdelenat H. Phytoestrogens and adjuvant endocrine treatment of breast cancer. *J Clin Oncol* 2000; 18: 2792-3.

[91] Tanos V, Brzezinski A, Drize O, Strauss N, Peretz T. Synergistic inhibitory effects of genistein and tamoxifen on human dysplastic and

malignant epithelial breast cells in vitro. *Eur J Obstet Gynecol Reprod Biol* 2002; 102: 188-94.
[92] Parvez S, Tabassum H, Rehman H, Banerjee BD, Athar M, Raisuddin S. Catechin prevents tamoxifen-induced oxidative stress and biochemical perturbations in mice. *Toxicology* 2006; 225: 109-18.
[93] Tabassum H, Parvez S, Rehman H, Banerjee BD, Raisuddin S. Catechin as an antioxidant in liver mitochondrial toxicity: Inhibition of tamoxifen-induced protein oxidation and lipid peroxidation. *J Biochem Mol Toxicol* 2007; 21: 110-7.
[94] Chen Y, Jia X, Chen J, Wang J, Hu M. The pharmacokinetics of raloxifene and its interaction with apigenin in rat. *Molecules* 2010; 15: 8478-87.
[95] Stuart EC, Rosengren RJ. The combination of raloxifene and epigallocatechin gallate suppresses growth and induces apoptosis in MDA-MB-231 cells. *Life Sci* 2008; 82: 943-8.
[96] Tian DD, Kellogg JJ, Okut N, Oberlies NH, Cech NB, Shen DD, McCune JS, Paine MF. Identification of intestinal UDP-glucuronosyltransferase inhibitors in green tea (Camellia sinensis) using a biochemometric approach: Application to raloxifene as a test drug via in vitro to in vivo extrapolation. *Drug Metab Dispos* 2018; 46: 552-60.
[97] Kaushik S, Shyam H, Agarwal S, Sharma R, Nag TC, Dwivedi AK, Balapure AK. Genistein potentiates centchroman induced antineoplasticity in breast cancer via PI3K/Akt deactivation and ROS dependent induction of apoptosis. *Life Sci* 2019; 239: 117073.
[98] Shelton P, Sausville E, Nakanishi T, Brodie A, Belosay A, LoRusso P, Njar V, Burger A. Breast cancer cells resistant to anti-hormone treatments retain sensitivity to aminoflavone (NSC 686288). *Mol Cancer Ther* 2007; 6Suppl11: PR-4.
[99] Rahideh ST, Shidfar F, Nourbakhsh M, Hoseini M, Koohdani F, Entezam M, Keramatipour M. The individual or combinational effects of hesperetin and letrozole on the activity and expression of aromatase in MCF-7 cells. *Cell Mol Biol* 2016; 62: 38-43.
[100] Rahideh ST, Keramatipour M, Nourbakhsh M, Koohdani F, Hoseini M, Shidfar F. The effects of nobiletin, hesperetin, and letrozole in a combination on the activity and expression of aromatase in breast cancer cells. *Cell Mol Biol* 2017; 63: 9-13.
[101] Selim ME, Aleisa NA, Daghestani MH. Evaluation of the possible protective role of quercetin on letrozole-induced testicular injury in male albino rats. *Ultrastruct Pathol* 2013; 37: 204-17.
[102] Morrissey C, Brown M, O`Sullivan J, Weathered N, Watson RW, Tenniswood M. Epigallocatechin-3-gallate and bicalutamide cause

growth arrest and apoptosis in NRP-152 and NRP-154 prostate epithelial cells. *Int J Urol* 2007; 14: 545-51.

[103] Naiki-Ito A, Naiki T, Kato H, Iida K, Etani T, Nagayasu Y, Suzuki S, Yamashita Y, Inaguma S, Onishi M, Tanaka Y, Yasui T, Takahashi S. Recruitment of miR-8080 by luteolin inhibits androgen receptor splice variant 7 expression in castration-resistant prostate cancer. *Carcinogenesis* 2020; 41: 1145-57.

[104] Arya A, Khandelwal K, Singh A, Ahmad H, Agarwal S, Khatik R, Mittapelly N, Dwivedi AK. Validation of RP-HPLC method for simultaneous quantification of bicalutamide and hesperetin in polycaprolactone-bicalutamide-hesperetin-chitosan nanoparticles. *J Chromatogr Sci* 2015; 53: 1485-90.

[105] Tummala R, Lou W, Gao AC, Nadiminty N. Quercetin targets hnRNPA1 to overcome enzalutamide resistance in prostate cancer cells. *Mol Cancer Ther* 2017; 16: 2770-9.

[106] Lateef A, Khan AQ, Tahir M, Khan R, Rehman MU, Ali F, Hamiza OO, Sultana S. Androgen deprivation by flutamide modulates uPAR, MMP-9 expressions, lipid profile, and oxidative stress: amelioration by daidzein. *Mol Cell Biochem* 2013; 374: 49-59.

[107] Ma ZS, Huynh TH, Ng CP, Do PT, Nguyen TH, Huynh H. Reduction of CWR22 prostate tumor xenograft growth by combined tamoxifen-quercetin treatment is associated with inhibition of angiogenesis and cellular proliferation. *Int J Oncol* 2004; 24: 1297-304.

[108] Arya A, Khandelwal K, Ahmad H, Laxman TS, Sharma K, Mittapelly N, Agrawal S, Bhatta RS, Dwivedi AK. Co-delivery of hesperetin enhanced bicalutamide induced apoptosis by exploiting mitochondrial membrane potential via polymeric nanoparticles in a PC-3 cell line. *RSC Adv* 2016; 6: 5925.

[109] Arya A, Ahmad H, Tulsankar S, Agrawal S, Mittapelly N, Boda R, Bhatta RS, Mitra K, Dwivedi AK. Bioflavonoid hesperetin overcome bicalutamide induced toxicity by co-delivery in novel SNEDDS formulations: Optimization, in vivo evaluation and uptake mechanism. *Mater Sci Eng C Mater Biol Appl* 2017; 71: 954-64.

[110] Li Q, Deng Q, Chao HP, Liu X, Lu Y, Lin K, Liu B, Tang GW, Zhang D, Tracz A, Jeter C, Rycaj K, Calhoun-Davis T, Huang J, Rubin MA, Beltran H, Shen J, Chatta G, Puzanov I, Mohler JL, Wang J, Zhao R, Kirk J, Chen X, Tang DG. Linking prostate cancer cell AR heterogeneity to distinct castration and enzalutamide responses. *Nat Commun* 2018; 9: 3600.

[111] Ray S, Chowdhury P, Pandit B, Ray SD, Das S. Exploring the antiperoxidative potential of morin on cyclophosphamide and flutamide-induced lipid peroxidation and changes in cholesterol profile in rabbit model. *Acta Pol Pharm* 2010; 67: 35-44.

# Chapter 4

# Plant Flavonoids Affect the Outcome of Targeted Biological Cancer Therapies

As conventional cytotoxic therapies act upon malignant cells as well as rapidly dividing normal cells, their administration is associated with severe side effects and significant morbidity in cancer patients, being often of limited benefit for survival [1]. In addition, the therapeutic failing may be related also to intrinsic or acquired resistance, and drug-resistant disease recurrence [2, 3]. Therefore, the need for improved anticancer strategies has remained that could specifically and effectively target malignant cells while minimizing the toxicity to healthy tissues [1, 2, 4].

Targeted biological cancer therapies focus on unique molecular changes in proteins and signaling pathways that are essential for cell survival and progression of certain cancer types. In other words, biological therapies affect specific cellular targets of neoplastic processes by using small selective inhibitory molecules and biological drugs such as monoclonal antibodies (like cetuximab, trastuzumab and rituximab) [2, 5]. As overexpression and/or aberrant activation of receptor tyrosine kinases (RTKs) play a major role in cancer development, progression and spread, selective tyrosine kinase inhibitors (TKIs) have been developed to target RTKs and treat different tumor types [2, 3, 6]. For example, several small molecule tyrosine kinase specific agents, like erlotinib, gefitinib, lapatinib, afatinib and osimertinib, block HER (ErbB) family proteins (EGFR, HER2) [7, 8]. Sorafenib and sunitinib possess anti-VEGF activity, crizotinib targets the ALK, temsirolimus and everolimus are mTOR inhibitors, vemurafenib and dabrafenib target the BRAF protein, and bortezomib inhibits proteasome machinery [2]. Rapid development of targeted anticancer therapies in the last few decades, made possible through an improved understanding of molecular carcinogenesis and cancer-associated signaling pathways, has significantly increased treatment efficacy and allowed personalized, highly efficient and less toxic therapeutic approach for individual patients [1, 2, 7, 9, 10]. In fact, more than 100 molecularly targeted agents have been approved by the FDA for treatment of different types of malignancies to date

[7]. However, the initial favorable response to treatment with targeted anticancer drugs is often followed by the development of resistance that severely limits therapeutic efficacy, and leads to cancer relapse and recurrence [2, 7, 8]. The complexity of resistance mechanisms to TKIs monotherapy is usually related to the occurrence of many cancer mutations, making such neoplasms less reliant on a single oncogenic event and more dependent on dynamic interconnected signaling pathways and molecular heterogeneity of tumor cell population, particularly in an advanced and metastatic stage [2, 3, 7]. Therefore, improvement of cancer management by applying plant-derived flavonoids which sensitize malignant cells to targeted agents can further progress current biological cancer therapy, enabling a personalized approach to patients suffering from different tumor types. Specific combinations with flavonoids could attack mutated targets and pathways related to drug resistance, thereby potentiating the efficacy of targeted therapies and enhancing clinical outcomes [2].

In the Chapter 4, the current knowledge about co-effects of targeted drugs and structurally different flavonoids is presented, focusing besides natural flavonoids also on their semisynthetic and synthetic derivatives, and also flavonoid-rich plant extracts. As combinational approach has been studied only for a limited number of targeted agents approved for the clinical use in oncology and hematology, other promising biological drugs are not covered in this book. In combinational investigation, both pharmacodynamic as well as pharmacokinetic interactions are under discussion to highlight the most efficient combinations for further *in vivo* studies and clinical trials. However, as can be seen from the following sections, several combinations between specific TKIs and certain widely used flavonoids may lead also to undesired results, attenuating or even abolishing anticancer activities of targeted drugs, occurring through different molecular mechanisms. Therefore, it is highly important for cancer patients under targeted biological therapies to consume only those dietary supplements which safety or improved efficacy in combinational treatment regimens is scientifically proven. The inadvisable and potentially hazardous combinations are indicated also in the end of each subchapter, together with highlighting the most attractive combinations resulting in synergistic anticancer effects in preclinical studies and deserving initiation of clinical trials.

## 4.1. Interfering of Flavonoids with Anticancer Monoclonal Antibodies

### 4.1.1. Influence of Flavonoids on Therapeutic Action of Monoclonal Antibodies Prescribed in Oncology

#### *4.1.1.1. Cetuximab*

Cetuximab (Erbitux) is a monoclonal antibody targeting epidermal growth factor receptor (EGFR), a transmembrane protein tyrosine kinase with pleiotropic intracellular effects [1, 2, 11]. This drug binds directly and specifically to the extracellular domain of the EGFR on the cell surface, and prevents ligand (EGF) binding and receptor dimerization, thereby leading to inactivation of a series of downstream intracellular signaling pathways, ultimately restraining tumor growth and progression [1, 11, 12]. Cetuximab is used for the treatment of cancers with EGFR overexpression, especially for recurrent and/or metastatic colorectal cancer, and head and neck cancers such as nasopharyngeal carcinoma or oral squamous cell carcinoma [1, 2, 7, 11, 12]. EGFR is indeed highly expressed in more than 80% of nasopharyngeal cancer patients, whereas tumors with EGFR overexpression tend to be more aggressive, chemoresistant and with worse prognosis [11]. The expression of EGFR is abnormally high also in colon cancers, where its levels have been related to progression of the disease [12]. Although cetuximab has significantly advanced the treatment of these tumors, the drug resistance can still develop and limit its use [11]. In addition, even though combining with conventional chemotherapy and/or radiotherapy has been shown to expand the applications of cetuximab in oncology, toxicities related to these treatment modalities on normal tissues can confine their administration [1, 11, 12]. Therefore, combination of cetuximab with a natural and safe agent would be highly attractive for enhancing the treatment efficacy of EGFR-overexpressed tumors.

##### *4.1.1.1.1. Effects of Flavonoids on Anticancer Potential of Cetuximab*

In the last decade, potential co-effects of cetuximab and a few flavonoids have been investigated with the results summarized in Table 4.1. The naturally abundant flavone apigenin (50 μM) was shown to remarkably strengthen cetuximab-induced antiproliferative and anticlonogenic activities in two human nasopharyngeal carcinoma cell lines (HONE1 and CNE2). This effect was achieved through enhancement of arrest of the cell cycle progression at G2/M phase and potentiation of apoptosis by suppressing EGFR signaling pathway. Moreover, apigenin augmented anticancer capacity of cetuximab also in nasopharyngeal carcinoma xenografts in mice, reducing tumor growth and inducing smaller tumors with lower weight. Therefore, combination of apigenin and cetuximab may upgrade the therapeutic level and represent a promising new approach for more efficient treatment of nasopharyngeal carcinoma [11]. Addition of another flavone-type compound, methylated chrysin or tectochrysin (18.6 μM), led to a synergistic increase in cetuximab-induced growth inhibition and apoptotic death in human colon cancer cells (HCT116 and SW480). Combined treatment of cells with cetuximab and tectochrysin suppressed the expression of phosphorylated EGFR (p-EGFR), cyclooxygenase-2 (COX-2) and interleukin-8 (IL-8), all of which are important factors for colon cancer development and growth. Elevation of COX-2 expression through EGFR-mediated signaling is indeed characteristic for colon cancer patients, whereas increased levels of IL-8 have been associated with higher stage and metastatic potential of colon neoplasms, indicating worse survival of colon cancer patients. Augmented blocking of EGFR pathway by combination of cetuximab and tectochrysin also led to a significant inhibition of NF-κB and AP-1 activities, thereby providing a useful strategy for management of colonic cancers with higher efficacy and less toxicity [12]. Furthermore, low micromolar doses of soy isoflavone genistein, known as a protein tyrosine kinase inhibitor, additively enhanced cetuximab-induced growth inhibition and apoptosis in human oral squamous cell carcinoma cells (HSC3 and KB); with elevating the potency of cetuximab to suppress EGFR pathway and downstream Akt signaling in HSC3 cells, but not in KB cells. Combined treatment with cetuximab and genistein caused a substantial tumor growth delay in both HSC3 and KB xenografts-bearing mice, while each single agent exerted no significant effect on tumor growth. Also, exposure of cancer-inoculated mice to combined treatment led to the lowest level of proliferating cells and microvessel density in xenografted tumors, clearly indicating that selective molecular targeting of distinct cellular pathways is required for effective clinical response. As no serious side effects were observed, combination of cetuximab and genistein could be considered as a potential novel treatment option for oral cancer [1]. However, in A431 human epidermoid carcinoma-bearing mice, addition of genistein did not remarkably affect cetuximab-induced decrease in tumor growth, as well as did not cause any significant differences in cellular metabolic profiles of malignant tissue [13].

**Table 4.1.** Effects of flavonoids on anticancer action of cetuximab

| Flavonoid and its dosage | Cetuximab and its dosage | Biological system | Assay method and time | Effect | Mechanisms | Ref. |
|---|---|---|---|---|---|---|
| FLAVONES | | | | | | |
| Apigenin; 50 µM | Cetuximab; 0.13-1 mg/ml | HONE1 human nasopharyngeal carcinoma cells | MTT; 24h. Colony assay; 2 weeks | Increase in antiproliferative effect of cetuximab, decrease in colony numbers | Increase in G2/M arrest and apoptosis (elevation of Bax/Bcl-2, cleavage of caspase-3). Downregulation of p-EGFR, p-Akt, p-Stat3, cyclin D1 | [11] |
| Apigenin; 50 µM | Cetuximab; 0.13-1 mg/ml | CNE2 human nasopharyngeal carcinoma cells | MTT; 24h. Colony assay; 2 weeks | Increase in antiproliferative effect of cetuximab, decrease in colony numbers | Increase in G2/M arrest and apoptosis (elevation of Bax/Bcl-2, cleavage of caspase-3). Downregulation of p-EGFR, p-Akt, p-Stat3, cyclin D1 | [11] |
| Apigenin; 50 mg/kg/day, i.p. injection, 2h after cetuximab | Cetuximab; 0.8 mg/mouse/day, i.p. injection | HONE1 cells injected s.c. into the left forelimb of SPF male nude mice | 4 weeks | Strengthening of cetuximab-induced decrease in tumor growth, reduction of tumor weight | | [11] |
| Apigenin; 50 mg/kg/day, i.p. injection, 2h after cetuximab | Cetuximab; 0.8 mg/mouse/day, i.p. injection | CNE2 cells injected s.c. into the left forelimb of SPF male nude mice | 4 weeks | Strengthening of cetuximab-induced decrease in tumor growth, reduction of tumor weight | | [11] |
| Tectochrysin; 5 µg/ml (18.6 µM) | Cetuximab; 30 µg/ml | SW480 human colon cancer cells | MTT; 24h | Synergistic inhibition of cell growth (CI 0.533) | Increase in apoptosis. Decrease in IL-8, p-EGFR and COX-2 expression; inhibition of AP-1 and NF-κB activities | [12] |
| Tectochrysin; 5 µg/ml (18.6 µM) | Cetuximab; 30 µg/ml | HCT116 human colon cancer cells | MTT; 24h | Synergistic inhibition of cell growth (CI 0.572) | Increase in apoptosis. Decrease in IL-8, p-EGFR and COX-2 expression; inhibition of AP-1 and NF-κB activities | [12] |

**Table 4.1.** (Continued)

| Flavonoid and its dosage | Cetuximab and its dosage | Biological system | Assay method and time | Effect | Mechanisms | Ref. |
|---|---|---|---|---|---|---|
| ISOFLAVONES | | | | | | |
| Genistein; 5 μM | Cetuximab; 25 μg/ml | HSC3 human oral squamous cell carcinoma cells | SRB; 48h | Additive increase in cell growth inhibition | Increase in apoptosis. Downregulation of p-EGFR and p-Akt expression | [1] |
| Genistein; 10, 20 μM | Cetuximab; 50, 100 μg/ml | KB human oral squamous cell carcinoma cells | SRB; 48h | Additive increase in cell growth inhibition | Increase in apoptosis | [1] |
| Genistein; 1 mg/kg, i.p. injection on days 1-5 each week | Cetuximab; 1 mg/kg, i.p. injection on days 2 and 5 each week | HSC3 cells inoculated s.c. into the right flank of 6-8 w-old female BALB/c nude mice | 30 days | Inhibition of tumor growth (no effect with either agent alone) | Lowering of proliferating cells (PCNA), decrease in MVD (CD31) | [1] |
| Genistein; 1 mg/kg, i.p. injection on days 1-5 each week | Cetuximab; 1 mg/kg, i.p. injection on days 2 and 5 each week | KB cells inoculated s.c. into the right flank of 6-8 w-old female BALB/c nude mice | 30 days | Inhibition of tumor growth (no effect with either agent alone) | Lowering of proliferating cells (PCNA), decrease in MVD (CD31) | [1] |
| Genistein; 500 mg/kg/day, p.o. | Cetuximab; 1 mg, i.p., every third day | A431 human epidermoid carcinoma cells inoculated s.c. into the upper right flank of 6-7 w-old female NMRI nu/nu mice | 12 days | No effect on cetuximab-induced decrease in tumor growth | No significant differences in [$^{18}$F]FLT, [$^{18}$F]FDG or [$^{64}$Cu]NODAGA-cetuximab uptake in tumors; no extensive metabolic differences as compared to cetuximab alone-treated mice | [13] |

#### *4.1.1.2. Trastuzumab*

Trastuzumab (Herceptin) is a monoclonal antibody directed against human epidermal growth factor receptor 2 (HER2, ErbB2) [14, 15]. This drug binds to domain IV of the extracellular segment of HER2 protein, reducing receptor activation and leading to blockage of downstream signaling pathways [16, 17]. Trastuzumab is used for the treatment of HER2-positive mammary tumors, constituting an essential part of today`s arsenal of breast cancer management [14, 18]. Receptor tyrosine kinase, HER2, has been found to be overexpressed in about 20-30% of all human breast cancer cases, being associated with aggressive tumor phenotype and poor clinical outcome, making HER2 an important therapeutic target [14-16, 18]. Although trastuzumab has been shown to improve survival in advanced metastatic breast cancer patients either as a single agent or combined with traditional chemotherapeutics, the outcome has remained unsatisfactory because of frequent development of drug resistance, disease recurrence and an elevated risk of cardiac dysfunctions associated with the use of trastuzumab [15, 18]. Therefore, there is a high need for development of an adjuvant natural agent that can be combined with trastuzumab to improve the efficacy and safety of this anti-HER2 monoclonal antibody [18]. This necessity is urgent also due to a continuous rise of new breast cancer cases each year [16].

##### *4.1.1.2.1. Effects of Flavonoids on Anticancer Potential of Trastuzumab*

To date, only a few flavonoids have been studied in combination with trastuzumab treatment in different human breast cancer preclinical models with the results presented in Table 4.2. Soy isoflavone genistein (10 μM) was shown to be able to significantly enhance the growth inhibitory effect of trastuzumab in HER2-overexpressing ERα/β-positive human breast cancer cells BT-474, accompanied by an additively increased expression of variant 2 of putative tumor suppressor ERβ, i.e., ERβ2. However, no such potentiating action was detected in HER2-overexpressing ERα-negative SK-BR-3 cells as well as in MDA-MB-231 cells that are negative for both ERα and HER2 receptors. These data indicate that combined treatment with genistein and trastuzumab might be beneficial for women with HER2-overexpressing and ERα/β-positive breast tumors, but their relevance must be first verified in animal studies and clinical settings [14]. In addition, anthocyanin cyanidin 3-glucoside (11.1 μM) was found to synergistically increase the antitumor action of trastuzumab in human HER2-positive breast cancer lines (BT474, HCC1569, MDA-MB-453), decreasing the percentage of viable cells and increasing apoptosis. These effects were achieved through suppression of HER2 activation and blocking of its downstream Akt and ERK1/2 pathways. Moreover, combined treatment of BT474 xenografts-bearing mice with trastuzumab and cyanidin 3-glucoside led to a significant increase in tumor growth inhibition as compared to the monoclonal antibody alone, by downregulating activated HER2 levels in malignant tissues. Further detailed studies are needed to examine the therapeutic potential of this combination, especially as no apparent signs of toxicity were detected in the co-treated mice [16]. The chalcone-type compound, flavokawain A, could also augment trastuzumab-induced growth inhibition in HER2-overexpressing MCF7/HER2 cells (ER-positive) as well as SKBR3 breast cancer cells (ER-negative), through downregulating the expression of antiapoptotic proteins (survivin, XIAP) and Cdc2 inhibitors (Myt1, Wee1). Therefore, flavokawain A may be another natural sensitizer for trastuzumab-based therapies against HER2-overexpressing breast tumors, definitely deserving further *in vivo* investigations [18].

Besides natural plant-derived flavonoids, the effect of a synthetic derivative, flavopiridol, has also been studied on antitumor action of anti-HER2 monoclonal antibody trastuzumab in human breast cancer cells. Combined treatment with flavopiridol and trastuzumab at the fixed dose ratios of 1:2.91 or 1:5.82 (nM: ng/ml) resulted in a synergistic cytotoxic action and reduced clonogenicity in HER2-overexpressing BT-474 and SKBR3 cells, independent on the sequence of administration of the two drugs. In SKBR3 cells, this combination induced an increase in inhibition of ERK1/2 and Akt pathways, decrease in cyclin D1 protein and Cdk2/4 abundance, and retardation of S-phase progression, as compared to the single-agent treatments [17]. However, at different dose ratios, somewhat different results have been reported, as diverse cellular mechanisms seem to be affected. Actually, combined treatment of BT474 cells with flavopiridol and trastuzumab at the dose ratio of 1:1.67 (nM: ng/ml) revealed no synergism in cytotoxicity, being attributed to the high levels of EGFR in these cells [15]. In other HER2-overexpressing breast cancer lines SKBR3 and MDA-MB-453, flavopiridol and trastuzumab at the dose ratio of 1:3.33 (nM: ng/ml) synergistically suppressed cellular proliferation and survival [19], whereas the mechanisms under these interactions mainly involved enhanced apoptosis with a marked suppression of both HER2 as well as EGFR proteins [15, 19]. As expected, no synergistic cytotoxicity was observed when flavopiridol and trastuzumab were co-applied in MCF7 cells that express only low or no endogenous HER2 [17, 19]. Therefore, the progress of targeted biological therapies can be possible when therapeutic efficacy of drugs will be improved through addition of natural or semisynthetic agents in their best combinations.

### 4.1.2. Influence of Flavonoids on Therapeutic Action of Monoclonal Antibodies Prescribed in Hematology

#### *4.1.2.1. Rituximab*

Rituximab is the anti-CD20 antibody used for the treatment of CD20-positive non-Hodgkin lymphoma (NHL), including diffuse large B-cell lymphoma (DLBCL) as the most common type of NHL [20]. Although combined treatment regimen of rituximab with conventional chemotherapeutics (cyclophosphamide, hydroxy-doxorubicin, vincristine and prednisone) has significantly improved clinical responses and survival rates, treatment with rituximab can still fail in about 30% of patients due to acquired resistance and low responses [20]. Therefore, identification of novel and safe natural compounds as potent adjuvant agents for rituximab treatment is urgently needed for improvement of therapeutic efficacy and prolongation of patients` survival; especially considering the worldwide increase in incidence of NHL [20].

##### *4.1.2.1.1. Effects of Flavonoids on Anticancer Potential of Rituximab*

To this day, only one study has been reported about combining rituximab with flavonol quercetin in two human DLBCL cell lines (WSU-DLCL2 and SUDHL4) (Table 4.3). In this work, addition of quercetin (20 μM) synergistically enhanced the growth inhibitory effect of rituximab and potentiated rituximab-induced apoptosis of malignant cells through inhibition of STAT3 pathway and downregulation of several survival-related genes (Mcl-1, survivin, Bcl-xl). Therefore, combining rituximab with quercetin may present a novel and attractive way to improve the treatment efficacy of DLBCL, whereas STAT3 can be considered as a new target for management of NHL [20].

**Table 4.2.** Effects of flavonoids on anticancer action of trastuzumab in breast tumor models

| Flavonoid and its dosage | Trastuzumab and its dosage | Biological system | Assay method and time | Effect | Mechanisms | Ref. |
|---|---|---|---|---|---|---|
| ISOFLAVONES | | | | | | |
| Genistein; 10 μM | Trastuzumab; 1, 10 μg/ml | BT-474 human breast cancer cells, ERα+, ERβ1/2+, overexpressing HER2 | CellTiter-Blue; 5, 6 days | Increase in trastuzumab-induced cell growth inhibition | Additive elevation of ERβ2 mRNA levels | [14] |
| Genistein; 10 μM | Trastuzumab; 1, 10 μg/ml | SK-BR-3 human breast cancer cells, ERα-, ERβ1/2+, overexpressing HER2 | CellTiter-Blue; 3-6 days | No effect on trastuzumab-induced cell growth inhibition | | [14] |
| Genistein; 10 μM | Trastuzumab; 1, 10 μg/ml | MDA-MB-231 human breast cancer cells, ERα-, ERβ1/2+, HER2- | CellTiter-Blue; 3-6 days | No potentiating effect on cell growth | | [14] |
| ANTHOCYANIDINS | | | | | | |
| Cyanidin 3-glucoside; 5 μg/ml (11.1 μM) | Trastuzumab; 5 μg/ml | BT474 human breast cancer cells, HER2+ | Alamar Blue; 24, 48h | Synergistic decrease in viable cells (CI<1) | Induction of apoptosis (increase in caspase-3/7 activity). Down-regulation of p-HER2, p-Akt and p-p44/42 MAPK levels | [16] |
| Cyanidin 3-glucoside; 5 μg/ml (11.1 μM) | Trastuzumab; 5 μg/ml | HCC1569 human breast cancer cells, HER2+ | Alamar Blue; 24, 48h | Synergistic decrease in viable cells (CI<1) | Induction of apoptosis (increase in caspase-3/7 activity). Down-regulation of p-HER2, p-Akt and p-p44/42 MAPK levels | [16] |

| Flavonoid and its dosage | Trastuzumab and its dosage | Biological system | Assay method and time | Effect | Mechanisms | Ref. |
|---|---|---|---|---|---|---|
| Cyanidin 3-glucoside; 5 μg/ml (11.1 μM) | Trastuzumab; 5 μg/ml | MDA-MB-453 human breast cancer cells, HER2+ | Alamar Blue; 24, 48h | Synergistic decrease in viable cells (CI<1) | Induction of apoptosis (increase in caspase-3/7 activity). Down-regulation of p-HER2, p-Akt and p-p44/42 MAPK levels | [16] |
| Cyanidin 3-glucoside; 6 mg/kg, i.p. injection twice a week | Trastuzumab; 6 mg/kg, i.p. injection twice a week | BT474 cells implanted s.c. into the flank region of 6-7 w-old female nude mice | 25 days | Increase in tumor growth inhibition, decrease in tumor volume and weight | Decrease in p-HER2 and Ki67 levels | [16] |
| CHALCONES | | | | | | |
| Flavokawain A; 2 μM | Trastuzumab; 0.5 μg/ml | MCF7/HER2 human breast cancer cells, ER+, overexpressing HER2 | MTT; 72h | Increase in trastuzumab-induced cell growth inhibition | Down-regulation of Myt1, Wee1, survivin and XIAP proteins | [18] |
| Flavokawain A; 2 μM | Trastuzumab; 0.5 μg/ml | SKBR3 human breast cancer cells, ER-, overexpressing HER2 | MTT; 72h | Increase in trastuzumab-induced cell growth inhibition | Down-regulation of Myt1, Wee1, survivin and XIAP proteins | [18] |
| SYNTHETIC FLAVONOIDS | | | | | | |
| Flavopiridol; ratio with trastuzumab of 25:1 or 50:1 (nM: nM) [1:5.82 or 1:2.91 (nM: ng/ml)] | Trastuzumab | BT-474 human breast cancer cells, overexpressing HER2 | MTS; 72h. Colony assay; 10 days | Synergism in cytotoxicity (CI<1). Decrease in colony formation | | [17] |

**Table 4.2.** (Continued)

| Flavonoid and its dosage | Trastuzumab and its dosage | Biological system | Assay method and time | Effect | Mechanisms | Ref. |
|---|---|---|---|---|---|---|
| Flavopiridol; ratio with trastuzumab of 1:1.67 (nM: ng/ml) | Trastuzumab | BT474 human breast carcinoma cells, overexpressing HER2, high levels of EGFR | Counting; 48h | No synergistic effect (CI 1.46) | Little effect on EGFR levels | [15] |
| Flavopiridol; ratio with trastuzumab of 25:1 or 50:1 (nM: nM) [1:5.82 or 1:2.91 (nM: ng/ml)] | Trastuzumab | SKBR3 human breast cancer cells, overexpressing HER2 | MTS; 72h. Colony assay; 10 days | Synergism in cytotoxicity (CI<1). Decrease in colony formation | Decrease in S phase progression. Reduction of cyclin D1 and Cdk2/4 proteins; decrease in pRB phosphorylation. Down-regulation of p-ERK1/2, MEK1 and p-Akt | [17] |
| Flavopiridol; ratio with trastuzumab of 1:3.33 (nM: ng/ml) | Trastuzumab | SKBR3 human breast carcinoma cells, overexpressing HER2 | Counting; 48h. Colony assay; 7 days | Synergistic inhibition of cell proliferation and survival (CI<1) | Decrease in HER2 protein levels | [19] |
| Flavopiridol; 10-300 nM | Trastuzumab; 50-200 ng/ml | SKBR3 human breast carcinoma cells, overexpressing HER2 | Apoptosis assay; 48h | | Increase in apoptosis. Suppression of EGFR protein expression | [15] |
| Flavopiridol; ratio with trastuzumab of 1:3.33 (nM: ng/ml) | Trastuzumab | MDA-MB-453 human breast carcinoma cells, overexpressing HER2 | Counting; 48h. Colony assay; 7 days | Synergistic inhibition of cell proliferation and survival (CI<1) | Decrease in HER2 protein levels | [19] |
| Flavopiridol; 10-300 nM | Trastuzumab; 50-200 ng/ml | MDA-MB-453 human breast carcinoma cells, overexpressing HER2 | Apoptosis assay; 48h | | Increase in apoptosis. Suppression of EGFR protein expression | [15] |

**Table 4.3.** Effects of flavonoids on anticancer action of rituximab in diffuse large B-cell lymphoma (DLBCL) models

| Flavonoid and its dosage | Rituximab and its dosage | Biological system | Assay method and time | Effect | Mechanisms | Ref. |
|---|---|---|---|---|---|---|
| FLAVONOLS | | | | | | |
| Quercetin; 20 µM | Rituximab; 5 µg/ml | WSU-DLCL2 human DLBCL cells | Alamar Blue; 48h | Synergistic increase in growth inhibition (CI 0.662) | Potentiation of rituximab-induced apoptosis. Suppression of STAT3 pathway (downregulation of Mcl-1, survivin and Bcl-xl) | [20] |
| Quercetin; 20 µM | Rituximab; 5 µg/ml | SUDHL4 human DLBCL cells | Alamar Blue; 48h | Synergistic increase in growth inhibition (CI 0.594) | Potentiation of rituximab-induced apoptosis. Suppression of STAT3 pathway, (downregulation of Mcl-1, survivin and Bcl-xl) | [20] |

### 4.1.3. Conclusions from Preclinical Knowledge with Dietary Recommendations to Patients under Anticancer Monoclonal Antibodies

According to the current limited data about combinational treatment of malignant cells with monoclonal antibodies and flavonoids, no negative effects of flavonoids on antitumor capacity of these biological drugs have been described to date. On the contrary, several natural flavonoids have been shown to remarkably augment the therapeutic capacity of monoclonal antibodies in preclinical experimental settings, providing therefore promising combinations for further *in vivo* studies and clinical trials.

- Based on *in vitro* and *in vivo* experiments, the antitumor efficacy of EGFR receptor-targeting drug CETUXIMAB can be potentiated by apigenin in nasopharyngeal carcinoma, tectochrysin in colon cancer, and genistein in oral squamous cell carcinoma models. If these results will be further confirmed in clinical trials, application of such combinations in clinical settings might allow to achieve significantly improved clinical outcomes with substantially lowered drug doses, providing better quality of life to patients. As the concept of combination treatment with anti-EGFR monoclonal antibodies seems to be a promising modality for improvement of anticancer efficacy, the spectrum of flavonoids should be expanded in combinational treatment studies with not only cetuximab, but also another EGFR-targeting antibody drug, i.e., panitumumab.
- Although soy isoflavone genistein has been shown to enhance the antitumor effect of HER2-directed monoclonal antibody TRASTUZUMAB in human breast cancer models, this potentiating action is strictly limited to specific tumor phenotypes (ERα/β-positive and HER2-overexpressing tumors that constitute about 10% of all breast cancer cases [21]) and must be verified in clinical settings. Also, anthocyanin cyanidin 3-glucoside and chalcone flavokawain A can be potential adjuvant agents for trastuzumab treatment of HER2-overexpressing breast cancers, both ER-positive and ER-negative neoplasms. If benefits of such combinational therapies will be confirmed in clinical trials, inclusion of proper natural agents in treatment regimens of specific breast cancer subtypes might not only improve therapeutic efficacy, but also allow to lower the doses of trastuzumab and thereby reduce the risks of

cardiac dysfunctions. Moreover, such approach might make cancer treatment even more personalized in the future.

- Quercetin might present a potent adjuvant agent for improvement of therapeutic efficacy of anti-CD20 monoclonal antibody RITUXIMAB in treatment of diffuse large B-cell lymphomas, if the respective preliminary *in vitro* results will be verified *in vivo* studies and clinical trials.

## 4.2. Interfering of Flavonoids with Pharmacological Inhibitors

### 4.2.1. Influence of Flavonoids on Therapeutic Action of Pharmacological Inhibitors Prescribed in Oncology

- **Inhibitors of membrane receptors: EGFR TKIs**

The epidermal growth factor receptor (EGFR, ErbB1, HER1), a member of receptor tyrosine kinase (RTK) family, is significantly overexpressed and upregulated in the majority of solid tumors, playing critical roles in the formation and progression of several human cancers [1, 12, 22]. Upon ligand binding to the extracellular domain of the EGFR, autophosphorylation is initiated through the intracellular tyrosine kinase domains, activating the subsequent downstream signaling cascades, which in turn trigger the transcription of genes responsible for cell survival, growth and proliferation, angiogenesis, metastasis and therapeutic resistance [7, 23, 24]. Aberrant activation of EGFR can therefore lead to uncontrolled growth, impaired apoptosis and metastatic spread of malignant cells [8]. Thus, EGFR tyrosine kinase inhibitors (TKIs) have been developed to suppress prosurvival signals and arrest problematic growth, resulting in a significant improvement in the treatment outcome of patients harboring specific mutations in EGFR gene, such as a deletion in exon 19 (del E746-A750) or a point mutation L858R in exon 21 [22, 25-27]. The discovery that somatic activating EGFR mutations are correlated with clinical benefits was an important milestone for personalized lung cancer therapy, implicating a radical advance in treatment options of patients, as such mutations can enhance EGF signaling and confer susceptibility of tumors to specific EGFR inhibitors [26, 28]. Today, EGFR is commonly considered as an addictive oncogene in non-small cell lung cancer (NSCLC); the leading cause of cancer-related mortality worldwide [28-30]. In 2020, there were almost 2.21 million new lung cancer cases globally, with 1.80 million deaths constituting 18.0% of all cancer-related mortality [31]. Over 80% of lung cancer cases are NSCLC, whereas the five-year survival rate of patients has remained unacceptably low, being only about 10% [29, 32, 33]. The first-generation EGFR-TKIs, like erlotinib and gefitinib (Figure 4.1), have been recommended as the second- or third-line therapy for NSCLC treatment, after failure of the first-line chemotherapy; or as standard first-line drugs for treatment of mutant EGFR NSCLC [25, 32, 34]. Interestingly, these gain-of-function mutations occur more often in Asian patients (30-50%) than in Caucasians (10%), which may explain also the differences in responsiveness to EGFR-targeted TKIs [27, 29, 30]. Clinical trials have indeed demonstrated that EGFR-targeted therapy with TKIs tended to result in longer progression-free survival than the mainstay platinum-based chemotherapy [28, 34, 35]. In addition, it is well known that EGFR-TKIs are generally less toxic than conventional cytotoxic chemotherapeutics [25, 35].

| PHARMACOLOGICAL INHIBITORS PRESCRIBED IN CANCEROLOGY | |
|---|---|
| Inhibitors of membrane receptors: EGFR TKIs | |
| 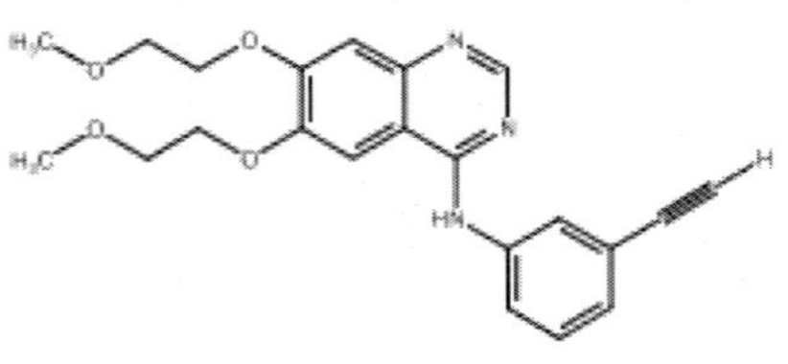<br>Erlotinib<br>(first generation EGFR TKI) | 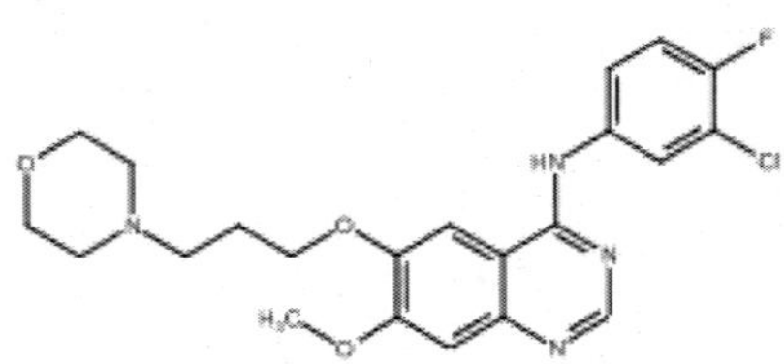<br>Gefitinib<br>(first generation EGFR TKI) |
| 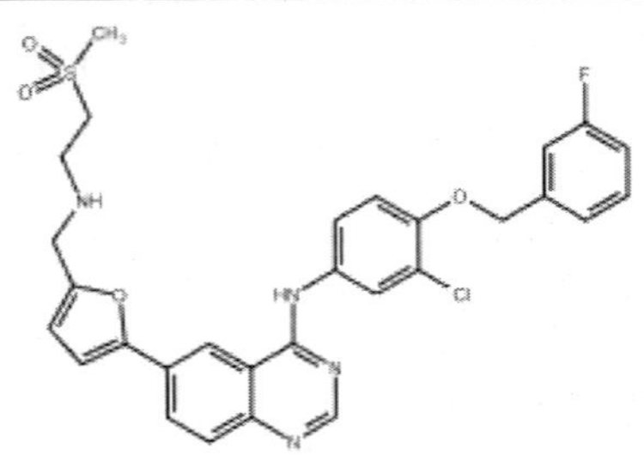<br>Lapatinib<br>(first generation EGFR TKI) | 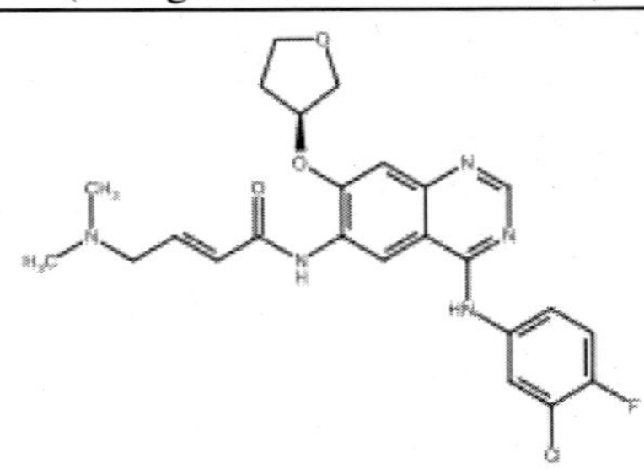<br>Afatinib<br>(second generation EGFR TKI) |

**Figure 4.1.** (Continued).

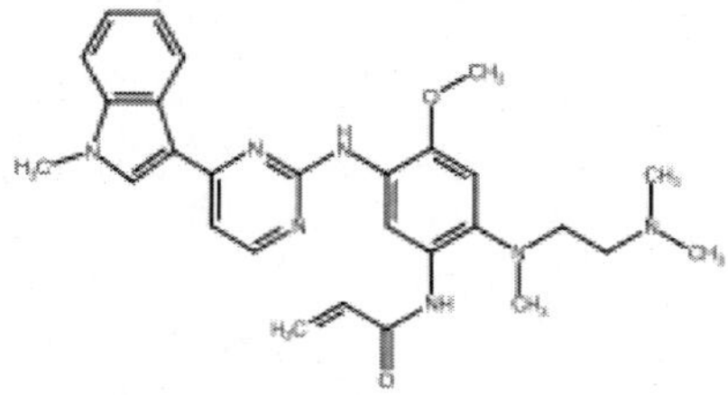

Osimertinib (third generation EGFR TKI)

Inhibitors of membrane receptors: small-molecule multikinase inhibitors

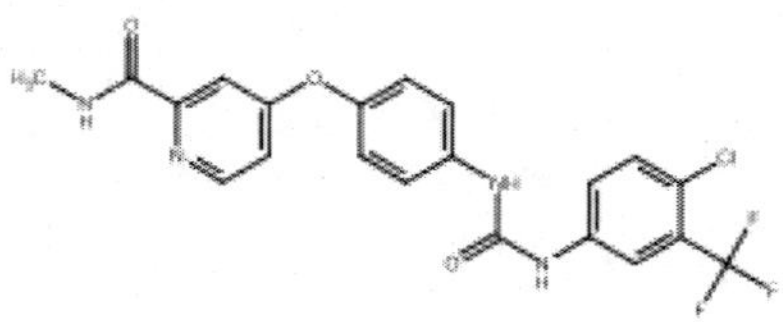

Sorafenib (multitarget protein kinase inhibitor)

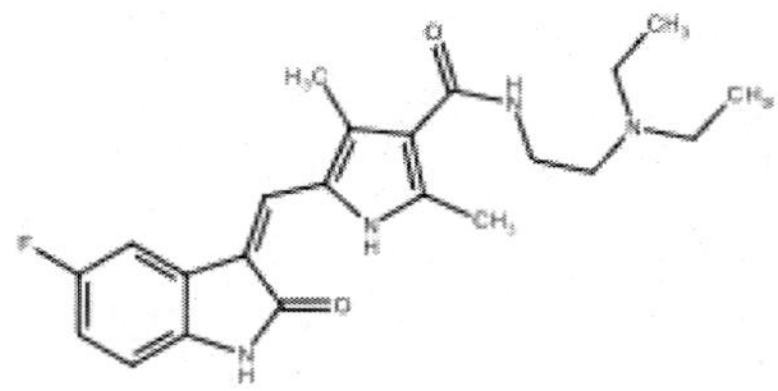

Sunitinib (multitarget RTK inhibitor)

Inhibitors with an intracellular target

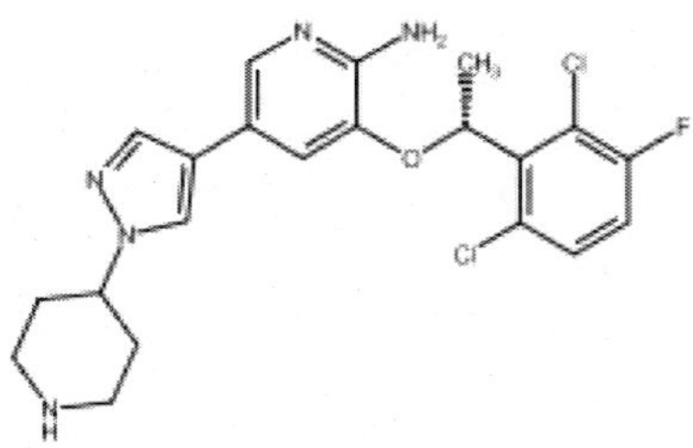

Crizotinib (ALK inhibitor)

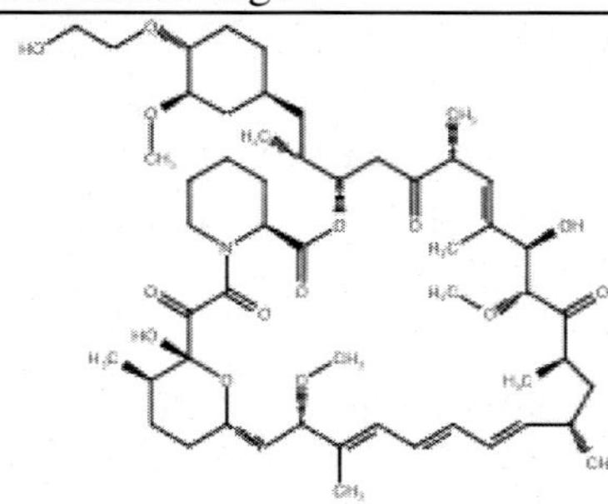

Everolimus (mTOR inhibitor)

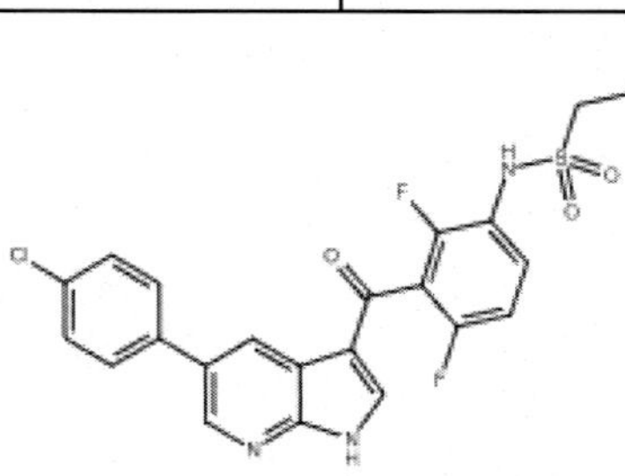

Vemurafenib (BRAF inhibitor)

**Figure 4.1.** Structural formulas of pharmacological inhibitors prescribed in cancerology, studied in combination with flavonoids.

However, although treatment with TKIs has achieved some favorable initial results, the tumor eventually relapses in almost all patients because of the emergence of acquired resistance to TKIs after a duration of response for about 10-12 months, making overall survival not significantly different as compared to standard chemotherapy [25, 27, 28, 34-36]. There is a variety of molecular mechanisms underlying development of resistance to EGFR-TKIs, summarized in Figure 4.2. In about half of the cases, the reason for acquired resistance can be attributed to secondary mutations in EGFR tyrosine kinase domain, mainly replacing threonine at position 790 with methionine in exon 20 (T790M) or the so-called gatekeeper mutation, that abrogates the inhibitory activity of TKIs [25, 26, 28]. As both erlotinib and gefitinib interfere with the ATP-binding pocket of EGFR catalytic domain to inhibit receptor phosphorylation [8, 23], T790M mutation is suggested to sterically hinder the binding of TKI and increase the affinity of ATP to activated EGFR mutants, thereby triggering EGFR pathway [28, 34, 36]. Another major mechanism of acquired resistance to EGFR-TKIs involves the amplification of the MET receptor tyrosine kinase gene and activation of c-Met receptor, which triggers downstream intracellular signaling independently on EGFR [26, 29, 36]. These two mechanisms account for approximately 60-70% of all known causes of acquired resistance to erlotinib and gefitinib, whereas they are not mutually exclusive and in a smaller number of cases, both of these two mechanisms, i.e., second-site EGFR mutation and MET amplification, can be detected coincidently [26, 36]. In addition, hyperactivation of downstream signaling molecules of EGFR can essentially contribute to acquired drug resistance. Among them, constitutively activated PI3K/Akt pathway has been shown to confer acquired EGFR-TKI resistance [22, 28]. mTOR, a downstream target of Akt, is another key molecule in the EGFR signaling that is important in cell proliferation and survival [28]. Also, ERK signaling cascade has a critical role in cell growth and tumorigenesis, being activated in a variety of malignant cells which are resistant to EGFR inhibitors [25]. Thus, targeting PI3K/Akt/mTOR or Raf/MEK/ERK pathway simultaneously with administration of EGFR-TKIs has attracted wide attention as a potentially effective therapeutic option for overcoming drug resistance [22, 25, 28]. The development of therapies that can simultaneously inhibit multiple signaling pathways seems therefore to be necessary in the fight against malignant neoplasms with dysregulated intracellular cascades upon targeting of HER family membrane receptors [29]. Furthermore, epithelial-mesenchymal transition (EMT) has also been proven as one of the mechanisms for acquired resistance to EGFR-TKIs, as mesenchymal phenotype of malignant cells is closely associated with the lack of responsiveness to EGFR-targeted drugs. An EMT signature can indeed predict the resistance of malignant cells to EGFR-directed inhibitors, regardless of receptor mutation status [22, 26, 37]. Therefore, suppression or reversal of EMT can ameliorate the resistance to EGFR-TKIs, enabling the development of novel approaches to optimize the efficacy of EGFR-TKIs and improve the therapeutic outcomes of patients [22, 37]. It is also possible that formation of subpopulations of malignant cells characterized by specific cancer stem cell (CSC)-related signatures might present an additional mechanism for stopping responsiveness of EGFR-mutant cells to EGFR-directed inhibitors [35]. Last but not least, metabolic changes and elevated levels of autophagy can also influence the treatment outcome of TKIs, causing acquired resistance. Inhibition of autophagy might therefore be an additional new means to govern drug resistance and improve the efficacy of cancer treatment [25]. Nevertheless, once the patients have developed resistance to EGFR-TKIs, there are no further effective therapies currently available [25, 29, 32]. Although second- and third-generation EGFR-TKIs, such as afatinib and osimertinib, respectively (Figure 4.1), may be able to overcome T790M-mediated resistance through forming irreversible covalent bonds with EGFR, their efficacy has still not been verified in clinical studies [34, 36]. In addition, resistance to these irreversible inhibitors has also been described [29]. Moreover, more potent TKIs may exert also more severe adverse events in patients [28]. Therefore, there is an urgent need to identify novel natural and safe adjuvant agents for controlling resistance and improving the efficacy of EGFR-targeted pharmacological inhibitors in combinational treatment regimens.

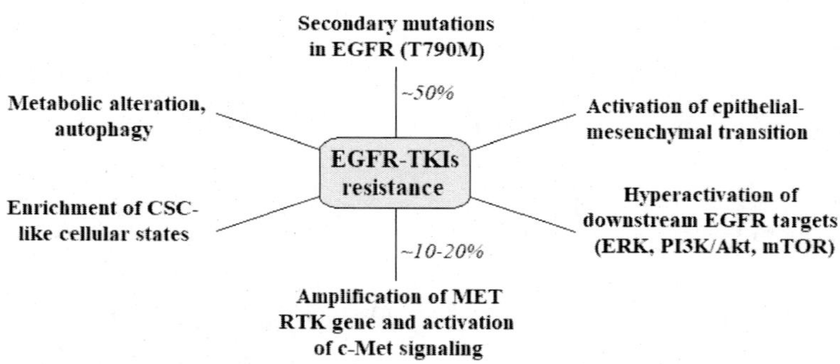


**Figure 4.2.** Overview of the most common mechanisms of acquired resistance to EGFR-TKIs.

#### *4.2.1.1. Erlotinib*

Erlotinib (Tarceva) is a potent tyrosine kinase inhibitor (TKI) that primarily targets EGFR, abrogates its tyrosine kinase activity and leads to blocking of EGFR-related signal transduction pathways [8, 23, 38] (Figure 4.1). This agent has revealed strong antitumor activities in a variety of cancer types in numerous investigational studies [38, 39]. Currently, erlotinib is approved by the FDA for treatment of non-small cell lung cancer (NSCLC) with activating EGFR mutations, and as a second-line therapy for locally advanced or metastatic pancreatic cancer in combination with gemcitabine-based chemotherapy [23, 35, 40, 41]. EGFR has been indeed reported to be frequently overexpressed in human pancreatic cancers, whereas its expression was inversely correlated with the survival rate of patients [41]. However, the use of erlotinib in clinical settings is usually limited by the presence of primary resistance or development of acquired resistance, providing only a minimal survival advantage for patients with advanced NSCLC [32, 35, 40]. The drug efficacy is unsatisfactory also in the treatment of pancreatic cancer, due to activation of alternative survival pathways that bypass the EGFR signaling, reduce sensitivity to erlotinib and promote cancer progression [41]. Therefore, identification of novel agents to overcome the resistance of malignant cells to erlotinib through simultaneously targeting different molecular mechanisms in combinational approach is highly important to enhance the drug efficacy and improve clinical outcomes. In the recent years, a number of studies have been devoted to find natural adjuvants for erlotinib, investigating into polyphenolic compounds synthesized by terrestrial plants.

##### *4.2.1.1.1. Effects of Flavonoids on Anticancer Potential of Erlotinib*

The summary of results obtained by combining erlotinib with structurally different flavonoids in diverse human cancer models is presented in Table 4.4. These studies clearly demonstrate the high potency of phytochemicals to improve the responses of malignant cells to erlotinib, opening new opportunities to overcome erlotinib resistance.

Specifically, combination of erlotinib with the most abundant green tea flavanol, EGCG (2.5-40 μM), was shown to result in greater inhibition of cellular proliferation and/or colony formation than either agent alone in several human NSCLC cell lines that harbor wild-type (wt) EGFR and are both erlotinib-sensitive (H2122) as well as erlotinib-resistant (H358, H460). EGCG was found to suppress c-Met activation in all these cell lines, showing that erlotinib-resistant cells might be sensitized to this drug by inhibiting another signaling pathway that can bypass the need for EGFR activity. Also, this combination caused a significant decrease in growth rate of H460 xenografts in mice leading to tumors with lower volume and weight, while no significant effects were observed with individual treatments. Addition of EGCG can thus confer sensitization of lung tumors to erlotinib therapy and control cancer progression, definitely deserving further clinical studies [29]. In addition, EGCG potentiated anticancer action of erlotinib also in a variety of human head and neck squamous cell carcinoma (HNSCC) cells derived from different tumor sites. It is well known that EGFR is overexpressed in about 80-90% of HNSCC cases, correlating with low treatment responses, poor disease-free and overall survival, and enhanced risk of disease recurrence and metastasis [7, 24, 38, 39]. However, only a very small percentage of HNSCC patients (less than 5%) responded to erlotinib in clinical trials [39]. Therefore, there is a great need to find novel adjuvant agents for potentiating erlotinib responses in malignant neoplasms developing in oral cavity, larynx and pharynx, widening the treatment options for this highly aggressive disease; especially considering that overall survival rate of HNSCC has not significantly improved during the past several decades [38, 39]. As a result, combining EGFR-targeted pharmacological inhibitor erlotinib with EGCG led to a synergistic growth inhibition in five HNSCC cell lines (Tu212, Tu177, 886LN, SQCCY1, 38), accompanied by increase in suppression of EGFR and Akt activation and induction of intrinsic apoptotic death. While erlotinib alone inhibited EGFR phosphorylation and stabilized the receptor at plasma membrane of Tu212 cells, combined treatment with EGCG resulted in internalization of EGFR with subsequent receptor degradation, thereby impairing EGFR signaling. In addition, an increase in cell cycle arrest at G0/G1 phase was observed in Tu212 and Tu177 lines as compared to the treatment with erlotinib alone. EGCG augmented anticancer action of erlotinib also in Tu212 xenografts-bearing nude mice, leading to delay in tumor progression through inhibition of proliferation and promotion of apoptosis in malignant cells via downregulation of EGFR signaling. Most importantly, no significant adverse effects were detected in mice undergone this combinational therapy [38]. The sensitizing effects of EGCG (30 μM) on erlotinib therapy were confirmed also in another study with several human HNSCC cell lines (Tu686, 686LN, 1986LN, SQCCY1), showing that addition of EGCG significantly suppressed erlotinib-induced expression of cell cycle regulatory proteins p21 and p27, mediated via p53, in the cells with wt p53. While combined treatment with erlotinib and EGCG inhibited NF-κB pathway, in a p53-dependent manner, leading to promotion of apoptosis in Tu686 cells; in p53-negative M4e line, no effects on p21 and p27 proteins were detected after the cells were exposed to either single or combined treatments, revealing also resistance to apoptotic death. Thus, p53 plays a crucial role in antitumor responses of HNSCC cells to erlotinib, whereas addition of EGCG shifted the phenotype from erlotinib-induced growth arrest to apoptotic death [39]. Moreover, induction of apoptosis by combined treatment with erlotinib and EGCG (30 μM) involved also stabilization and upregulation of proapoptotic Bim protein through its posttranslational dephosphorylation, mediated via suppression of ERK activation, in Tu212 and Tu686 HNSCC cells, besides decrease in antiapoptotic Bcl-2 expression [7, 42]. Therefore, EGCG might be a useful agent to study as a potent adjunct for erlotinib treatment, providing novel promising regimens for future clinical management of NSCLC or HNSCC. This strategy definitely warrants further preclinical investigation and also initiation of clinical trials, being potentially of clinical relevance. In addition to the promising results demonstrated with monomeric EGCG, combination of erlotinib with hexameric proanthocyanidin (oligomer of the flavanols epicatechin and catechin; 0.5-30 μM) led to a synergistic decrease in cell viability through attenuating EGFR dimerization and phosphorylation in human colorectal adenocarcinoma line Caco-2. It is well accepted that overexpression and overactivation of the EGFR are implicated in the carcinogenic processes of intestinal epithelium, showing that combined targeting of colorectal cancer cells with EGFR-TKI and specific dietary components might be an attractive approach for retardation of malignant progression and optimization of therapeutic responses in colorectal cancer treatment [8].

Very recently, the flavonol kaempferol (48 μM) was shown to synergistically enhance erlotinib-induced cell growth inhibition and intrinsic apoptosis in two pancreatic cancer lines (BxPC-3 and PANC-1). This potentiating effect was achieved through dramatic decrease in expression of phosphorylated EGFR, AKT and ERK1/2. Moreover, kaempferol sensitized pancreatic cancer to erlotinib treatment also in PANC-1 xenografts-bearing mice, leading to tumors with lower volume and weight as compared to the treatment with erlotinib alone. Therefore, plant-derived kaempferol might be a promising therapeutic adjuvant for augmenting sensitivity of pancreatic cancer cells to erlotinib, being potentially of clinical importance and

**Table 4.4.** Effects of flavonoids on anticancer action of erlotinib (highlighted rows indicate undesired negative effects on anticancer efficacy)

| Flavonoid and its dosage | Erlotinib and its dosage | Biological system | Assay method and time | Effect | Mechanisms | Ref. |
|---|---|---|---|---|---|---|
| FLAVANOLS (monomers and oligomers) | | | | | | |
| EGCG; 2.5-40 μM | Erlotinib; 2 μM | H358 human NSCLC cells; wt EGFR, erlotinib-resistant | MTS; 72h | Additive inhibition of cell growth, increase in response to erlotinib | Suppression of c-Met and EGFR phosphorylation by EGCG | [29] |
| EGCG; 2.5-40 μM | Erlotinib; 2 μM | H460 human NSCLC cells; wt EGFR, erlotinib-resistant | MTS; 72h. Colony assay; 7 days | Additive inhibition of cell growth, increase in response to erlotinib. Suppression of colony formation, decrease in colony size | Suppression of c-Met phosphorylation by EGCG | [29] |
| EGCG; 2.5-40 μM | Erlotinib; 2 μM | H2122 human NSCLC cells; wt EGFR, erlotinib-sensitive | MTS; 72h | Additive inhibition of cell growth, increase in response to erlotinib | Suppression of c-Met phosphorylation by EGCG | [29] |
| EGCG; 15 mg/kg, p.o. (5-days-on, 2-days-off dosing) | Erlotinib; 10 mg/kg, p.o. (5-days-on, 2-days-off dosing) | H460 cells injected s.c. into the hind flank of 6-8 w-old male SCID/bg mice | 22 days | Reduction of tumor volume and weight (no significant effect with either agent alone) | | [29] |
| EGCG; at $IC_{50}$ dose (2-fold serial dilutions) | Erlotinib; at $IC_{50}$ dose (2-fold serial dilutions) | 38 human HNSCC cells; from tonsil fossa, chemoresistant | SRB; 72h | Synergistic inhibition of cell growth (CI<1) | | [38] |
| EGCG; 30 μM | Erlotinib; 0.5 μM | 686LN human HNSCC cells; from lymph node metastasis of tongue cancer, wt p53 | 72h | | Inhibition of erlotinib-induced p21 and p27 expression | [39] |

**Table 4.4.** (Continued)

| Flavonoid and its dosage | Erlotinib and its dosage | Biological system | Assay method and time | Effect | Mechanisms | Ref. |
|---|---|---|---|---|---|---|
| EGCG; 30 μM | Erlotinib; 2 μM | M4e human HNSCC cells; derived from 686LN, p53-null, erlotinib-resistant | Apoptosis assay; 120h | No antitumor effect | No induction of apoptosis (either by individual agents or combination) | [39] |
| EGCG; at $IC_{50}$ dose (2-fold serial dilutions) | Erlotinib; at $IC_{50}$ dose (2-fold serial dilutions) | 886LN human HNSCC cells; from lymph node metastasis of larynx tumor, EGFR-TKI-insensitive | SRB; 72h | Synergistic inhibition of cell growth (CI<1) only at relatively high doses | | [38] |
| EGCG; 30 μM | Erlotinib; 0.5 μM | 1986LN human HNSCC cells; from lymph node metastasis of tongue cancer, wt p53 | 24, 48h | | Inhibition of erlotinib-induced p21 and p27 expression | [39] |
| EGCG; at $IC_{50}$ dose (2-fold serial dilutions) | Erlotinib; at $IC_{50}$ dose (2-fold serial dilutions) | SQCCY1 human HNSCC cells; from oral cavity | SRB; 72h | Synergistic inhibition of cell growth (CI<1) | | [38] |
| EGCG; 30 μM | Erlotinib; 0.5 μM | SQCCY1 human HNSCC cells; from oral cavity, wt p53 | 24, 48h | | Inhibition of erlotinib-induced p21 and p27 expression | [39] |
| EGCG; at $IC_{50}$ dose (2-fold serial dilutions) | Erlotinib; at $IC_{50}$ dose (2-fold serial dilutions) | Tu177 human HNSCC cells; from laryngeal tumor, erlotinib-sensitive | SRB; 72h | Synergistic inhibition of cell growth (CI<1) | Additive arrest of cell cycle at G0/G1 phase; increase in apoptosis | [38] |

| Flavonoid and its dosage | Erlotinib and its dosage | Biological system | Assay method and time | Effect | Mechanisms | Ref. |
|---|---|---|---|---|---|---|
| EGCG; at $IC_{50}$ dose (2-fold serial dilutions) | Erlotinib; at $IC_{50}$ dose (2-fold serial dilutions) | Tu212 human HNSCC cells; from hypopharyngeal tumor, erlotinib-sensitive | SRB; 72h | Synergistic inhibition of cell growth (CI<1) | Additive arrest of cell cycle at G0/G1 phase; increase in apoptosis (cleavage of caspases-3, -9 and PARP). Downregulation of p-EGFR and p-Akt | [38] |
| EGCG; 30 μM | Erlotinib; 1 μM | Tu212 human HNSCC cells; from hypopharyngeal tumor | 48h | | Stabilization and upregulation of Bim through its dephosphorylation; decrease in Bcl-2 expression | [7] |
| EGCG; 30 μM | Erlotinib; 2 μM | Tu686 human HNSCC cells; from tongue cancer, wt p53 | Apoptosis assay; 120h | Increase in antitumor action of erlotinib | Potentiation of apoptosis. Increase in p-p53. Inhibition of erlotinib-induced p21 and p27 expression. Decrease in NF-κB (p65) and Bcl-2 | [39] |
| EGCG; 30 μM | Erlotinib; 1 μM | Tu686 human HNSCC cells; from tongue cancer | Apoptosis assay; 48h | | Induction of apoptosis (cleavage of PARP). Stabilization and upregulation of Bim through p-ERK inhibition-mediated Bim dephosphorylation; decrease in Bcl-2 expression | [7] |

**Table 4.4.** (Continued)

| Flavonoid and its dosage | Erlotinib and its dosage | Biological system | Assay method and time | Effect | Mechanisms | Ref. |
|---|---|---|---|---|---|---|
| EGCG; 125 mg/kg, p.o., 7 days before inoculation, continued 5 days a week for 7 weeks | Erlotinib; 50 mg/kg, p.o., 7 days before inoculation, continued 5 days a week for 7 weeks | Tu212 cells injected s.c. into the right flank of 4-6 w-old athymic nu/nu nude mice | 7 weeks | Suppression of tumor growth (no significant effect with either agent alone). Delay in tumor progression | Inhibition of proliferation (decrease in Ki67), induction of apoptosis. Downregulation of p-EGFR | [38] |
| Hexameric proanthocyanidin; 0.5-30 µM | Erlotinib; 5 µM | Caco-2 human colorectal adenocarcinoma cells | CellTiter-Glo; 72h | Synergistic decrease in cell growth (CI<1) | Augmentation of inhibition of EGFR phosphorylation | [8] |
| FLAVONES | | | | | | |
| Luteolin; 1-100 µM | Erlotinib; 1-100 µM | PC-3 human prostate cancer cells; EGFR wt | Counting; 24h | Increase in cell growth inhibition | | [43] |
| FLAVONOLS | | | | | | |
| Fisetin; 40 µM (10-120 µM, at 1:1 molar ratio with erlotinib) | Erlotinib; 15 µM (10-120 µM, at 1:1 molar ratio with fisetin) | HCC827-ER human NSCLC cells; erlotinib-resistant | MTT; 24, 48h | Synergistic inhibition of cell growth (CI<1), overcoming of erlotinib resistance | Potentiation of apoptosis (cleavage of caspases-3 and -8, release of cyt c, decrease in survivin). Downregulation of p-AXL, p-MAPK and p-Akt. Decrease in Snail, increase in E-cadherin | [32] |
| Kaempferol; 48 µM | Erlotinib; 8 µM | BxPC-3 human pancreatic cancer cells | CCK-8; 72h. Colony assay; 14 days | Synergistic inhibition of cell growth (CI 0.368). Suppression of colony formation | Potentiation of apoptosis (cleavage of caspase-9 and PARP, increase in Bax, decrease in Bcl-2). Downregulation of p-EGFR, p-Akt and p-ERK1/2 | [41] |

| Flavonoid and its dosage | Erlotinib and its dosage | Biological system | Assay method and time | Effect | Mechanisms | Ref. |
|---|---|---|---|---|---|---|
| Kaempferol; 48 μM | Erlotinib; 32 μM | PANC-1 human pancreatic cancer cells | CCK-8; 72h. Colony assay; 14 days | Synergistic inhibition of cell growth (CI 0.528). Suppression of colony formation | Potentiation of apoptosis (cleavage of caspase-9 and PARP, increase in Bax, decrease in Bcl-2). Downregulation of p-EGFR, p-Akt and p-ERK1/2 | [41] |
| Kaempferol; 100 mg/kg/day, i.p. injection | Erlotinib; 50 mg/kg/day, i.p. injection | PANC-1 cells (with Matrigel) inoculated s.c. into the right armpit of 4 w-old SPF-grade BALB/C female nude mice | 4 weeks | Potentiation of erlotinib-induced inhibition of tumor volume and weight | Suppression of p-EGFR, p-Akt and p-ERK1/2 expression | [41] |
| ISOFLAVONES | | | | | | |
| Genistein; 100 μM | Erlotinib; 10 μM | A431 human epithelial carcinoma cells | SRB; 72h (co- or serial incubation) | Antagonism in erlotinib-induced cytostatic effect (CI 1.90 at cotreatment) | Antagonistic effect on erlotinib-induced inhibition of EGFR phosphorylation | [23] |
| ANTHOCYANIDINS | | | | | | |
| Delphinidin; 10 μM | Erlotinib; 1 μM | A431 human epithelial carcinoma cells | SRB; 72h (co- or serial incubation) | Impairment of erlotinib-induced cell growth inhibition, increase in $IC_{50}$ of erlotinib | No effect on erlotinib-induced inhibition of EGFR phosphorylation | [23] |
| Delphinidin 3-O-glucoside (myrtillin); 10 μM | Erlotinib; 1 μM | A431 human epithelial carcinoma cells | SRB; 72h (co- or serial incubation) | Impairment of erlotinib-induced cell growth inhibition, increase in $IC_{50}$ of erlotinib | No interaction on EGFR phosphorylation inhibition | [23] |
| FLAVANONOLS | | | | | | |
| Ampelopsin; 20 μM | Erlotinib; 2.5 μM | H1650 human NSCLC cells; erlotinib-resistant | Counting; 72h | Synergistic inhibition of cell viability (CI 0.6845) | Upregulation of NOX2, accumulation of ROS, increase in apoptosis (increase in Bim, decrease in Mcl-1) | [40] |

**Table 4.4.** (Continued)

| Flavonoid and its dosage | Erlotinib and its dosage | Biological system | Assay method and time | Effect | Mechanisms | Ref. |
|---|---|---|---|---|---|---|
| Ampelopsin; 20 μM | Erlotinib; 2.5 μM | H1975 human NSCLC cells; erlotinib-resistant | Counting; 72h. Colony assay; 2 weeks | Synergistic inhibition of cell viability (CI 0.6733). Decrease in colony formation | Upregulation of NOX2, accumulation of ROS, increase in apoptosis (activation of caspases-8, -9 and -3; increase in Bim, decrease in Mcl-1) | [40] |
| FLAVONOLIGNANS | | | | | | |
| Silibinin; 50, 100 μM | Erlotinib; 1 μM | PC-9/ER human NSCLC cells; erlotinib resistant (EGFR T790M) | MTT; 72h. Colony assay; 7-10 days | Synergistic increase in growth inhibition (CI<1), overcoming erlotinib resistance. Decrease in colony size and number | Downregulation of p-EGFR and p-Akt expression | [36] |
| Silibinin; 200 mg/kg, p.o., 5 days a week | Erlotinib; 100 mg/kg, p.o., 5 days a week | PC-9/ER cells (with Matrigel) implanted into the flanks of 6 w-old female SCID mice | 24 days | Increase in tumor growth inhibition | Decrease in proliferation index (Ki67), increase in apoptosis index (TUNEL). Downregulation of p-EGFR and p-Akt | [36] |
| Silibinin (as silibinin-meglumine); 100 mg/kg, p.o., 5 days a week | Erlotinib; 100 mg/kg, p.o., 5 days a week | PC-9/Erl-R cells (EGFR del E746-A750, erlotinib-resistant) inoculated s.c. into 4-5 w-old female athymic mice | 35 days | Complete abrogation of tumor growth, dramatic decrease in mean tumor volume. Sensitization of tumors to erlotinib | Reversion of high miR-21/ low miR-200c signature; reversal of EMT phenotype (decrease in Snail1, Zeb1, Zeb2, N-cadherin) | [26] |

certainly requiring further clinical trials [41]. Another widely found natural flavonol, fisetin (40 μM), reversed acquired resistance to erlotinib in lung adenocarcinoma line HCC827-ER, through inhibition of aberrantly activated MAPK and AKT signaling pathways by suppressing RTK AXL activity. Combined treatment with erlotinib and fisetin yielded a synergistic decrease in cell viability and promoted apoptosis in these erlotinib-resistant NSCLC cells. Moreover, addition of fisetin to erlotinib treatment resulted also in suppression of the EMT process, by decreasing Snail and increasing E-cadherin expression. Thus, fisetin can make EGFR-TKI-resistant lung cancer cells vulnerable to the cytotoxic responses of erlotinib, providing a potential novel therapeutic strategy for NSCLC patients with acquired resistance to EGFR-TKIs. However, the precise molecular mechanisms underlying these effects are still needed to be unraveled in further preclinical studies [32]. In two other erlotinib-resistant human NSCLC cell lines (H1650 and H1975), addition of flavanonol ampelopsin (dihydromyricetin; 20 μM) to erlotinib also led to a synergistic inhibition of cell viability and colony formation. Combined treatment with erlotinib and ampelopsin caused an upregulation of nicotinamide adenine dinucleotide phosphate oxidase 2 (NOX2), resulting in accumulation of reactive oxygen species (ROS) and induction of oxidative stress that in turn led to increase in caspase-dependent apoptotic death. Therefore, ampelopsin could be an additional option for overcoming acquired resistance to erlotinib in EGFR-TKI-resistant NSCLC cells, making them again sensitive to anticancer action of erlotinib [40]. Furthermore, flavonolignan silibinin (50 or 100 μM) enhanced the ability of erlotinib to inactivate EGFR through suppression of receptor dimerization in erlotinib-resistant human NSCLC cells PC-9/ER harboring T790M mutation. Combined treatment of PC-9/ER cells with erlotinib and silibinin inhibited EGFR downstream Akt signaling, leading to synergistic cell growth inhibition and decrease in clonogenicity. Similarly, this combination potentiated tumor growth inhibition also in PC-9/ER xenografts-bearing mice, reducing proliferation and increasing apoptosis via downregulation of EGFR signaling in malignant tissues. Therefore, addition of silibinin to erlotinib treatment may overcome T790M-mediated resistance through restoration of the ability of erlotinib to suppress EGFR survival pathways, providing one more therapeutic option for NSCLC patients with acquired resistance to EGFR-TKIs. This novel combinational approach is especially compelling, considering that second- and third-generation irreversible EGFR-TKIs have still not allowed to circumvent acquired drug resistance following to development of secondary mutations in EGFR gene [36].

Benefits of silibinin were further confirmed also in another *in vivo* study, demonstrating that this milk thistle-derived flavonolignan could reverse acquired resistance and restore sensitivity to erlotinib in athymic mice implanted with erlotinib-refractory PC-9/Erl-R xenografts, harboring no T790M mutation. In this work, silibinin meglumine as a commercially used water-soluble formulation of silibinin complexed with the excipient amino-sugar meglumine was used, due to poor water solubility and low bioavailability of the parent silibinin. As a result, combined treatment with erlotinib and silibinin led to a complete abrogation of tumor growth with dramatic 85% decrease in tumor volume, achieved via a full reversion of the EMT-related high miR-21/low miR-200c signature and suppression of mesenchymal phenotype markers in erlotinib-refractory tumors. Recent studies have indeed demonstrated that the EMT-driving miR-21 expression confers tumor aggressiveness, anti-apoptotic and metastatic potential, while miR-200c can determine the responsiveness of malignant cells to EGFR-TKIs. Thus, silibinin could circumvent the EMT-driven acquired resistance to erlotinib in NSCLC xenografts, with no apparent signs of toxicity or adverse effects detected in the mice co-treated with erlotinib and silibinin [26]. Therefore, in the near future, clinical trials focusing on the combined treatment of EGFR-TKIs-resistant NSCLC patients with erlotinib and silibinin-rich milk thistle extract should be designed and conducted, aimed at preventing lung cancer progression after emergence of erlotinib resistance.

The above-described results may have implications in identification of naturally occurring and safe compounds that can synergize with erlotinib in inhibiting malignant progression and improving therapeutic outcome, thereby impacting future clinical approaches for several cancer types. As plant-derived flavonoids can simultaneously target multiple mechanisms involved in emergence of acquired resistance to erlotinib, the possibilities of malignant cells to bypass the need for several coincidently blocked survival pathways might be minimized, enhancing the likelihood to restore EGFR-TKIs sensitivity and enhance treatment responses (Figure 4.3). However, it is still needed to be aware that in human epithelial carcinoma cells A431, addition of isoflavone genistein (100 μM) or anthocyanidins delphinidin (10 μM) and delphinidin 3-O-glucoside (10 μM) was found to cause antagonism in erlotinib-induced cytostatic effects with impairment of cell growth inhibition. In doing so, soy isoflavone genistein could attenuate also erlotinib-mediated suppression of EGFR activation, while the two anthocyanidins showed no significant interactions in this regard, pointing to a different mechanism of interference [23]. Although the underlying molecular events have remained to be clarified, these rather surprising results still emphasize the necessity for a heightened caution when patients under erlotinib therapy decide to consume plant-derived supplements.

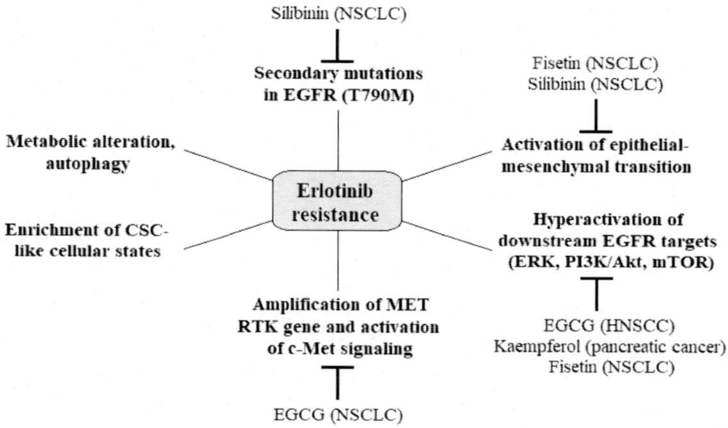


**Figure 4.3.** Overcoming erlotinib resistance and augmenting its antitumor action by flavonoids.

### *4.2.1.1.2. Effects of Flavonoid-Rich Natural Products on Anticancer Efficacy of Erlotinib*

As flavonoids occur in plants and plant-derived products usually in different combinations, it is important, besides studying the individual compounds, to know also the effects of herbal extracts on the antitumor action of EGFR-TKIs. As a result, it was reported that isoflavone-rich extracts derived from soy or red clover could significantly enhance antiproliferative action of erlotinib in three human NSCLC cell lines with different EGFR genotypes (A549, H1975, HCC827), showing that specific bioactive constituents of these natural products can augment the antitumor efficacy of erlotinib. Further studies are needed to elucidate these mechanisms and identify individual active flavonoids, in order to ultimately reduce the doses of erlotinib in combined treatment regimens [34] (Table 4.5). However, a recent study still surprisingly revealed that anthocyanins-rich bilberry extract (like its major constituents delphinidin and delphinidin 3-O-glucoside) could antagonize erlotinib-induced growth inhibition in human epithelial carcinoma line A431, with no interactions on EGFR activation [23]; indicating that specific flavonoids can not only augment but also abolish the antitumor activities of EGFR-TKIs on certain conditions.

**Table 4.5.** Effects of flavonoid-rich natural products on anticancer action of erlotinib (highlighted rows indicate undesired negative effects on anticancer efficacy)

| Flavonoid-rich natural product | Erlotinib and its dosage | Biological system | Assay method and time | Effect | Mechanisms | Ref. |
|---|---|---|---|---|---|---|
| Red clover extract | Erlotinib | A549 human NSCLC cells; EGFR wt | MTT, Crystal violet; 48h | Increase in antiproliferative activity, decrease in $IC_{50}$ of erlotinib | | [34] |
| Red clover extract | Erlotinib | H1975 human NSCLC cells; EGFR T790M | MTT, Crystal violet; 48h | Increase in antiproliferative activity, decrease in $IC_{50}$ of erlotinib | | [34] |
| Red clover extract | Erlotinib | HCC827 human NSCLC cells; EGFR del E746-A750 | MTT, Crystal violet; 48h | Increase in antiproliferative activity, decrease in $IC_{50}$ of erlotinib | | [34] |
| Soy extract | Erlotinib | A549 human NSCLC cells; EGFR wt | MTT, Crystal violet; 48h | Increase in antiproliferative activity, decrease in $IC_{50}$ of erlotinib | | [34] |
| Soy extract | Erlotinib | H1975 human NSCLC cells; EGFR T790M | MTT, Crystal violet; 48h | Increase in antiproliferative activity, decrease in $IC_{50}$ of erlotinib | | [34] |
| Soy extract | Erlotinib | HCC827 human NSCLC cells; EGFR del E746-A750 | MTT, Crystal violet; 48h | Increase in antiproliferative activity, decrease in $IC_{50}$ of erlotinib | | [34] |
| Bilberry extract; 250 ng/ml | Erlotinib; 250 nM | A431 human epithelial carcinoma cells | SRB; 72h | Antagonistic effect on erlotinib-induced cell growth inhibition, increase in $IC_{50}$ of erlotinib | No interaction on EGFR phosphorylation inhibition | [23] |

#### *4.2.1.2. Gefitinib*

Gefitinib (Iressa) is another first-generation EGFR TKI that acts through competitive inhibition of autophosphorylation of the intracellular catalytic domain of the receptor [24, 25, 44] (Figure 4.1). Targeting of the EGFR further results in inactivation of its downstream signaling pathways, ultimately leading malignant cells to apoptotic death [30, 45]. In preclinical settings, gefitinib has been shown to exert antitumor activity against many types of malignancies, including NSCLC, HNSCC, colon, breast, ovarian and prostate cancer [24, 44, 46]. Although gefitinib has revealed therapeutic promise for the management of numerous human cancers, this EGFR-TKI is currently approved by the FDA for the first-line treatment of patients with metastatic NSCLC whose tumors harbor activating EGFR mutations (L858R or del E746-A750) [22, 33, 46]. Nevertheless, despite improving the tumor responses and prolonging the progression-free survival, gefitinib has still not shown the ability to enhance overall survival rate of patients [30]. In fact, clinical application of gefitinib is limited by acquired resistance that inevitably occurs after a period of exposure leading to disease recurrence, as well as severe drug-related adverse effects, including gastrointestinal diseases, hepatobiliary diseases, metabolic and nutritional disorders, and skin and subcutaneous diseases [22, 33, 45-47]. Therefore, it is highly important to develop new strategies for overcoming gefitinib resistance, and identify novel safe and efficient compounds for sensitizing NSCLC cells to gefitinib-based therapies [33]. Plant-derived flavonoids represent attractive candidates for implementation of this task, being commonly non-toxic and exhibiting a wide range of bioactivities.

##### *4.2.1.2.1. Effects of Flavonoids on Anticancer Potential of Gefitinib*

To date, the possible role of structurally diverse flavonoids on antitumor efficacy of gefitinib has been reported only in a few studies. The results of these works are summarized in Table 4.6 and discussed more closely below.

In fact, the most abundant green tea flavanol EGCG (34 μM) was found to synergistically enhance the sensitivity to gefitinib treatment in human NSCLC cells A549 by augmenting the suppression of cellular proliferation and promoting cell death. This effect was achieved through inhibition of gefitinib-induced autophagy and suppression of ERK signaling pathway. Moreover, combined treatment of A549 xenografts-bearing nude mice with gefitinib and EGCG significantly potentiated tumor growth suppression as compared to either single agent alone, besides prolonging also the survival rate of experimental animals [25]. EGCG (20 μM) in combination with gefitinib increased cytotoxicity also in benzo[a]pyrene (BaP)-transformed human normal lung epithelial BEAS-2B cells (BEAS-$2B_{BaP}$) that are tumorigenic and overexpress EGFR, through regulation of several signaling pathways. Combined treatment of transformed cells with gefitinib and EGCG resulted in a significant decrease in EGFR, activated Akt, cyclin D1 and survivin expression, with reducing also the levels of phase I and II metabolic enzymes (CYP1A1, CYP1B1, COMT) thereby slowing elimination of gefitinib from the cells and extending its intracellular activities [30]. Moreover, it was only very recently reported that a natural derivative of EGCG containing 6-methoxycarbonyl moiety, i.e., 2R,3R-6-methoxycarbonyl-gallocatechin-3-O-gallate (10-40 μM), derived from Anhua dark tea could also potently alleviate gefitinib resistance in gefitinib-refractory human NSCLC cells HCC827-Gef, leading to a synergistic decrease in cellular proliferation and clonogenicity and increase in apoptotic death. This sensitizing effect to EGFR-TKI was achieved through inactivation of PI3K/Akt/mTOR signaling and suppression of the EMT process, accompanied by significantly impaired migratory and invasive potential [22]. Addition of EGCG (25-100 μM) to gefitinib treatment was reported to synergistically reduce cellular migration and invasion also in human HNSCC line CAL-27, restricting aggressive behavior and metastatic ability of these oral cancer cells. Combined treatment with gefitinib and EGCG augmented the suppression of phosphorylation of EGFR and its several downstream targets, including MAPKs (ERK, JNK, p38) and Akt [24]; providing thereby a novel promising approach for future management of not only NSCLC but also HNSCC.

Two common flavone-type compounds, apigenin and luteolin, have also been studied in combination with gefitinib in some preclinical malignant models. As a result, apigenin (20-80 μM) was found to synergistically inhibit the viability and clonogenicity of EGFR-TKIs-resistant human NSCLC cells H1975 harboring both activating EGFR mutations as well as T790M, but exerted no beneficial responses in human lung cancer line 95-D with wt EGFR. In H1975 cells, combined treatment with gefitinib and apigenin led to a remarkable decrease in multiple oncogenic drivers, including p-EGFR, hypoxia-inducible factor 1α (HIF-1α) and c-Myc, downregulated the expression of glucose transporters (Gluts) and monocarboxylate transporter 1

(MCT1), and inactivated AMP-activated protein kinase (AMPK) signaling that regulates glucose uptake and maintains energy metabolism, altogether resulting in an impaired energy utilization, severe metabolic stress and attenuated malignant behavior in EGFR-mutant NSCLC cells. Although it is possible that crosstalk between glucose metabolism and oncogenic pathways could provide new strategies for mitigating TKI resistance in NSCLC, EGFR-directed pharmacological inhibitors alone have been shown to be insufficient in suppressing glucose uptake, indicating the necessity for combinational therapies. Co-exposure of H1975 cells to gefitinib and apigenin was indeed demonstrated to augment the damage of glucose metabolism, block autophagy flux and induce apoptotic death. In addition, combined treatment caused also G0/G1 phase arrest in the cell cycle progression and restricted migratory potential of H1975 cells. Therefore, combination of apigenin and gefitinib might present a very attractive approach for future management of NSCLC patients with acquired resistance to EGFR-TKIs [27]. Addition of another naturally abundant flavone, luteolin, led to an enhanced cell growth arrest and apoptosis in human prostate cancer line PC-3 as compared to the treatment with gefitinib alone [43, 48]; at least in part, through reduction of protein expression of cyclin G-associated kinase (GAK) and androgen receptor. Downregulation of GAK was achieved via miRNA-mediated translational inhibition and was further shown to disturb proper activation of EGFR-mediated intracellular signaling. The level of GAK has been indeed correlated with the severity of the disease and poor prognosis in prostate cancer patients [43]. However, co-administration of gefitinib and luteolin (60 μM) restricted the cellular growth also in EGFR-deficient human osteosarcoma line U2OS with overexpressed GAK levels, showing that GAK might serve as a new target for the combined treatment of not only hormone-refractory prostate cancers but also osteosarcomas, although the precise molecular mechanisms have remained elusive [43].

To investigate the possible effects of common dietary flavonol quercetin on antitumor action of gefitinib, different types of nanoparticles were prepared and characterized. In consequence, it was demonstrated that co-loading gefitinib and quercetin into PLGA-PEG nanocarriers led to a markedly higher cellular uptake and cell growth inhibition in human NSCLC line PC-9 than administration of individual drug-loaded nanoparticles. Co-loaded nanopreparation of gefitinib and quercetin enhanced tumor growth inhibition also in PC-9 xenografts-bearing nude mice, reducing tumor volume *in vivo* [47]. In addition, incorporating gefitinib and quercetin into PVP-functionalized graphene oxide (GO) nanovehicles (GO-PVP) led to a significant increase in cytotoxicity in human ovarian cancer cells PA-1 as compared to the treatment with single drug-loaded nanosystems [44]. Although these results demonstrate the great benefits accompanying with the use of nanomaterial-based drug delivery systems in combined anticancer therapy, the molecular mechanisms underlying these potentiating activities have still remained to be unraveled. Likewise, entrapping of flavanone naringenin into biotin-modified PEG-PCL nanoparticles significantly enhanced the antiproliferative and cytotoxic effects of respective gefitinib nanoparticles in human NSCLC cells A549, through strengthening the cell cycle arrest at G2/M phase and promoting apoptotic death. Moreover, combined treatment with naringenin nanoparticles and gefitinib nanoparticles led to a superior antitumor action also in urethane-induced lung cancers-bearing Albino wistar rats, reducing both tumor volume as well as the number of tumors in lungs. These effects were accompanied by restoring the biochemical parameters and serum metabolites to an almost normal level, besides regaining normal structural integrity of lung tissue. Concomitant downregulation of antiapoptotic proteins and upregulation of proapoptotic proteins were also observed. Most importantly, animal death rate of experimental rats was significantly declined during the dual treatment regimen with nanoparticulated system [45].

Combination of gefitinib with the most important soy isoflavone, genistein (10-320 μM), was reported to induce synergistic cell growth inhibition in human EGFR-TKIs-resistant NSCLC line H1975, carrying T790M mutation. In doing so, genistein potentiated gefitinib-induced apoptosis through suppression of activation of EGFR and its downstream targets Akt and mTOR, but not Erk1/2. Moreover, combination of gefitinib and genistein augmented tumor growth inhibition also in H1975 xenografts-bearing mice, leading to tumors with significantly lower volume, while causing no treatment-related adverse events. Therefore, as gefitinib alone exerts only a limited therapeutic effect against NSCLC with an acquired resistance to EGFR-TKIs, addition of genistein might lead to synergistic therapeutic responses by surmounting the threshold that cancer cells could tolerate [28]. In similar way, milk thistle flavonolignan silibinin (50, 100 μM) could synergistically increase the growth inhibitory and anticlonogenic effects of gefitinib in EGFR-TKIs-resistant human NSCLC lines H1975 and PC-9/GR, both harboring T790M mutation. Addition of silibinin enhanced the ability of gefitinib to inactivate EGFR signaling through suppression of receptor dimerization and disruption of preformed dimers, leading to downregulation of activated Akt. Therefore, supplementation with silibinin may overcome secondary mutation-mediated drug resistance of NSCLC to gefitinib, providing a promising therapeutic option for patients with acquired resistance to this EGFR-directed pharmacological inhibitor, but also for those harboring preexisting T790M mutant tumors [36]. Moreover, combined treatment with gefitinib and silibinin augmented antitumor activities and delayed malignant growth also in PC-9 xenografts-implanted mice, resulting in tumors with significantly smaller volumes, in the apparent absence of toxicity. These sensitizing effects were achieved through impeding the EMT process and reversal of gefitinib-induced mesenchymal phenotype of tumor cells, thereby suppressing one of the major resistance mechanisms that bypasses the therapeutic effects of EGFR-TKIs in NSCLC. The upregulated expression of mesenchymal marker N-cadherin has been indeed consistently found in most biopsy specimens obtained from NSCLC patients progressed under EGFR TKI-based therapies. As an active agent, oral milk thistle extract formulation that was enriched with a water-soluble form of silibinin, complexed with the amino-sugar meglumine, was used in this study, allowing to surmount the issue of low aqueous solubility and bioavailability of the parent silibinin. Thus, silibinin might serve as an attractive adjuvant agent for gefitinib treatment of NSCLC, providing a novel promising approach for preventing acquired resistance to EGFR-TKIs and improving therapeutic outcomes [37]. Furthermore, combination of gefitinib and silibinin (100 μM) was found to increase the growth inhibition and decrease colony formation also in two human hepatocellular carcinoma lines (SNU761 and Huh-BAT), via downregulation of EGFR-dependent Akt signaling in SNU761 cells. These results altogether suggest that silibinin might represent a potent adjunct to gefitinib for the treatment of not only EGFR-mutant NSCLC but also other EGFR-overexpressed tumors like HCC [49].

In brief, it appears that specific flavonoids can play a pivotal role in the treatment of tumors with overexpressed/ overactivated EGFR, being potentially useful as adjuvant agents for sensitizing the therapeutic responses to EGFR-targeted drug gefitinib. For better characterization of the acting modes of these natural phytochemicals in combination with gefitinib, further preclinical as well as clinical studies are required to be performed (Figure 4.4).

**Table 4.6.** Effects of flavonoids on anticancer action of gefitinib

| Flavonoid and its dosage | Gefitinib and its dosage | Biological system | Assay method and time | Effect | Mechanisms | Ref. |
|---|---|---|---|---|---|---|
| FLAVANOLS | | | | | | |
| EGCG; 20 μM | Gefitinib; 2-32 μM | BEAS-$2B_{BaP}$ BaP-transformed human lung epithelial cells; overexpressing EGFR | MTT; 24, 48h | Increase in gefitinib-induced cytotoxicity | Modulation of phase I/II metabolism (decrease in gefitinib-induced CYP1A1/1B1 and COMT). Downregulation of EGFR, cyclin D1, p-Akt and survivin, upregulation of p-p53 expression | [30] |
| EGCG; 34 μM | Gefitinib; 1.87 μM | A549 human NSCLC cells; gefitinib-resistant | MTS; 48h | Synergistic inhibition of proliferation (CI<1), overcoming of gefitinib resistance | Increase in TUNEL-positive, decrease in Ki67-positive cells. Inhibition of gefitinib-induced autophagy (decrease in LC3-II/I and ATG5, increase in p62). Downregulation of p-ERK1/2 and p-MEK1/2 | [25] |
| EGCG; 200 mg/kg/day, p.o. | Gefitinib; 10 mg/kg/day, p.o. | A549 cells injected s.c. into the left flanks of 7-8 w-old BALB/C male nude mice | 21 days | Potentiation of tumor growth suppression, decrease in tumor volume. Increase in survival rate of mice (60 days assay) | | [25] |
| EGCG; 25-100 μM | Gefitinib; 10 μM | CAL-27 human HNSCC cells; from oral cancer | 48h | | Synergistic inhibition of migration and invasion (decrease in MMP-2 expression and activity, increase in TIMP-2). Downregulation of p-EGFR, p-ERK, p-JNK, p-p38, p-Akt and PKCα | [24] |

| Flavonoid and its dosage | Gefitinib and its dosage | Biological system | Assay method and time | Effect | Mechanisms | Ref. |
|---|---|---|---|---|---|---|
| 2R,3R-6-methoxycarbonyl-gallocatechin-3-O-gallate; 10-40 μM | Gefitinib; 1.25-5.0 μM | HCC827-Gef human NSCLC cells, gefitinib-resistant | MTT; 72h. Colony assay; 10 days | Synergistic inhibition of proliferation (CI<1), increase in gefitinib potency. Suppression of colony formation | Enhancement of apoptosis (cleavage of caspase-3 and PARP). Restraining EMT (increase in E-cadherin, decrease in vimentin and MMP-9), suppression of migration and invasion. Downregulation of p-PI3K, p-Akt and p-mTOR | [22] |
| FLAVONES | | | | | | |
| Apigenin; 20-80 μM | Gefitinib; 20-80 μM | H1975 human NSCLC cells; EGFR L858R, del E746-A750, T790M, EGFR-TKIs-resistant | CCK-8; 48h (co- or serial incubation). Colony assay (8 days) | Synergistic decrease in cell viability at co-incubation (no significant interaction at serial incubation). Inhibition of colony formation | Damaging glucose uptake and utilization through inhibition of oncogenic drivers (c-Myc, HIF-1α, EGFR), decrease in Gluts and MCT1 expression, and inactivation of AMPK signaling. Blocking of autophagy flux (decrease in LC3-II/I, increase in p62), leading to increase in apoptosis (cleavage of caspase-3 and PARP-1, decrease in Bcl-2). Induction of G0/G1 phase arrest (downregulation of cyclin D1, CDK4), inhibition of cell migration (decrease in E-cadherin, MMP-2/9) | [27] |
| Apigenin; 20-80 μM | Gefitinib; 20-80 μM | 95-D human lung SCC cells; highly metastatic, EGFR wt | CCK-8; 72h | No synergistic decrease in cell viability | | [27] |

**Table 4.6.** (Continued)

| Flavonoid and its dosage | Gefitinib and its dosage | Biological system | Assay method and time | Effect | Mechanisms | Ref. |
|---|---|---|---|---|---|---|
| Luteolin; 60 μM | Gefitinib; 60 μM | PC-3 human prostate cancer cells; EGFR wt | Counting; 24, 48, 72h | Cumulative inhibitory effect on cell growth | Induction of apoptosis (cleavage of caspase-3, increase in subG1 cells). Reduction of GAK and AR proteins | [43] |
| Luteolin; 17.5, 35 μM | Gefitinib; 22, 44 μM | PC-3 human prostate cancer cells | Apoptosis assay; 24h | | Decrease in gefitinib-induced G0/G1, increase in G2/M phase arrest. Small increase in apoptosis | [48] |
| Luteolin; 60 μM | Gefitinib; 20 μM | U2OS human osteosarcoma cells; EGFR-deficient | Counting; 72h | Increase in gefitinib-induced reduction of cell viability | | [43] |
| FLAVONOLS | | | | | | |
| Quercetin (co-loaded with gefitinib to PLGA-PEG NPs); 0.05-20 μg/ml | Gefitinib (co-loaded with quercetin to PLGA-PEG NPs); 0.05-20 μg/ml | PC-9 human lung cancer cells | MTT; 24h | Increase in cell growth inhibition (compared to single drug-loaded NPs) | | [47] |
| Quercetin (co-loaded with gefitinib to PLGA-PEG NPs); 20 mg/kg, via tail vein on days 1, 4, 7, 10 and 13 | Gefitinib (co-loaded with quercetin to PLGA-PEG NPs); 20 mg/kg, via tail vein on days 1, 4, 7, 10 and 13 | PC-9 cells injected s.c. into the right flank of 4-5 w-old male BALB/c nude mice | 28 days | Increase in tumor growth inhibition, decrease in tumor volume (compared to single drug-loaded NPs) | | [47] |
| Quercetin (co-loaded with gefitinib to GO-PVP nanocomplex); 10 μg/ml | Gefitinib (co-loaded with quercetin to GO-PVP nanocomplex); 10 μg/ml | PA-1 human ovarian cancer cells | SRB; 48h | Increase in cytotoxic activity (compared to single drug-loaded nanosystems) | | [44] |

| Flavonoid and its dosage | Gefitinib and its dosage | Biological system | Assay method and time | Effect | Mechanisms | Ref. |
|---|---|---|---|---|---|---|
| Quercetin (co-loaded with gefitinib to GO-PVP nanocomplex); 10 μg/ml | Gefitinib (co-loaded with quercetin to GO-PVP nanocomplex); 10 μg/ml | PA-1 human ovarian cancer cells | SRB; 48h | Increase in cytotoxic activity (compared to single drug-loaded nanosystems) | | [44] |
| FLAVANONES | | | | | | |
| Naringenin (as biotinylated PEG-PCL NPs); ratio with gefitinib NPs of 1:2 | Gefitinib (as biotinylated PEG-PCL NPs) | A549 human NSCLC cells | MTT, AlamarBlue; 48h | Increase in cytotoxic and antiproliferative action of gefitinib | Increase in G2/M phase arrest, enhancement of apoptosis. Increase in ROS inhibition | [45] |
| Naringenin (as biotinylated PEG-PCL NPs); 30 mg/kg, i.p., every 3 days | Gefitinib (as biotinylated PEG-PCL NPs); 20 mg/kg, i.v. tail injection, every 3 days | Urethane (1 g/kg, i.p.)-induced lung cancers in male and female Albino wistar rats | 4 weeks | Superior antitumor activity, reduction of tumor nodules and tumor volume. Decline in animal death (16 weeks assay) | Regaining normal structure of lung tissue. Restoring TBARS, PC, SOD, CAT and GSH levels to almost normal values. Decrease in Bcl-2, increase in P-16 and caspase-9 | [45] |
| ISOFLAVONES | | | | | | |
| Genistein; 10-320 μM, ratio with gefitinib of 10:1 | Gefitinib; 1-32 μM | H1975 human NSCLC cells; EGFR L858R and T790M, gefitinib-resistant | MTT; 72h | Synergistic inhibition of cell growth (CI<1) | Potentiation of apoptosis (cleavage of caspase-3 and PARP). Downregulation of p-EGFR, p-Akt and p-mTOR | [28] |
| Genistein; 100 mg/kg | Gefitinib; 50 mg/kg, p.o. | H1975 cells inoculated s.c. into 4-6 w-old female nude BALB/c mice | 5 weeks | Augmentation of decrease in tumor volume, slowing the tumor growth | | [28] |

**Table 4.6.** (Continued)

| Flavonoid and its dosage | Gefitinib and its dosage | Biological system | Assay method and time | Effect | Mechanisms | Ref. |
|---|---|---|---|---|---|---|
| FLAVONOLIGNANS | | | | | | |
| Silibinin; 50, 100 µM | Gefitinib; 1 µM | H1975 human NSCLC cells; EGFR T790M | MTT; 72h. Colony assay; 7-10 days | Synergistic increase in growth inhibition (CI<1); overcoming of gefitinib resistance. Decrease in colony size and number | Downregulation of p-EGFR and p-Akt expression | [36] |
| Silibinin; 50, 100 µM | Gefitinib; 1 µM | PC-9/GR human NSCLC cells; EGFR T790M, gefitinib-resistant | MTT; 72h. Colony assay; 7-10 days | Synergistic increase in growth inhibition (CI<1); overcoming of gefitinib resistance. Decrease in colony size and number | Downregulation of p-EGFR and p-Akt expression | [36] |
| Silibinin (as silibinin meglumine); 100 mg/kg, p.o., 5 days a week | Gefitinib; 100 mg/kg, p.o., 5 days a week | PC-9-derived cells (EGFR del E746-A750) inoculated s.c. into NOD/SCID mice | 35 days | Potentiation of gefitinib-induced tumor growth inhibition, decrease in tumor volume | Reversal of gefitinib-induced mesenchymal phenotype, prevention of gefitinib-upregulated Twist1 and N-cadherin expression | [37] |
| Silibinin; 100 µM | Gefitinib; 1 µM | Huh-BAT human HCC cells | MTT, counting; 72h. Colony assay; 2 weeks | Additive increase in growth inhibition. Decrease in colony numbers | Inhibition of EGFR activity | [49] |
| Silibinin; 100 µM | Gefitinib; 1 µM | SNU761 human HCC cells | MTT, counting; 72h. Colony assay; 2 weeks | Synergistic increase in growth inhibition (CI<1). Decrease in colony numbers | Inhibition of EGFR and Akt activities | [49] |

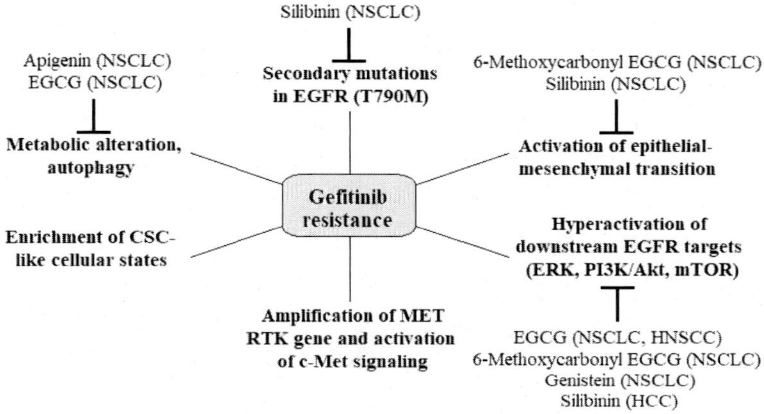


**Figure 4.4.** Overcoming gefitinib resistance and augmenting its antitumor action by flavonoids.

### *4.2.1.2.2. Effects of Flavonoid-Rich Natural Products on Anticancer Efficacy of Gefitinib*

Besides individual flavonoids, different natural mixtures and herbal extracts that are rich in these polyphenolic phytochemicals have also been studied in combination with EGFR-targeted drug gefitinib in some preclinical malignant models. These results are summarized in Table 4.7 and discussed more closely in this subsection.

As a result, isoflavone rich extracts derived from soy or red clover were shown to significantly increase the antiproliferative activity of gefitinib in a range of genotypically different human NSCLC lines, harboring either wt EGFR (A549), EGFR with activating mutation (del E746-A750; HCC827) or EGFR with acquired resistance-related secondary mutation T790M (H1975) [34]. The mixture of flavonoids derived from clover plants (*Trifolium* L.) potentiated gefitinib-induced growth inhibitory and apoptotic activities also in EGFR-TKIs-resistant human NSCLC line PC-9R, sensitizing the cells to gefitinib [33]. It is possible that soy and red clover isoflavones in combination with gefitinib might represent a potential new strategy to contribute to arresting the growth of NSCLC, thereby allowing to reduce also the drug doses required for achieving therapeutic responses. However, precise molecular mechanisms under these effects have remained to be unraveled in further preclinical studies. In addition, a mixture of grape polyphenols consisting of two flavonoids, catechin and quercetin, and a stilbenoid resveratrol augmented gefitinib-induced decrease in cellular viability in EGFR-overexpressing human breast cancer line, MDA-MB-231.

**Table 4.7.** Effects of flavonoid-rich natural products on anticancer action of gefitinib

| Flavonoid-rich natural product | Gefitinib and its dosage | Biological system | Assay method and time | Effect | Mechanisms | Ref. |
|---|---|---|---|---|---|---|
| Red clover extract | Gefitinib | A549 human NSCLC cells; EGFR wt | Crystal violet; 48h | Increase in antiproliferative activity, decrease in $IC_{50}$ of gefitinib | | [34] |
| Red clover extract | Gefitinib | H1975 human NSCLC cells; EGFR T790M | Crystal violet; 48h | Increase in antiproliferative activity, decrease in $IC_{50}$ of gefitinib | | [34] |
| Red clover extract | Gefitinib | HCC827 human NSCLC cells; EGFR del E746-A750 | Crystal violet; 48h | Increase in antiproliferative activity, decrease in $IC_{50}$ of gefitinib | | [34] |
| Soy extract | Gefitinib | A549 human NSCLC cells; EGFR wt | Crystal violet; 48h | Increase in antiproliferative activity, decrease in $IC_{50}$ of gefitinib | | [34] |
| Soy extract | Gefitinib | H1975 human NSCLC cells; EGFR T790M | Crystal violet; 48h | Increase in antiproliferative activity, decrease in $IC_{50}$ of gefitinib | | [34] |
| Soy extract | Gefitinib | HCC827 human NSCLC cells; EGFR del E746-A750 | Crystal violet; 48h | Increase in antiproliferative activity, decrease in $IC_{50}$ of gefitinib | | [34] |
| Trifolium flavonoids; 5-50 μM | Gefitinib; 8, 17 μM | PC-9R human NSCLC cells; gefitinib-resistant | MTT; 24h | Potentiation of gefitinib-induced cell growth inhibition; sensitization to gefitinib | Augmentation of gefitinib-induced apoptosis (cleavage of caspases-3, -9, -8 and PARP; decrease in Bcl-2 and Mcl-1) | [33] |

| Flavonoid-rich natural product | Gefitinib and its dosage | Biological system | Assay method and time | Effect | Mechanisms | Ref. |
|---|---|---|---|---|---|---|
| Grape polyphenols (resveratrol, quercetin, catechin); 5 μM | Gefitinib; 30 μM | MDA-MB-231 human breast cancer cells; overexpressing EGFR, gefitinib-resistant | Counting; 48h | Potentiation of decrease in cell viability | Inhibition of Akt, activation of AMPK, decrease in p70S6K activity | [46] |
| Grape polyphenols (resveratrol, quercetin, catechin); 5 mg/kg bw, p.o., every other day 7 days a week (alternate days of gefitinib) | Gefitinib; 200 mg/kg bw, p.o., every other day 7 days a week | GFP-MDA-MB-231 cells (with Matrigel) injected into the fourth right mammary fat pad of 5-6 w-old hairless SCID female mice | 84 days | Inhibition of tumor growth (no decrease in tumor size with either treatment alone) | Reduction of metastases in lung, liver and kidneys | [46] |

This effect was achieved via inhibition of Akt and elevation of AMPK activities by one or more bioactive constituents. Moreover, the same mixture of grape polyphenols suppressed the tumor growth also in MDA-MB-231 xenografts-bearing mice, besides reducing the metastasis to the lungs, liver and kidneys. The relevance of these results becomes obvious through the reports revealing about 45% of breast cancer patients to be EGFR-positive [46]. Therefore, potentiating role of flavonoids towards the antitumor action of EGFR-targeted drug gefitinib might not be restricted to NSCLC, being potentially important also in some other tumor types with overexpressed/ overactivated EGFR, highlighting the power of inclusion of specific phytochemicals in combined treatment regimens for sensitizing tumors to EGFR-directed inhibitors and impeding the malignant progression.

#### ***4.2.1.3. Lapatinib***

Lapatinib is the first-generation TKI that besides blocking the activation of EGFR (HER1, ErbB1) inhibits also the HER2 (ErbB2) tyrosine kinase activity, leading to inactivation of their downstream signaling pathways and suppression of cellular proliferation and survival [50] (Figure 4.1). Lapatinib is approved by the FDA for the treatment of breast cancer patients with HER2-overexpressing tumors, in combination with either capecitabine for patients with advanced tumors that have progressed after previous chemotherapy or letrozole for postmenopausal women with hormone receptor-positive metastatic breast cancer [51]. HER2 is overexpressed in about 20-25% of breast cancer patients, where lapatinib alone can achieve an efficiency of more than 28% [50]. Moreover, as this small orally active drug can penetrate the blood-brain barrier, it is effective also for breast cancer patients with metastases in the brain [50]. In 2020, there were more than 2.26 million new breast cancer cases in the whole world, with almost 685,000 new cancer-related deaths, accounting for 24.5% of all new cancer cases in females [31]. Therefore, new strategies for more efficient treatment of breast cancer patients are highly needed, with combination therapies that coincidently target several cellular pathways being especially attractive.

##### *4.2.1.3.1. Effects of Flavonoids on Anticancer Potential of Lapatinib*

To date only one natural flavonoid, i.e., flavone luteolin, has been tested in combination with lapatinib therapy in some HER2-positive human breast cancer preclinical models. The results of this work are presented in Table 4.8. Specifically, the combination of luteolin (50 μM) and lapatinib increased the sensitivity of BT-474, SKBR-3 and ZR-75-1 cells to the HER1/2-targeted drug, by potentiating proapoptotic, antimigratory and antiinvasive properties of lapatinib. These sensitizing effects were achieved through upregulation of the expression of FOXO3a and NQO1 proteins and their downstream target genes related to apoptotic death and tumor suppression. Moreover, in mice transplanted with BT-474 or ZR-75-1 cells, combined treatment with lapatinib and luteolin led to a significant inhibition of subcutaneous tumor growth, with decrease in the tumor volume and increase in the expression levels of FOXO3a and NQO1 in malignant tissues [50].

In addition, semisynthetic flavonoid flavopiridol was also tested in combination with lapatinib to study their potential co-effects in several breast cancer lines as well as colon cancer models. As a result, flavopiridol could synergistically enhance the cytotoxicity of lapatinib in HER2-overexpressing human breast cancer cells (SKBR3 and BT474), but also HER2-negative MCF-7 where co-exposure to dual agents further led to radiosensitization of malignant cells. In SKBR3 cells, combined treatment with lapatinib and flavopiridol induced suppression of EGFR, Akt and ERK1/2 activation, resulting in several apoptosis-related changes and rendering the cells more susceptible to tumor cell death. Moreover, addition of flavopiridol enhanced lapatinib-induced cytotoxic responses also in human colon cancer cells HCT116, with contribution to overcoming the drug resistance in lapatinib-resistant HCT116 subline, HCT116-AD [51]. Further studies are required to investigate the possibilities to include different flavonoids in lapatinib-based therapeutic strategies for more efficient management of breast cancer in the future.

#### *4.2.1.4. Afatinib*

Afatinib (Gliotrif) is the second-generation EGFR inhibitor that can form irreversible covalent bonds with EGFR to overcome T790M-mediated acquired resistance [34] (Figure 4.1). This drug is approved by the FDA as a first- or second-line treatment for EGFR mutant metastatic NSCLC.

##### *4.2.1.4.1. Effects of Flavonoid-Rich Natural Products on Anticancer Efficacy of Afatinib*

Both soy as well as red clover extracts rich in isoflavones were shown to enhance afatinib-induced antiproliferative activities in human NSCLC lines harboring genotypically different EGFR, i.e., EGFR wt (A549), EGFR with activating mutation (del E746-A750; HCC827) and EGFR with secondary mutation (T790M; H1975). Molecular mechanisms under these beneficial effects as well as their possible translation into *in vivo* systems have remained to be unraveled in further works [34] (Table 4.9).

**Table 4.8.** Effects of flavonoids on anticancer action of lapatinib

| Flavonoid and its dosage | Lapatinib and its dosage | Biological system | Assay method and time | Effect | Mechanisms | Ref. |
|---|---|---|---|---|---|---|
| FLAVONES | | | | | | |
| Luteolin; 50 μM | Lapatinib; 0.16-10 uM | BT-474 human breast ductoma cells; HER2+ | CCK-8; 24h | Increase in sensitivity of lapatinib, decrease in $IC_{50}$ of lapatinib | Increase in apoptosis, potentiation of lapatinib-induced inhibition of migration and invasion. Upregulation of FOXO3a and NQO1, and their downstream target genes Bim, GADD45, P21; decrease in FOXO3a phosphorylation | [50] |
| Luteolin; 50 μM | Lapatinib; 0.16-10 μM | SKBR-3 human breast cancer cells; HER2+ | CCK-8; 24h | Increase in sensitivity to lapatinib | Increase in apoptosis, potentiation of lapatinib-induced inhibition of migration and invasion. Upregulation of FOXO3a and NQO1, and their downstream target genes Bim, GADD45, P21; decrease in FOXO3a phosphorylation | [50] |
| Luteolin; 50 μM | Lapatinib; 0.16-10 μM | ZR-75-1, human breast cancer cells; HER2+ | CCK-8; 24h | Increase in sensitivity of lapatinib, decrease in $IC_{50}$ of lapatinib | Increase in apoptosis, potentiation of lapatinib-induced inhibition of migration and invasion. Upregulation of FOXO3a and NQO1, and their downstream target genes Bim, GADD45, P21; decrease in FOXO3a phosphorylation | [50] |
| Luteolin; 100 mg/kg | Lapatinib; 100 mg/kg | BT-474 cells inoculated s.c. into mice | 28 days | Inhibition of tumor growth rate, decrease in tumor volume | Upregulation of FOXO3a and NQO1 expression | [50] |
| Luteolin; 100 mg/kg | Lapatinib; 100 mg/kg | ZR-75-1 cells inoculated s.c. into mice | 28 days | Inhibition of tumor growth rate, decrease in tumor volume | Upregulation of FOXO3a and NQO1 expression | [50] |

| Flavonoid and its dosage | Lapatinib and its dosage | Biological system | Assay method and time | Effect | Mechanisms | Ref. |
|---|---|---|---|---|---|---|
| SYNTHETIC FLAVONOIDS | | | | | | |
| Flavopiridol; 50 nM | Lapatinib; 1 μM | BT474 human breast cancer cells; overexpressing HER2 | Counting; 48h | Greater than additive increase in cell viability reduction | | [51] |
| Flavopiridol; 50 nM | Lapatinib; 1 μM | MCF7 human breast cancer cells | Counting; 48h | Greater than additive increase in cell viability reduction | Increase in sensitivity to radiotherapy of combination-treated cells | [51] |
| Flavopiridol; 25-75 nM | Lapatinib; 0.5-1.5 μM | SKBR3 human breast cancer cells; overexpressing HER2 | Counting; 12, 24, 48h. Colony assay; 10-14 days | Synergistic increase in cell viability reduction (CI<1) | Downregulation of p-ErbB1 (p-EGFR), p-Akt and p-ERK1/2; decrease in Mcl-1, increase in Bax and Bak | [51] |
| Flavopiridol; 100 nM | Lapatinib; 100-200 nM | HCT116 human colon cancer cells | Counting; 48h | Increase in cell viability reduction | | [51] |
| Flavopiridol; 100 nM | Lapatinib; 100-200 nM | HCT116-AD human colon cancer cells; lapatinib-adapted | Counting; 48h | Increase in cell viability reduction; partial circumvention of lapatinib resistance | | [51] |

**Table 4.9.** Effects of flavonoid-rich natural products on anticancer action of afatinib

| Flavonoid-rich natural product | Afatinib and its dosage | Biological system | Assay method and time | Effect | Ref. |
|---|---|---|---|---|---|
| Red clover extract | Afatinib | A549 human NSCLC cells; EGFR wt | MTT, Crystal violet; 48h | Increase in antiproliferative activity, decrease in $IC_{50}$ of afatinib | [34] |
| Red clover extract | Afatinib | H1975 human NSCLC cells; EGFR T790M | MTT, Crystal violet; 48h | Increase in antiproliferative activity, decrease in $IC_{50}$ of afatinib | [34] |
| Red clover extract | Afatinib | HCC827 human NSCLC cells; EGFR del E746-A750 | MTT, Crystal violet; 48h | Increase in antiproliferative activity, decrease in $IC_{50}$ of afatinib | [34] |
| Soy extract | Afatinib | A549 human NSCLC cells; EGFR wt | MTT, Crystal violet; 48h | Increase in antiproliferative activity, decrease in $IC_{50}$ of afatinib | [34] |
| Soy extract | Afatinib | H1975 human NSCLC cells; EGFR T790M | MTT, Crystal violet; 48h | Increase in antiproliferative activity, decrease in $IC_{50}$ of afatinib | [34] |
| Soy extract | Afatinib | HCC827 human NSCLC cells; EGFR del E746-A750 | MTT, Crystal violet; 48h | Increase in antiproliferative activity, decrease in $IC_{50}$ of afatinib | [34] |

#### *4.2.1.5. Osimertinib*

Osimertinib (Tagrisso) is the third-generation irreversible EGFR inhibitor that was developed to combat the resistance emerged after the use of first- and second-generation EGFR-TKIs [34] (Figure 4.1). This drug is approved by the FDA as a first-line treatment for locally advanced and metastatic NSCLC with activating mutations in the EGFR gene (del E746-A750 or L858R) or for metastatic NSCLC harboring T790M after progression under EGFR-TKIs.

##### *4.2.1.5.1. Effects of Flavonoid-Rich Natural Products on Anticancer Efficacy of Osimertinib*

As in the experiments with first- and second-generation EGFR-TKIs, soy and red clover isoflavone extracts potentiated the cell growth inhibitory effects also in combination with osimertinib, leading to a significant decrease in the half-maximal inhibitory concentrations ($IC_{50}$) of the drug in a panel of different human NSCLC cells (A549, H1975, HCC827). Thus, one or more bioactive constituents of these herbal products may synergize the antitumor efficacy of osimertinib. The specific bioactive compound, its action mechanisms as well as potential activities in combined treatment regimens with osimertinib should be clarified in further studies [34] (Table 4.10).

- **Inhibitors of membrane receptors: small-molecule multikinase inhibitors**

Multiple protein kinases, both serine/threonine kinases and receptor tyrosine kinases (RTKs), are related to a wide range of vital cellular functions, including growth, proliferation, survival and apoptosis. Moreover, diverse intracellular pathways induced by activated RTKs control also malignant processes, regulating tumor formation, development, growth and metastasis, but also complex angiogenic events [52-54]. Therefore, antagonizing these RTKs and suppressing their signaling routes by multikinase inhibitors, is a promising targeted therapeutic strategy in oncology. Recently, a number of multikinase inhibitors have been developed and tested against different tumors, leading some of them to approval for the treatment of specific cancer types. However, the expected therapeutic success has still not been achieved by applying these multitargeted agents in clinical practice, remaining an important challenge and indicating that new strategies to optimize the efficacy of these drugs are urgently required.

**Table 4.10.** Effects of flavonoid-rich natural products on anticancer action of osimertinib

| Flavonoid-rich natural product | Osimertinib and its dosage | Biological system | Assay method and time | Effect | Ref. |
|---|---|---|---|---|---|
| Red clover extract | Osimertinib | A549 human NSCLC cells; EGFR wt | MTT, Crystal violet; 48h | Increase in antiproliferative activity, decrease in $IC_{50}$ of osimertinib | [34] |
| Red clover extract | Osimertinib | H1975 human NSCLC cells; EGFR T790M | MTT, Crystal violet; 48h | Increase in antiproliferative activity, decrease in $IC_{50}$ of osimertinib | [34] |
| Red clover extract | Osimertinib | HCC827 human NSCLC cells; EGFR del E746-A750 | MTT, Crystal violet; 48h | Increase in antiproliferative activity, decrease in $IC_{50}$ of osimertinib | [34] |
| Soy extract | Osimertinib | A549 human NSCLC cells; EGFR wt | MTT, Crystal violet; 48h | Increase in antiproliferative activity, decrease in $IC_{50}$ of osimertinib | [34] |
| Soy extract | Osimertinib | H1975 human NSCLC cells; EGFR T790M | MTT, Crystal violet; 48h | Increase in antiproliferative activity, decrease in $IC_{50}$ of osimertinib | [34] |
| Soy extract | Osimertinib | HCC827 human NSCLC cells; EGFR del E746-A750 | MTT, Crystal violet; 48h | Increase in antiproliferative activity, decrease in $IC_{50}$ of osimertinib | [34] |

#### *4.2.1.6. Sorafenib*

Sorafenib (Nexavar), an orally active small-molecule multikinase inhibitor, impedes diverse oncogenic pathways by affecting specific molecular targets, to restrict the growth and induce apoptosis of malignant cells [52, 55, 56] (Figure 4.1). This drug represses proliferation of tumor cells through inhibition of rapidly accelerated fibrosarcoma (Raf) serine/threonine kinases-dependent signaling pathway (Raf/MEK/ERK), whereas sorafenib can suppress both the c-Raf as well as wild-type and mutant B-Raf kinases including the highly oncogenic V600E isoform [3, 9, 57, 58]. Additionally, sorafenib acts also by suppressing tumor angiogenesis via blocking multiple RTKs, including vascular endothelial growth factor receptors (VEGFRs), platelet-derived growth factor receptor β (PDGFRβ), fibroblast growth factor receptor (FGFR), FMS-like tyrosine kinase 3 (FLT3), c-KIT protein as well as RET receptor tyrosine kinase [9, 57-61]. Moreover, sorafenib can restrict also cell migration and invasion through suppression of the EMT process in malignant cells, conferring impediment of metastatic spread of cancerous neoplasms [55].

Although sorafenib has been shown to exert its antitumor potential against various tumor types in numerous preclinical and clinical investigations [3, 5, 6, 55, 60], this drug is approved by the FDA for treatment of advanced renal cell carcinoma (RCC), unresectable hepatocellular carcinoma (HCC) and metastatic differentiated thyroid cancer [5, 6, 57, 62, 63]. Differentiated thyroid carcinoma, including both papillary and follicular thyroid carcinomas, is the most common endocrine-related malignancy occurring about three times more often in women than in men [63]. Treatment with sorafenib has shown a notable prolongation in the survival of patients with radioactive iodine-refractory thyroid carcinoma [63]. In hepatocellular carcinoma (HCC), sorafenib is currently the only approved agent for systemic treatment of advanced disease, being commonly used as the front-line therapy [52, 57, 64, 65]. HCC is the major type of primary liver cancer, accounting for about 70-90% of all cases of this highly aggressive tumor [52, 65, 66]. In 2020, there were more than 905,000 new liver cancer cases worldwide with over 830,000 deaths, representing the sixth most prevalent malignancy and the third most frequent cause of cancer-related mortality worldwide [31]. Unfortunately, the incidence and mortality rates of HCC have been continuously rising in the recent decades, with the hepatitis B or C virus infections, hepatic cirrhosis and hemochromatosis as the most common risk factors [52, 64, 66, 67]. Vascularization level is dramatically high in HCC and proteins related to Raf/MAPK pathways are significantly more expressed and activated as compared to non-tumorigenic liver tissues, being associated with poor prognosis, and representing effective cellular targets for antiangiogenic and antiproliferative effects of sorafenib [52, 57, 68, 69]. However, although sorafenib has shown significant therapeutic benefits in advanced HCC patients, revealing some improvement in both progression-free survival as well as median overall survival (nearly 3-months prolongation) in several phase III clinical trials [9, 59, 60, 68, 70-72], only about 20-40% of patients respond to this drug and get clinical benefit, with the five-year survival rate of HCC patients remaining disappointingly low [54, 61, 65]. Such unsatisfactory outcomes of sorafenib therapy can be caused by two major reasons. Firstly, HCC cells are prone to develop resistance to sorafenib treatment, greatly limiting its clinical efficacy [59, 72, 73]. Most of the patients gain resistance to this multikinase inhibitor within six months, resulting in a treatment failure and tumor progression [52, 61, 70]. The mechanisms under acquired sorafenib resistance are diverse, complex and largely elusive, comprising the continuous activation of Raf/MEK/ERK pathway, abnormal activation of the STAT3 signaling, presence of cancer stem cells (CSCs), activation of hypoxia-inducible pathways and the EMT process [9, 57, 61, 69, 72]. Another important mechanism under acquired resistance to sorafenib includes enhanced efflux of the drug by transporters, particularly Breast Cancer Resistance Protein (BCRP), resulting in the inability of sorafenib to achieve sufficient intracellular levels to be efficient in malignant cells [5, 9, 71]. Secondly, the large doses of sorafenib needed to be taken by patients for therapeutic responses, exert toxic effects also on healthy cells, inducing a variety of adverse reactions including lymphopenia, hypophosphatemia, hemorrhage, vomiting, nausea, diarrhea, jaundice, weight loss, fatigue, rash/desquamation, hand-foot skin reactions, alopecia and hypertension, but also secondary malignancies, pleural effusion and dyspnea [49, 52, 61-63, 73]. Moreover, a wide application of the drug at its high doses presents a considerable burden also to healthcare budgets [73, 74]. Therefore, further research and development must be focused on elucidation of resistance mechanisms under sorafenib therapy and identification of safe and efficient adjuvant agents to improve cancer cells sensitivity to this multikinase inhibitor, allowing to enhance clinical outcomes besides reducing also undesirable side effects via decrease in therapeutically efficient drug doses [9, 57, 59, 74]. Natural plant-derived flavonoids represent excellent candidates for this task, being commonly non-toxic and exerting a wide range of anticancer bioactivities [62, 67].

#### *4.2.1.6.1. Effects of Flavonoids on Pharmacokinetics of Sorafenib*

An important mechanism of sorafenib resistance is related to enhanced efflux by transporters, so that concentrations of this multikinase inhibitor cannot reach therapeutically efficient levels in malignant cells. Sorafenib has been reported to be mainly the substrate of BCRP/ATP-binding cassette transporter G2 (ABCG2), whereas overexpression of this protein was found to confer decrease in sorafenib efficacy [5, 9]. To overcome efflux transporter-mediated sorafenib resistance, combined administration of this drug with a few flavonoids as potential efflux transporter inhibitors has been investigated. Results of these works are presented in Table 4.11 and discussed more closely below.

In detail, methoxylated flavone, 5,7-dimethoxyflavone, remarkably changed the pharmacokinetic parameters of sorafenib, by significantly enhancing the plasma concentration (AUC value) and reducing the systemic clearance of the drug in male mice. A great increase in sorafenib AUC was detected also in the most collected tissues, including lung, gut, muscle, fat and kidney. These effects were attributed to potent inhibition of BCRP-mediated sorafenib efflux by 5,7-dimethoxyflavone, as this natural agent could significantly enhance the intracellular level of sorafenib in MDCK-II/Bcrp1 cells *in vitro*. Therefore, co-administration of sorafenib and 5,7-dimethoxyflavone might result in increased exposure of plasma and tissues to this targeted drug, indicating that 5,7-dimethoxyflavone could represent a promising sensitizing agent for overcoming BCRP-mediated sorafenib resistance [5]. In addition, the methylated flavonol, rhamnetin, was very recently shown to be able to delay the metabolism and clearance rate of sorafenib in human HCC cells HepG2 and MHCC97-H with prolongation of the half-life of the drug, by suppressing the expression of CYP3A4 and P-gp proteins in a p53-dependent manner. Deceleration of sorafenib metabolic clearance by rhamnetin was further confirmed also in HepG2 and MHCC97-H xenografts-bearing mice [73]. However, as can be seen, the current knowledge on pharmacokinetic *in vivo* interactions of phytochemicals with TKIs is still very limited. Further studies are urgently needed to better understand the potential effects of specific dietary flavonoids on pharmacokinetic profile and tissue distribution of multikinase inhibitors. It is highly possible that the results of these works might lead to identification of novel potent BCRP inhibitors and hence development of new strategies that allow to reduce the efficient doses of targeted drugs.

**Table 4.11.** Effects of flavonoids on pharmacokinetic parameters of sorafenib

| Flavonoid and its dosage | Sorafenib and its dosage | Biological system | Effects | Purported mechanism | Ref. |
|---|---|---|---|---|---|
| FLAVONES | | | | | |
| 5,7-Dimethoxyflavone; 50 mg/kg p.o. 30 min before and 25 mg/kg i.p. 4-5 min before sorafenib | Sorafenib; 10 mg/kg, i.v. as bolus injection under light anesthesia | Male ND4 Swiss Webster mice | Increase in sorafenib AUC in plasma, decrease in sorafenib systemic clearance. Increase in sorafenib AUC in lung, gut, muscle, fat and kidney | Inhibition of BCRP-mediated sorafenib efflux | [5] |
| FLAVONOLS | | | | | |
| Rhamnetin; 1 μM | Sorafenib; 1 μM | HepG2 human HCC cells | Deceleration of elimination or clearance of sorafenib, prolongation of $t_{1/2}$ of sorafenib | Decrease in CYP3A4 and P-gp expression | [73] |
| Rhamnetin; 1 μM | Sorafenib; 1 μM | Huh7 human HCC cells; p53-deficient | No effect on metabolism or clearance of sorafenib | No effect on CYP3A4 and P-gp expression | [73] |
| Rhamnetin; 1 μM | Sorafenib; 1 μM | MHCC97-H human HCC cells; highly aggressive | Deceleration of elimination or clearance of sorafenib, prolongation of $t_{1/2}$ of sorafenib | Decrease in CYP3A4 and P-gp expression | [73] |
| Rhamnetin | Sorafenib; injected into tumors | HepG2 cells seeded s.c. into 4-5 w-old Bal B/$c^{null}$ nude mice | Deceleration of elimination or clearance of sorafenib, prolongation of $t_{1/2}$ of sorafenib | | [73] |
| Rhamnetin | Sorafenib; injected into tumors | MHCC97-H cells seeded s.c. into 4-5 w-old Bal B/$c^{null}$ nude mice | Deceleration of elimination or clearance of sorafenib, prolongation of $t_{1/2}$ of sorafenib | | [73] |

On the other hand, it is also possible that such studies will identify those plant-derived compounds consuming of which with sorafenib can lower the drug uptake in malignant cells by promoting the expression and activity of efflux transporters. These situations are definitely needed to be ascertained in further studies.

*4.2.1.6.2. Effects of Flavonoids on Anticancer Potential of Sorafenib*

Unlike pharmacokinetic research, much higher preclinical interest has been shown in investigation of possible effects of structurally diverse flavonoids on antitumor potential of sorafenib, both *in vitro* as well as *in vivo* models of different cancer types. The results of these works are summarized in Table 4.12 and thoroughly discussed in the further subsections.

The most abundant green tea flavanol, EGCG (25 μM), was recently reported to increase sorafenib-induced cell growth inhibition in two high-glycolytic sorafenib-resistant human HCC lines (HCC-LM3 and HepG2) through augmentation of suppression of phosphofructokinase (PFK) expression and inhibition of tumor glycolysis. PFK, an essential metabolic sensor in the glycolytic pathway, is highly expressed in human carcinomas including HCC, representing a potentially important target for depriving cancer cells from their essential energy. Both growth-inhibitory as well as proapoptotic activities of sorafenib were enhanced by EGCG also in HCC-LM3 xenografts-bearing nude mice, leading to tumors with significantly smaller sizes and showing the potential value of EGCG as an adjuvant agent for treatment of advanced HCC with sorafenib [64].

The naturally abundant flavone-type compound, apigenin (50 μM), augmented growth inhibitory, anticlonogenic and proapoptotic activities of sorafenib in human HCC cells HepG2. Apigenin additionally enhanced sorafenib-induced suppression of cell migration and invasion, thereby conferring antimetastatic potential of this multikinase inhibitor [52]. The sugar-conjugated derivative of apigenin, i.e., apigenin 8-C-glucoside or vitexin (50 μM), also potentiated proapoptotic effects and anticancer potential of sorafenib in HepG2 cells [66]. Bis-apigenin or amentoflavone (75 μM) promoted sorafenib-induced cytotoxicity and apoptosis not only in sorafenib-resistant human HCC line Sk-Hep1R by reducing the levels of antiapoptotic proteins (XIAP, Mcl-1, c-FLIP) and triggering proapoptotic proteins [70], but potentiated tumor growth inhibition also in Sk-Hep1 xenografts-bearing nude mice [75]. The latter effect was achieved through

**Table 4.12.** Effects of flavonoids on anticancer action of sorafenib (highlighted rows indicate undesired negative effects on anticancer efficacy)

| Flavonoid and its dosage | Sorafenib and its dosage | Biological system | Assay method and time | Effect | Mechanisms | Ref. |
|---|---|---|---|---|---|---|
| FLAVANOLS | | | | | | |
| EGCG; 25 μM | Sorafenib; 5 μM | HCC-LM3 human HCC cells; sorafenib-resistant | CCK-8; 24h | Increase in sorafenib-induced growth inhibition; improvement of resistance to sorafenib | Increase in sorafenib-induced inhibition of PFK expression | [64] |
| EGCG; 25 μM | Sorafenib; 5 μM | HepG2 human HCC cells; sorafenib-resistant | CCK-8; 24h | Increase in sorafenib-induced growth inhibition; improvement of resistance to sorafenib | Increase in sorafenib-induced inhibition of PFK expression | [64] |
| EGCG; 10 mg/kg bw, i.p. injection once daily | Sorafenib; 10 mg/kg bw, daily p.o. administration | HCC-LM3 cells injected s.c. into the upper flank of 4 w-old male athymic BALB/C nu/nu mice | 30 days | Increase in sorafenib-induced tumor growth inhibition, decrease in tumor size | Increase in sorafenib-induced apoptosis | [64] |
| FLAVONES (monomers and oligomers) | | | | | | |
| Apigenin; 50 μM | Sorafenib; 5 μM | HepG2 human HCC cells | XTT; 48h. Colony assay; 14 days | Increase in cell growth inhibition, potentiation of sorafenib cytotoxicity. Repression of colony formation | Potentiation of apoptosis (increase in caspases-3, -8, -10). Increase in sorafenib-induced inhibition of migration and invasion. Increase in BID, p21 and p16 expression | [52] |

| Flavonoid and its dosage | Sorafenib and its dosage | Biological system | Assay method and time | Effect | Mechanisms | Ref. |
|---|---|---|---|---|---|---|
| Chrysin; 25 μM | Sorafenib; 5 μM | Hep3B human HCC cells | Crystal violet; 1 day. MTT; 3 days | Augmentation of anticancer activity, decrease in $IC_{50}$ of sorafenib | Blocking of BCRP/ABCG2 activity, no recovery of ERK1/2 phosphorylation from inhibition by sorafenib. Increase in PARP cleavage | [9] |
| Chrysin; 25 μM | Sorafenib; 5 μM | Hep3B human HCC cells | Crystal violet; 2 days | Increase in sorafenib-mediated inhibition of cell viability | Induction of sustained phosphorylation of ERK1/2 by chrysin | [57] |
| Chrysin; 25 μM | Sorafenib; 5 μM | HepG2 human HCC cells | Crystal violet; 1 day. MTT; 3 days | Augmentation of anticancer activity, decrease in $IC_{50}$ of sorafenib | Blocking of BCRP/ABCG2 activity, no recovery of ERK1/2 phosphorylation from inhibition by sorafenib. Increase in PARP cleavage | [9] |
| Chrysin; 25 μM | Sorafenib; 5 μM | HepG2 human HCC cells | Crystal violet; 2 days | Increase in sorafenib-mediated inhibition of cell viability | Induction of sustained phosphorylation of ERK1/2 by chrysin | [57] |
| Chrysin; 25 μM | Sorafenib; 5 μM | Huh-7 human HCC cells | Crystal violet; 2 days. MTT; 3 days | Augmentation of anticancer activity, decrease in $IC_{50}$ of sorafenib | Blocking of BCRP/ABCG2 activity, no recovery of ERK1/2 phosphorylation from inhibition by sorafenib | [9] |
| Nobiletin; 10, 20 μM | Sorafenib; 0.5-2.5 μM | PC-3 human prostate cancer cells | WST-1; 24h | Synergistic inhibition of cell viability (CI<1) | Induction of G0/G1 phase arrest; increase in apoptosis. Upregulation of Bax, Rb1, CDKN1A genes | [6] |
| Vitexin; 50 μM | Sorafenib; 3 μM | HepG2 human HCC cells | Apoptosis assay; 24h | Augmentation of anticancer potential of sorafenib | Increase in sorafenib-induced apoptosis | [66] |

**Table 4.12.** (Continued)

| Flavonoid and its dosage | Sorafenib and its dosage | Biological system | Assay method and time | Effect | Mechanisms | Ref. |
|---|---|---|---|---|---|---|
| Wogonin; 10-40 µM | Sorafenib; 2-4 µM | Bel-7402 human HCC cells | LDH release; 72h | Synergistic cytotoxicity (CI<1). Sensitization of cells to sorafenib | Inhibition of sorafenib-induced cytoprotective autophagy (decrease in LC3-II expression); potentiation of sorafenib-induced apoptosis (increase in PARP cleavage) | [59] |
| Wogonin; 10-40 µM | Sorafenib; 2-4 µM | Hep3B human HCC cells | LDH release; 72h | Synergistic cytotoxicity (CI<1). Sensitization of cells to sorafenib | Potentiation of sorafenib-induced apoptosis (increase in PARP cleavage) | [59] |
| Wogonin; 5-20 µM | Sorafenib; 4 µM | HepG2 human HCC cells | LDH release; 72h | Synergistic cytotoxicity (CI<1). Sensitization of cells to sorafenib | | [59] |
| Wogonin; 10, 20 µM | Sorafenib; 2-6 µM | SMMC-7721 human HCC cells | LDH release; 72h | Synergistic cytotoxicity (CI<1). Sensitization of cells to sorafenib | | [59] |
| Amentoflavone (bis-apigenin); 75 µM | Sorafenib; 10-25 µM | Sk-Hep1R human HCC cells; sorafenib-resistant | MTT; 24h | Increase in sorafenib-induced cytotoxicity | Potentiation of sorafenib-induced apoptosis (enhancement of $\Delta\Psi m$ loss and DNA fragmentation; decrease in XIAP, Mcl-1, c-FLIP; increase in cleaved caspases-3 and -8, release of cyt c) | [70] |

| Flavonoid and its dosage | Sorafenib and its dosage | Biological system | Assay method and time | Effect | Mechanisms | Ref. |
|---|---|---|---|---|---|---|
| Amentoflavone (bis-apigenin); 50 mg/kg/day, p.o. | Sorafenib; 10 mg/kg/day, p.o. | Sk-Hep1 cells inoculated s.c. in the right legs of 6 w-old nude mice | 14 days | Potentiation of sorafenib-induced tumor growth inhibition, decrease in tumor volume | Downregulation of p-Akt and p-ERK. Decrease in Mcl-1, c-FLIP and XIAP expression. Activation of caspases-9, -8 and -3 | [75] |
| FLAVONOLS | | | | | | |
| Fisetin; 20 μM | Sorafenib; 5, 10 μM | A375 human malignant melanoma cells; BRAF-mutated | MTT; 48h. Colony assay; 2 weeks | Synergistic increase in growth inhibition (CI<1); decrease in colony number and size | Augmentation of apoptosis (cleavage of caspase-3 and PARP, decrease in Bcl-2 and Mcl-1, increase in Bax and Bak). Downregulation of MEK1/2, ERK1/2, AKT and mTOR phosphorylation, decrease in PI3K, increase in PTEN | [58] |
| Fisetin; 10, 20 μM | Sorafenib; 2, 5 μM | A375 human malignant melanoma cells; BRAF-mutated | 24, 48h | | Potentiation of sorafenib-induced inhibition of migration and invasion. Modulation of EMT markers (decrease in N-cadherin, vimentin, fibronectin; increase in E-cadherin), reduction of EMT-inducing transcription factors (Snail1, Twist1, Slug, ZEB1) | [55] |
| Fisetin; 20 μM | Sorafenib; 5, 10 μM | RPMI-7951 human malignant melanoma cells; BRAF-mutated | MTT; 48h. Colony assay; 2 weeks | Synergistic increase in growth inhibition (CI<1); decrease in colony number and size | | [58] |

**Table 4.12.** (Continued)

| Flavonoid and its dosage | Sorafenib and its dosage | Biological system | Assay method and time | Effect | Mechanisms | Ref. |
|---|---|---|---|---|---|---|
| Fisetin; 20 μM | Sorafenib; 5, 10 μM | SK-MEL-28 human malignant melanoma cells; BRAF-mutated | MTT; 48h. Colony assay; 2 weeks | Synergistic increase in growth inhibition (CI<1); decrease in colony number and size | Augmentation of apoptosis (cleavage of caspase-3 and PARP, decrease in Bcl-2 and Mcl-1, increase in Bax and Bak). Downregulation of MEK1/2, ERK1/2, AKT and mTOR phosphorylation, decrease in PI3K, increase in PTEN | [58] |
| Fisetin; 10, 20 μM | Sorafenib; 2, 5 μM | SK-MEL-28 human malignant melanoma cells; BRAF-mutated | 24, 48h | | Potentiation of sorafenib-induced inhibition of migration and invasion. Modulation of EMT markers (decrease in N-cadherin, vimentin, fibronectin; increase in E-cadherin), reduction of EMT-inducing transcription factors (Snail1, Twist1, Slug, ZEB1) | [55] |
| Fisetin; 45 mg/kg, p.o., thrice per week | Sorafenib; 45 mg/kg, p.o., thrice per week | A375 cells inoculated s.c. into each flank of 5 w-old female athymic nude mice | 16 days | Potentiation of sorafenib-induced tumor growth inhibition, decrease in tumor volume (augmentation of antitumor activity of sorafenib against growing as well as pre-existing xenograft tumors) | Augmentation of sorafenib-induced reduction of PCNA, Ki67 and cyclin D1; increase in cleaved caspase-3 and PARP, decrease in Bcl-2, increase in Bax. Potentiation of reduction of MEK1/2, ERK1/2, AKT and mTOR phosphorylation, decrease in PI3K, increase in PTEN expression. Decrease in CD31 and VEGF | [58] |

| Flavonoid and its dosage | Sorafenib and its dosage | Biological system | Assay method and time | Effect | Mechanisms | Ref. |
|---|---|---|---|---|---|---|
| Fisetin; 45 mg/kg, p.o., thrice per week | Sorafenib; 45 mg/kg, p.o., thrice per week | A375 cells transplanted s.c. into 5 w-old female athymic nude mice | | | Potentiation of sorafenib-induced decrease in N-cadherin, vimentin, fibronectin; increase in E-cadherin. Increase in reduction of EMT-inducing transcription factors (Snail1, Twist1, Slug, ZEB1). Decrease in MMP-2/9 proteins | [55] |
| Fisetin; 45 mg/kg bw, p.o., thrice per week | Sorafenib; 45 mg/kg bw, p.o., thrice per week | EGFP/luciferase reporter A375 cells injected via lateral tail vein into 6 w-old athymic nude mice | 2-4 weeks | Potentiation of reduction of lung metastases formation and progression | | [55] |
| Fisetin; 45 mg/kg, p.o., thrice per week | Sorafenib; 45 mg/kg, p.o., thrice per week | SK-MEL-28 cells inoculated s.c. into each flank of 5 w-old female athymic nude mice | 48 days | Potentiation of sorafenib-induced tumor growth inhibition, decrease in tumor volume (augmentation of antitumor activity of sorafenib against growing as well as pre-existing xenograft tumors) | Augmentation of sorafenib-induced reduction of PCNA, Ki67 and cyclin D1; increase in cleaved caspase-3 and PARP, decrease in Bcl-2, increase in Bax. Potentiation of reduction of MEK1/2, ERK1/2, AKT and mTOR phosphorylation, decrease in PI3K, increase in PTEN expression. Decrease in CD31 and VEGF | [58] |

**Table 4.12.** (Continued)

| Flavonoid and its dosage | Sorafenib and its dosage | Biological system | Assay method and time | Effect | Mechanisms | Ref. |
|---|---|---|---|---|---|---|
| Fisetin; 45 mg/kg, p.o., thrice per week | Sorafenib; 45 mg/kg, p.o., thrice per week | SK-MEL-28 cells transplanted s.c. into 5 w-old female athymic nude mice | | | Potentiation of sorafenib-induced decrease in N-cadherin, vimentin, fibronectin; increase in E-cadherin. Increase in reduction of EMT-inducing transcription factors (Snail1, Twist1, Slug, ZEB1). Decrease in MMP-2/9 proteins | [55] |
| Fisetin; 40 µM | Sorafenib; 2.5, 5 µM | HeLa human cervical cancer cells | MTT; 24h | Potentiation of decrease in cell viability | Augmentation of apoptosis (increase in DR5 expression, activation of caspases-8 and -3, cleavage of PARP; increase in Bax/Bcl-2 ratio, loss of $\Delta\Psi m$) | [60] |
| Fisetin; 4 mg/kg, p.o., twice per week | Sorafenib; 10 mg/kg, p.o., twice per week | HeLa cells injected s.c. into the right flank of 5 w-old BALB/c female mice | 5 weeks | Increase in tumor growth inhibition, decrease in tumor volume and weight | Reduction of Ki67 expression; increase in DR5, cleaved caspases-3 and -8, and cleaved PARP levels | [60] |
| Kaempferol; 2.5 µM | Sorafenib; 2.5 µM | HepG2 human liver cancer cells | MTT; 72h | Increase in sorafenib-induced cytotoxicity, sensitization to sorafenib | | [67] |
| Kaempferol; 2.5 µM | Sorafenib; 2.5 µM | N1S1 murine liver cancer cells | MTT; 72h | Increase in sorafenib-induced cytotoxicity, sensitization to sorafenib | | [67] |

| Flavonoid and its dosage | Sorafenib and its dosage | Biological system | Assay method and time | Effect | Mechanisms | Ref. |
|---|---|---|---|---|---|---|
| Quercetin (as free mixture or co-loaded with sorafenib into lipid coated PLGA NPs); 1-50 μM | Sorafenib (as free mixture or co-loaded with quercetin into lipid coated PLGA NPs); 1-50 μM | HepG2 human HCC cells | MTT; 48h | Increase in sorafenib-induced anticancer efficacy, decrease in cell viability (compared to the single drug formulations in NPs or solution) | | [65] |
| Quercetin (as free mixture or co-loaded with sorafenib into lipid coated PLGA NPs); 20 mg/kg, i.v. injection on days 0, 7, 14 and 21 | Sorafenib (as free mixture or co-loaded with quercetin into lipid coated PLGA NPs); 10 mg/kg, i.v. injection on days 0, 7, 14 and 21 | HepG2 cells injected into the right flank of 4-6 w-old BALB/c nude mice | 24 days | Increase in sorafenib-induced tumor growth inhibition (compared to the single drug formulations in NPs or solution) | | [65] |
| Quercetin; 25 μM | Sorafenib; 0.1 μM | BCPAP human papillary thyroid cancer cells | MTT; 24h | Augmentation of cell proliferation inhibition | Potentiation of reduction of cell adhesion and migration; increase in E-cadherin expression | [62] |
| Quercetin; 25 μM | Sorafenib; 0.1 μM | K1 human papillary thyroid cancer cells | MTT; 24h | Augmentation of cell proliferation inhibition | Potentiation of reduction of cell adhesion and migration; increase in E-cadherin, decrease in N-cadherin expression | [62] |
| Quercetin; 30 μM | Sorafenib; 0.75 μM | MOGGCCM human anaplastic astrocytoma cells | Apoptosis assay; 24h | | Potentiation of proapoptotic properties of sorafenib (increase in cyt c in cytoplasm, activation of caspases -3 and -9). Downregulation of Hsp27, Hsp72, Ras and Raf | [56] |

**Table 4.12.** (Continued)

| Flavonoid and its dosage | Sorafenib and its dosage | Biological system | Assay method and time | Effect | Mechanisms | Ref. |
|---|---|---|---|---|---|---|
| Quercetin; 50 µM | Sorafenib; 0.75 µM | T98G human glioblastoma cells | Apoptosis assay; 48h | | Decrease in sorafenib-induced autophagy in favor of apoptosis (increase in cyt c in cytoplasm, activation of caspases-3 and -9). Downregulation of Hsp27, Hsp72, Ras and Raf | [56] |
| Rhamnetin; 3 µM | Sorafenib; 0.01-10 µM | HepG2 human HCC cells | MTT; 48h. Colony assay; 3 weeks | Increase in antitumor efficacy, decrease in $IC_{50}$ of sorafenib. Decrease in colony numbers | Enhancement of sorafenib-induced apoptosis. Increase in sorafenib-induced inhibition of cell migration and invasion. Increase in miR-34a, inhibition of Notch-1 pathway (decrease in survivin and cIAP1/2) | [54] |
| Rhamnetin; 1 µM | Sorafenib; 0.01-10 µM | HepG2 human HCC cells | MTT; 48h | Increase in sensitivity to sorafenib, decrease in $IC_{50}$ of sorafenib | Potentiation of sorafenib-induced inhibition of migration and invasion. Increase in miR-148a expression, suppression of PXR activation, downregulation of P-gp and CYP3A4 | [73] |
| Rhamnetin; 3 µM | Sorafenib; various | HepG2/ADR human HCC cells; drug-resistant | MTT; 48h | Increase in antitumor effect, decrease in $IC_{50}$ of sorafenib | Increase in miR-34a, inhibition of Notch-1. Decrease in P-gp and BCRP expression | [54] |
| Rhamnetin; 1 µM | Sorafenib | Huh7 human HCC cells; p53-deficient | | | No effect on expression of miR-148a and PXR | [73] |
| Rhamnetin; 3 µM | Sorafenib; various | L-02 human HCC cells | MTT; 48h | Increase in antitumor effect, decrease in $IC_{50}$ of sorafenib | | [54] |

| Flavonoid and its dosage | Sorafenib and its dosage | Biological system | Assay method and time | Effect | Mechanisms | Ref. |
|---|---|---|---|---|---|---|
| Rhamnetin; 1 μM | Sorafenib; 0.01-10 μM | MHCC97-H human HCC cells; highly aggressive | MTT; 48h | Increase in sensitivity to sorafenib, decrease in $IC_{50}$ of sorafenib | Potentiation of sorafenib-induced inhibition of migration and invasion. Increase in miR-148a expression, suppression of PXR activation, downregulation of P-gp and CYP3A4 | [73] |
| Rhamnetin; 3 μM | Sorafenib; various | MHCC-97L human HCC cells | MTT; 48h | Increase in antitumor effect, decrease in $IC_{50}$ of sorafenib | | [54] |
| Rhamnetin; 200 μg/kg bw, i.p. administration daily for 20 days | Sorafenib; 10 mg/kg, p.o., once daily for 18 days | HepG2 cells injected into 4-5 w-old male SCID mice | 20 days | Increase in sorafenib-induced inhibition of tumor volumes and weight. Sensitization of tumors to sorafenib | Increase in miR-34a, decrease in Notch-1 expression (by rhamnetin) | [54] |
| Rhamnetin; via tail-vein injection, once every two days | Sorafenib; p.o., once every two days | HepG2 cells seeded s.c. into 4-5 w-old Bal B/$c^{null}$ nude mice | 3 weeks | Enhancement of antitumor effect of sorafenib on tumor volumes and weights, decrease in $IC_{50}$s of sorafenib | Suppression of PXR activation | [73] |
| Rhamnetin; via tail-vein injection, once every two days | Sorafenib; p.o., once every two days | MHCC97-H cells seeded s.c. into 4-5 w-old Bal B/$c^{null}$ nude mice | 3 weeks | Enhancement of antitumor effect of sorafenib on tumor volumes and weights, decrease in $IC_{50}$s of sorafenib | Suppression of PXR activation | [73] |

**Table 4.12.** (Continued)

| Flavonoid and its dosage | Sorafenib and its dosage | Biological system | Assay method and time | Effect | Mechanisms | Ref. |
|---|---|---|---|---|---|---|
| Rhamnetin; via tail-vein injection | Sorafenib; p.o. | MHCC97-H cells injected directly into the livers of 4-5 w-old Bal $B/c^{null}$ nude mice | | Enhancement of antitumor effect of sorafenib | Increase in miR-148a expression, suppression of PXR activation | [73] |
| ISOFLAVONES | | | | | | |
| Biochanin A; 0.15-50 µM, ratio with sorafenib of 50:1 | Sorafenib; 0.003-1 µM | HepG2 human HCC cells | SRB; 72h | Synergistic cytotoxicity (CI<1); decrease in $IC_{50}$ of sorafenib | Increase in cell cycle arrest at pre-G, decrease in S phase (compared to the drug alone). Increase in sorafenib-induced Bax, upregulation of caspases-9 and -3, downregulation of survivin and Ki67 | [74] |
| Biochanin A; ratios with sorafenib of 16:1 and 50:1 | Sorafenib | Huh-7 human HCC cells | WST-1; 72h | Increase in cytotoxicity; decrease in $IC_{50}$ of sorafenib | | [74] |
| Biochanin A; ratios with sorafenib of 16:1 and 50:1 | Sorafenib | SNU449 human HCC cells | SRB; 72h | Increase in cytotoxicity; decrease in $IC_{50}$ of sorafenib | Increase in sorafenib-induced caspase-3 level | [74] |
| Genistein; 1, 10 µM | Sorafenib; 0-200 µM | HepG2 human HCC cells | MTT; 48h with genistein, followed by 16h with sorafenib | Decrease in sorafenib efficacy. Enhancement of resistance to sorafenib cytotoxicity, increase in $IC_{50}$ of sorafenib | Increase in P-gp and MRP2 protein expression and activity by genistein (decrease in miR-379 upregulating MRP2, increase in PXR upregulating P-gp and MRP2) | [71] |

| Flavonoid and its dosage | Sorafenib and its dosage | Biological system | Assay method and time | Effect | Mechanisms | Ref. |
|---|---|---|---|---|---|---|
| Genistein; 1, 10 µM | Sorafenib; 0-200 µM | Huh7 human HCC cells | MTT; 48h with genistein, followed by 16h with sorafenib | Decrease in sorafenib efficacy. Enhancement of resistance to sorafenib cytotoxicity, increase in $IC_{50}$ of sorafenib | Increase in P-gp and MRP2 protein expression and activity by genistein | [71] |
| Genistein; 50 µM | Sorafenib; 10 µM | Primary human papillary thyroid cancer cells | WST-1, counting; 4h | Synergistic increase in antiproliferative activity (CI 0.89). No genotoxicity, no loss of DNA integrity | | [76] |
| Genistein; 25 µM | Sorafenib; 2.5 µM | SH-SY5Y human malignant neuroblastoma cells | MTT; 24h | Synergistic decrease in cell viability (CI 0.886) | Increase in G0/G1, decrease in G2/M phase arrest. Potentiation of sorafenib-induced apoptosis (activation of caspase-8, cleavage of Bid to tBid, upregulation of p53 and p21, decrease in Mcl-1, increase in Bax/Bcl-2 ratio, increase in cytosolic cyt c and Smac, activation of calpain and caspase-3). Downregulation of MDR, hTERT, N-Myc, VEGF, FGF-2, NF-κB, p-Akt and c-IAP2 | [77] |

**Table 4.12.** (Continued)

| Flavonoid and its dosage | Sorafenib and its dosage | Biological system | Assay method and time | Effect | Mechanisms | Ref. |
|---|---|---|---|---|---|---|
| Genistein; 25 μM | Sorafenib; 2.5 μM | SK-N-DZ human malignant neuroblastoma cells | MTT; 24h | Synergistic decrease in cell viability (CI 0.366) | Decrease in G0/G1 phase arrest. Potentiation of sorafenib-induced apoptosis (activation of caspase-8, cleavage of Bid to tBid, upregulation of p53 and p21, decrease in Mcl-1, increase in Bax/Bcl-2 ratio, increase in cytosolic cyt c and Smac, activation of calpain and caspase-3). Downregulation of MDR, hTERT, N-Myc, VEGF, FGF-2, NF-κB, p-Akt and c-IAP2 | [77] |
| FLAVONOLIGNANS | | | | | | |
| Silibinin; 100, 200 μM | Sorafenib; 2.5-10 μM | Bel-7404 human HCC cells | MTT; 72h. Colony assay; 7 days | Synergistic cytotoxicity (CI<1), decrease in survival. Decrease in clonogenicity | Synergistic increase in apoptosis (decrease in Mcl-1 and Bcl-2, increase in caspase-3 and PARP cleavage). Decrease in STAT3, AKT, p38 MAPK and ERK phosphorylation | [61] |
| Silibinin; 100 μM | Sorafenib; 5 μM | CSCs from Bel-7404, human HCC cells-induced stem cells | Counting; 72h | Inhibition of self-renewal, increase in sorafenib-induced blocking of spherogenesis | Increase in sorafenib-induced inhibition of STAT3 phosphorylation, decrease in KLF4 and β-catenin expression | [61] |

| Flavonoid and its dosage | Sorafenib and its dosage | Biological system | Assay method and time | Effect | Mechanisms | Ref. |
|---|---|---|---|---|---|---|
| Silibinin; 100 µM | Sorafenib; 5 µM | CSCs from Hepa 1-6, mouse HCC cells-induced stem cells | Counting; 72h | Inhibition of self-renewal, increase in sorafenib-induced blocking of spherogenesis | Inhibition of tumor cell stemness (decrease in expression of HCC stem cell markers CD133, CD13 and EpCAM) | [61] |
| Silibinin; 100, 200 µM | Sorafenib; 2.5-10 µM | HepG2 human HCC cells | MTT; 72h | Synergistic cytotoxicity (CI<1), decrease in survival | | [61] |
| Silibinin; 100 µM | Sorafenib; 2 µM | Huh7 human HCC cells | MTT, counting; 72h. Colony assay; 2 weeks | Increase in sorafenib-induced growth inhibition. Decrease in colony numbers | | [49] |
| Silibinin; 100 µM | Sorafenib; 5 µM | CSCs from Huh7, human HCC cells-induced stem cells | Counting; 72h | Inhibition of self-renewal, increase in sorafenib-induced blocking of spherogenesis | | [61] |
| Silibinin; 100 µM | Sorafenib; 2 µM | Huh-BAT human HCC cells | MTT; 72h | Increase in sorafenib-induced growth inhibition | | [49] |
| Silibinin; 100, 200 µM | Sorafenib; 2.5-10 µM | MHCC97L human HCC cells | MTT; 72h | Synergistic cytotoxicity (CI<1), decrease in survival | | [61] |
| Silibinin; 100 µM | Sorafenib; 2 µM | PLC/PRF5 human HCC cells | MTT; 72h | Increase in sorafenib-induced growth inhibition | | [49] |
| Silibinin; 100, 200 µM | Sorafenib; 2.5-10 µM | SMMC-7721 human HCC cells | MTT; 72h | Synergistic cytotoxicity (CI<1), decrease in survival | | [61] |

**Table 4.12.** (Continued)

| Flavonoid and its dosage | Sorafenib and its dosage | Biological system | Assay method and time | Effect | Mechanisms | Ref. |
|---|---|---|---|---|---|---|
| Silibinin; 100 μM | Sorafenib; 2 μM | SNU761 human HCC cells | MTT, counting; 72h. Colony assay; 2 weeks | Increase in sorafenib-induced growth inhibition. Decrease in colony numbers | | [49] |
| Silibinin; 200 mg/kg, i.v., every day | Sorafenib; 10 mg/kg, i.p., every day | Bel-7404 cells injected s.c. into the right foreleg of 5 w-old male athymic BALB/c nu/nu mice | 15 days | Increase in tumor growth inhibition, decrease in tumor volume and weight | Reduction of proportion of proliferative cells (decrease in Ki67, PCNA), increase in apoptotic cells. Inhibition of STAT3 and ERK phosphorylation; decrease in Mcl-1, Bcl-2, KLF4 and SOX2 levels | [61] |
| CHALCONES | | | | | | |
| Licochalcone A; 10 μM | Sorafenib; 2.5, 5 μM | Huh-7 human HCC cells | 24h | | Potentiation of sorafenib-induced inhibition of migration and invasion | [68] |
| Licochalcone A; 10 μM | Sorafenib; 2.5, 5 μM | SK-Hep-1 human HCC cells | 24h | | Potentiation of sorafenib-induced inhibition of migration and invasion (decrease in uPA). Downregulation of p-MEK4 and p-JNK | [68] |
| Licochalcone A; 10 mg/kg bw, p.o., daily | Sorafenib; 20 mg/kg bw, p.o., daily | SK-Hep-1 cells injected into the tail vein of immunodeficient nude mice | 2 months | Potentiation of sorafenib-induced inhibition of lung metastasis, decrease in the number of lung nodules | | [68] |

| Flavonoid and its dosage | Sorafenib and its dosage | Biological system | Assay method and time | Effect | Mechanisms | Ref. |
|---|---|---|---|---|---|---|
| Phloretin; 6.25-100 μM | Sorafenib; 1.25-20 μM | Hep3B2.1-7 human HCC cells | MTT; 48h | Potentiation of sorafenib-induced suppression of cell proliferation | Augmentation of apoptosis. Increase in SHP-1 activity, decrease in p-STAT3 | [69] |
| Phloretin; 6.25-100 μM | Sorafenib; 1.25-20 μM | HepG2 human HCC cells | MTT; 48h | Potentiation of sorafenib-induced suppression of cell proliferation | Augmentation of apoptosis. Increase in SHP-1 activity, decrease in p-STAT3 | [69] |
| Phloretin; 50 μM | Sorafenib; 10 μM | $HepG2^{SR}$ human HCC cells; sorafenib-resistant | Colony assay; 2 weeks | Potentiation of antitumor efficacy of sorafenib; inhibition of colony forming ability | Increase in SHP-1 activity. Downregulation of p-STAT3 and downstream signal proteins (Mcl-1, cyclin D1, survivin). Cleavage of caspases-3 and -9, increase in DNA fragmentation | [69] |
| Phloretin; 50 μM | Sorafenib; 10 μM | $Huh7^{SR}$ human HCC cells; sorafenib-resistant | Colony assay; 2 weeks | Potentiation of antitumor efficacy of sorafenib; inhibition of colony forming ability | Increase in SHP-1 activity. Downregulation of p-STAT3 and downstream signal proteins (Mcl-1, cyclin D1, survivin). Cleavage of caspases-3 and -9, increase in DNA fragmentation | [69] |
| Phloretin; 6.25-100 μM | Sorafenib; 1.25-20 μM | SK-Hep1 human HCC cells | MTT; 48h | Potentiation of sorafenib-induced suppression of cell proliferation | Augmentation of apoptosis. Increase in SHP-1 activity, decrease in p-STAT3 | [69] |
| Phloretin; 50 mg/kg, i.p. injection, 5 times a week for 3 weeks | Sorafenib; 20 mg/kg | HepG2 cells inoculated s.c. into the posterior flank of nude mice | 30 days | Additive decrease in tumor volume | Increase in SHP-1 activity. Downregulation of p-STAT3, Mcl-1 and survivin expression | [69] |

**Table 4.12.** (Continued)

| Flavonoid and its dosage | Sorafenib and its dosage | Biological system | Assay method and time | Effect | Mechanisms | Ref. |
|---|---|---|---|---|---|---|
| Phloretin; 50 mg/kg | Sorafenib; 20 mg/kg | $HepG2^{SR}$ cells inoculated s.c. into the posterior flank of nude mice | 30 days | Additive decrease in tumor volume and weight | Increase in SHP-1 activity. Downregulation of p-STAT3, Mcl-1 and survivin. Decrease in Ki67 and CD31, increase in caspase-3 | [69] |
| Phloretin; 50 mg/kg | Sorafenib; 20 mg/kg | $Huh7^{SR}$ cells inoculated s.c. into the posterior flank of nude mice | 30 days | Additive decrease in tumor volume and weight | Increase in SHP-1 activity. Downregulation of p-STAT3, Mcl-1 and survivin. Decrease in Ki67 and CD31, increase in caspase-3 | [69] |
| Phloretin; 50 mg/kg, i.p. injection, 5 times a week for 3 weeks | Sorafenib; 20 mg/kg | SK-Hep1 cells inoculated s.c. into the posterior flank of nude mice | 30 days | Additive decrease in tumor volume | Increase in SHP-1 activity | [69] |
| SYNTHETIC FLAVONOIDS | | | | | | |
| 8-Bromo-7-methoxychrysin; 5 μM | Sorafenib; 5-45 μM | Stem cells from SMMC-7721, human HCC cells-derived sphere-forming cells | Counting the number of spheroids; 5 days | Increase in inhibition of self-renewal capacity and stem cell biomarkers (CD133, CD44, ALDH1) expression | Enhancement of apoptosis. Potentiation of inhibition of migration, invasion and EMT (increase in E-cadherin, decrease in N-cadherin and Twist1). Downregulation of HIF-1α, suppression of sorafenib-upregulated NF-κB expression and activity | [72] |

| Flavonoid and its dosage | Sorafenib and its dosage | Biological system | Assay method and time | Effect | Mechanisms | Ref. |
|---|---|---|---|---|---|---|
| 7-(O)-carboxymethyl daidzein conjugated to N-t-boc-hexylenediamine; 0.3 μM | Sorafenib; 20 μg/ml (43 μM) | Cultured human papillary thyroid carcinoma cells | $[^3H]$thymidine incorporation; 24h | Amplification of sorafenib-induced reduction of DNA synthesis (the strongest effect when 1,25-dihydroxyvitamin D3 included) | | [63] |
| Flavopiridol; 0.2 μM | Sorafenib; 1.25-100 μM | MCF-7 human breast cancer cells; ER+/PR+ | MTT; 72h | No synergism in cytotoxicity | | [3] |
| Flavopiridol; 0.2 μM (ratio with sorafenib of 1:6 to 1:25) | Sorafenib; 1.25-5 μM | MDA-MB-231 human breast cancer cells; triple-negative, KRAS G13D, BRAF G464V | MTT; 72h | Potentiation of sorafenib-induced cytotoxicity, synergism (CI<1) | Potentiation of sorafenib-induced apoptosis. Suppression of pRb, decrease in Mcl-1 expression | [3] |
| Flavopiridol; 0.2 μM (ratio with sorafenib of 1:6 to 1:25) | Sorafenib; 1.25-5 μM | MDA-MB-468 human breast cancer cells; overexpressing EGFR | MTT; 72h | Potentiation of sorafenib-induced cytotoxicity, synergism (CI<1) | Potentiation of sorafenib-induced apoptosis. Decrease in Mcl-1 expression | [3] |
| Flavopiridol; 0.2 μM (ratio with sorafenib of 1:6) | Sorafenib; 1.25 μM | SKBR3 human breast cancer cells; overexpressing HER2 | MTT; 72h | Potentiation of sorafenib-induced cytotoxicity, synergism (CI<1) | | [3] |
| Flavopiridol; 0.2 μM | Sorafenib; 1.25-100 μM | T47D human breast cancer cells; ER+/PR+ | MTT; 72h | No synergism in cytotoxicity | | [3] |

**Table 4.12.** (Continued)

| Flavonoid and its dosage | Sorafenib and its dosage | Biological system | Assay method and time | Effect | Mechanisms | Ref. |
|---|---|---|---|---|---|---|
| Flavopiridol; 3 mg/kg, i.p., every 2 days | Sorafenib; 30 mg/kg, p.o., every 2 days | MDA-MB-231 cells injected into the right inguinal mammary gland of mice | 28 days | Increase in tumor growth suppression. Decrease in metastatic tumor load in the lungs | Decrease in p-Erk, pRb and Mcl-1 levels. Reduction of CD31 expression | [3] |

inhibition of Akt and ERK phosphorylation and inducing apoptotic death [75]. While sorafenib acts by blocking Raf/MEK/ERK signaling, it does not affect PI3K/Akt pathway, showing that constitutive activation of Akt might contribute to acquired drug resistance and poor prognosis [9, 75]. Poor survival of HCC patients has been related also to the higher expression of antiapoptotic proteins XIAP, Mcl-1 and c-FLIP [75]. Thus, amentoflavone might serve as a potential candidate for sorafenib sensitizer to overcome resistance and enhance therapeutic responses to sorafenib. Another common flavone, chrysin (25 μM), augmented cytotoxicity and antitumor activity of sorafenib in three human HCC cell lines (Hep3B, HepG2 and Huh-7), with the mechanisms involving blockage of BCRP/ABCG2 efflux transporter activity, preventing recovery of ERK1/2 phosphorylation from inhibition by the drug. These data clearly indicate that BCRP/ABCG2 could be used as a potential biomarker for prediction of sorafenib sensitivity in HCC [9]. Moreover, the enhanced inhibition of cellular viability of Hep3B and HepG2 lines by combined treatment with sorafenib and chrysin was found to be associated also with the ability of chrysin to trigger sustained phosphorylation of ERK1/2 [57]. In addition, the presence of monomethylated flavone wogonin (10-40 μM) in sorafenib treatment resulted in synergistic cytotoxicity in several human HCC lines (Bel-7402, Hep3B, HepG2, SMMC-7721), with suppression of sorafenib-induced cytoprotective autophagy and potentiation of apoptotic death in Bel-7402 cells. Wogonin might be therefore another suitable candidate for increasing therapeutic efficacy of sorafenib in HCC, warranting further *in vitro* and *in vivo* studies [59]. Furthermore, combination of sorafenib and polymethoxylated flavone nobiletin (10 μM, 20 μM) resulted in a synergistic growth inhibition and apoptotic death in human metastatic prostate cancer cells PC-3, arresting also the cell cycle progression at G0/G1 phase. At the same time, nobiletin reduced sorafenib-induced toxicity in human umbilical vein endothelial cells (HUVECs), indicating that this combination might be useful also for the management of metastatic prostate cancer; especially considering the fact that the current treatment options for metastatic prostate cancer after the failure of chemotherapy are very limited [6].

Combinations of sorafenib with several flavonol-type phytochemicals have also been studied in different preclinical cancer models. Specifically, methylated flavonol rhamnetin (3 μM) enhanced antiproliferative, anticlonogenic and proapoptotic, but also antimigratory and antiinvasive activities of sorafenib in human HCC line HepG2, through miR-34a-mediated inhibition of Notch-1 pathway. Treatment with rhamnetin potentiated sorafenib-induced suppression of tumor growth also in HepG2 xenografts-bearing mice, accompanied by an increase in miR-34a and decrease in Notch-1 expression in malignant tissues. Moreover, addition of rhamnetin to the drug-resistant subline HepG2/ADR not only modulated miR-34a/Notch-1 pathway, but reduced also BCRP and P-gp expression, thereby increasing the susceptibility of HCC cells to sorafenib. Sorafenib cytotoxicity was similarly potentiated in two other human HCC lines, L-02 and MHCC-97L, by the presence of rhamnetin [54]. In addition, rhamnetin (1 μM) sensitized HepG2 and MHCC97-H cells to antiproliferative, antimigratory and antiinvasive effects of sorafenib also by increasing miR-148a level, followed by suppression of pregnane X receptor (PXR) activation and decrease in downstream drug resistance- and drug metabolism-related genes (P-gp and CYP3A4). This elevation of tumor suppressive miR-148a expression by rhamnetin was p53-dependent, occurring through repression of sirtuin 1 (Sirt1) activation to enhance P53 acetylation. No effects on PXR pathway were indeed observed in p53-deficient human HCC cells Huh7. Rhamnetin was further able to augment sorafenib-induced anticancer action in nude mice implanted with HepG2 or MHCC97-H cells, leading to tumors with smaller volumes and weights, by suppressing PXR activation. In this context, it is important to underline that both the median time to progression as well as overall survival were found to be significantly longer in sorafenib-treated advanced HCC patients with high miR-148a levels as compared to the low-miR-148a group [73]. Therefore, rhamnetin may provide a good basis for developing a novel sensitizer for sorafenib therapy to improve the treatment outcomes of HCC patients. Another common flavonol kaempferol (2.5 μM) could enhance sorafenib-induced cytotoxicity in both human HCC cells HepG2 as well as murine hepatoma cells N1S1 [67]. Likewise, the naturally abundant flavonol quercetin (1-50 μM) increased the susceptibility of HepG2 cells to sorafenib, applied either as free mixture of dual agents or co-loaded with sorafenib into lipid-coated PLGA nanoparticles. This sensitizing effect was further verified also in HepG2 xenografts-bearing nude mice, but the molecular mechanisms involved were remained elusive [65]. Moreover, quercetin (25 μM) was found to potentiate anticancer action of sorafenib also in two human papillary thyroid cancer lines, K1 and BCPAP, by suppressing cell proliferation, adhesion and migration through reduction of the EMT process, manifesting as a significant increase in E-cadherin and decrease in N-cadherin expression [62]. Quercetin (30 μM, 50 μM) augmented sorafenib-induced programmed cell death also in human malignant glioma lines MOGGCCM and T98G, with specifically suppressing the drug-induced autophagy in favor of intrinsic apoptosis in glioblastoma multiforme cells T98G [56]. These data clearly show that the combination of sorafenib and quercetin may provide a novel approach for overcoming sorafenib resistance and lowering effective drug doses in not only HCC but also some other tumor types. Further mechanistic studies both *in vitro* as well as *in vivo* models are therefore highly needed. Very attractive preclinical results have been reported also for combining multikinase inhibitor sorafenib with flavonol fisetin to enhance therapeutic responses. In detail, fisetin (20 μM) was found to synergistically increase the growth inhibitory, anticlonogenic and proapoptotic effects of sorafenib in several BRAF-mutated human malignant melanoma lines (A375, RPMI-7951, SK-MEL-28), through dual suppression of MEK/ERK and PI3K/AKT/mTOR signaling cascades in A375 and SK-MEL-28 cells [58]. As constitutively activated MAPK pathway has been associated with increased melanoma progression and activated (mutated) BRAF can propagate signals by phosphorylating MEK1/2 and ERK1/2 proteins, reduction of this pathway is critical for treatment of melanoma. However, MAPK pathway further cooperates with PI3K signaling in promoting melanoma initiation and progression, indicating that an efficient anti-melanoma strategy should simultaneously target both of these signaling pathways. In melanoma tissues, the presence of BRAF mutation is indeed often accompanied with the downregulation of PTEN, a negative regulator of PI3K signaling. Inactivation of PTEN has been actually observed in about 10-30% of late-stage melanomas, whereas overexpression of AKT as the PI3K downstream effector was found in even 50-75% of melanoma cases [55, 58]. Besides promising *in vitro* findings, combined treatment with sorafenib and fisetin led to a significant increase in tumor growth inhibition also in athymic nude mice harboring A375 or SK-MEL-28 xenografts as compared to the respective monotherapies, by augmenting antiproliferative, proapoptotic and antiangiogenic activities via repression of MEK/ERK and PI3K/AKT/mTOR pathways. In doing so, the combination therapy suppressed the growth of not only developing tumors but also pre-existing, established neoplasms [58]. Moreover, fisetin (10 μM, 20 μM) could potentiate also sorafenib-induced inhibition of migration and invasion through suppression of the EMT process (the cadherin switch) in both BRAF-mutated human malignant melanoma lines (A375 and SK-MEL-28) as well as A375 and SK-MEL-28 xenografts-bearing nude mice, thereby essentially contributing to the antimetastatic potential of combination therapy. Cotreatment of intravenous A375 melanoma model in mice with sorafenib and fisetin indeed induced a significantly greater decrease in pulmonary metastases formation and progression as compared to the antimetastatic effect of sorafenib alone, resulting in almost a halt in the progression of lung metastases [55]. Therefore, it is highly possible that combination of sorafenib and fisetin may represent a potential novel strategy for future treatment of patients with malignant melanoma, definitely requiring urgent initiation of clinical trials. In addition, besides melanoma, fisetin (40 μM) was shown to augment antitumor responses to sorafenib also in human cervical cancer cells HeLa, leading to suppression of cellular viability and augmentation of apoptosis through both intrinsic (mitochondria-mediated) as well as extrinsic (death receptor-dependent) pathways. Combined treatment with sorafenib and fisetin enhanced tumor growth inhibition also in HeLa xenografts-bearing nude mice, potentiating antiproliferative and proapoptotic properties of sorafenib, and resulting in tumors with remarkably smaller volume and weight [60]. Addition of fisetin to sorafenib treatment might be therefore attractive for improving the therapeutic efficacy in management of not only malignant melanomas, but also cervical carcinomas.

The potential role of isoflavones on antitumor efficacy of sorafenib has also been investigated in several preclinical studies. As a result, biochanin A was shown to increase antiproliferative and cytotoxic activities of sorafenib in several human HCC lines (HepG2, Huh-7, SNU449). Combined treatment of HepG2 cells with sorafenib and biochanin A led to both strengthening of the cell cycle arrest at pre-G phase as well as enhancement of apoptotic death via mitochondrial pathway as compared to sorafenib monotherapy [74]. However, pretreatment of HepG2 and Huh7 cells with the soy isoflavone genistein (1 μM, 10 μM) for 48h, followed by the treatment with sorafenib for further 16h, unexpectedly resulted in a significant reduction of the drug therapeutic efficacy and enhanced resistance to antitumor action of sorafenib. This undesired effect was accompanied by increase in the expression and activity of P-gp and MRP2 efflux transporters by genistein, modulated through downregulation of tumor suppressive miR-379 and upregulation of nuclear receptor PXR. Further *in vivo* studies are warranted to validate the translational power of these results in experimental animals, before making any extrapolating conclusions concerning the intake of genistein-rich soy products or dietary supplements prior to sorafenib therapy against HCC [71]. Unlike the data from HCC lines, cotreatment of primary human papillary thyroid cancer cells with sorafenib and genistein (50 μM) led to a synergistic decrease in cellular proliferation, paralleled by no loss of DNA integrity [76]. Likewise, combined treatment with sorafenib and genistein (25 μM) led to a synergistic decrease in cell viability in two human malignant neuroblastoma lines, SH-SY5Y and SK-N-DZ. This sensitizing effect was achieved via modulation of the cell cycle progression, promotion of both intrinsic and extrinsic apoptosis, and suppression of angiogenic and cell survival pathways. Malignant neuroblastoma is known as a highly vascularized tumor, whereas the significant repression of VEGF and FGF-2 expression levels by combination treatment could not only block tumor angiogenesis but also destroy tumor vessels. Combined therapy suppressed also the activation of Akt and its downstream survival factor NF-κB in both neuroblastoma lines, helping induction of apoptotic death. Therefore, combining sorafenib with genistein could present a novel promising strategy for improving therapeutic outcomes of this devastating childhood malignancy [77].

Milk thistle-derived flavonolignan silibinin (100 μM) was found to potentiate sorafenib-induced suppression of cell growth and colony formation in several human HCC lines (Huh7, Huh-BAT, PLC/PRF5, SNU761) [49]. Silibinin (100 μM, 200 μM) synergistically enhanced antiproliferative and cytotoxic properties of sorafenib also in many other human HCC lines (Bel-7404, HepG2, SMMC-7721, MHCC97L), verifying the great promise of this natural agent against hepatomas. Combined treatment of Bel-7404 cells with sorafenib and silibinin resulted in suppression of STAT3, AKT, ERK and p38 MAPK pathways, leading to decrease in clonogenicity and synergistic increase in apoptosis. Moreover, addition of silibinin enhanced also sorafenib-induced inhibition of formation and self-renewal of cancer stem cells (CSCs), observed in both human HCC lines Bel-7404 and Huh7 and murine HCC line Hepa 1-6, by downregulating different stemness-related proteins including Krueppel-like factor 4 (Klf4), β-catenin, CD133, CD13 and EpCAM. These promising *in vitro* results were further translated to *in vivo* HCC subcutaneous transplantation model, revealing a significant increase in tumor growth inhibition in Bel-7404 xenografts-bearing nude mice by cotreatment with sorafenib and silibinin as compared to sorafenib alone-treated animals. This sensitizing effect was accompanied by reduced proportion of proliferative cells and increased proportion of apoptotic cells in the malignant tissues, achieved through deactivation of STAT3 and ERK and inhibition of tumor cell stemness [61]. These promising findings may contribute to development of more effective clinical strategies for HCC therapy in future, by combining multikinase inhibitor sorafenib with plant-derived flavonoid-type agent silibinin, to improve treatment outcome, reduce cancer recurrence, decrease adverse side effects and overcome drug resistance.

A few chalcone-type natural agents have also been tested in combination with sorafenib in preclinical models of HCC. As a result, licochalcone A (10 μM) was found to potentiate antimigratory and antiinvasive activities of sorafenib in human HCC lines Huh-7 and SK-Hep-1, with no significant impact on cellular viability or growth arrest. This invasive motility-limiting action was accompanied by downregulation of MEK4/JNK pathway in HCC cells. Also, combination treatment of licochalcone A and sorafenib led to an enhanced suppression of pulmonary metastasis in SK-Hep-1 intravenous tumor model in nude mice, inducing a remarkably lower number of lung nodules as compared to sorafenib monotherapy, while exerting no effect on the body weight of mice [68]. Another natural chalcone, phloretin, augmented growth inhibitory and proapoptotic properties of sorafenib in human HCC lines Hep3B2.1-7, HepG2 and SK-Hep1, but also in sorafenib-resistant sublines HepG2$^{SR}$ and Huh7$^{SR}$. Combined treatment of these cells with sorafenib and phloretin led to a significant increase in tumor suppressor SHP-1 tyrosine phosphatase activity, further suppressing STAT3 pathway and its downstream antiapoptotic proteins (Mcl-1, survivin), thereby promoting apoptosis and reversing sorafenib resistance. Enhanced STAT3 activity has been indeed related to severe resistance to sorafenib therapy and poor prognosis in HCC patients. Moreover, phloretin potentiated sorafenib-induced inhibition of tumor growth also in nude mice subcutaneously implanted with HepG2, SK-Hep1, HepG2$^{SR}$ or Huh7$^{SR}$ cells, by regulating the SHP-1/STAT3 signaling pathway and resulting in antiproliferative, proapoptotic and antiangiogenic changes within the malignant tissues, with no apparent clinical signs of toxicity. Combination of sorafenib and phloretin might therefore hold a great promise for further improvement of therapeutic efficacy and treatment outcomes in HCC patients [69].

In addition to naturally occurring flavonoids, the effect of some semisynthetic flavonoid-type compounds has also been investigated in combination with sorafenib in preclinical cancer models. Specifically, a synthetic analog of the flavone chrysin, 8-bromo-7-methoxychrysin (5 μM), enhanced sorafenib-induced inhibition of self-renewal capacity and the expression of stemness markers (CD133, CD44, ALDH1) in sphere-forming cells derived from human HCC line SMMC-7721. Combined treatment of these liver cancer stem-like cells with sorafenib and chrysin analog led to a greater apoptosis than sorafenib treatment alone, with potentiating also antimigratory and antiinvasive properties of the drug through inhibition of the EMT process (cadherin switch). Moreover, the presence of 8-bromo-7-methoxychrysin exerted a significant antagonistic effect on sorafenib-upregulated protein expression and DNA binding activity of NF-κB, thereby suppressing stemness characteristics, overcoming sorafenib resistance and improving therapeutic effects [72]. Another synthetic flavonoid derivative, 7-(O)-carboxymethyl daidzein conjugated to N-t-boc-hexylenediamine (0.3 μM), potentiated sorafenib-induced decrease in DNA synthesis in human papillary thyroid carcinoma cells, whereas the strongest effect was observed when 1,25-dihydroxyvitamin D3 (calcitriol, 2.5 nM) was additionally included. This triple combination made it possible to use a ten-fold lower dose of sorafenib for receiving therapeutic effects observed with sorafenib alone, being achieved, at least in part, via increase in modulation of ERβ signaling by daidzein derivative after enhancement of ERβ expression by calcitriol. If these findings will be further reproduced *in vivo* settings, the dosage of sorafenib required for treatment of metastatic differentiated thyroid cancer might be reduced by the addition of low doses of synthetic daidzein analog and calcitriol [63]. Last but not least, semisynthetic flavonoid-type compound flavopiridol (0.2 μM) synergistically augmented sorafenib-induced cytotoxicity and apoptotic death in human breast cancer cells with constitutively active Ras/Raf/MEK/ERK signaling related to EGFR overexpression (MDA-MB-468), HER2 overexpression (SKBR3) or RAS/RAF mutations (MDA-MB-231), but revealed no synergistic interactions in hormone-dependent lines MCF-7 and T47D. Combination of sorafenib and flavopiridol enhanced tumor growth suppression also in MDA-MB-231 orthotopic xenograft-bearing mice, reducing not only primary tumor growth rates but also metastatic tumor burden in the lungs, as compared to the treatment with either agent alone. This increased antitumor action was accompanied by significant decrease in p-ERK, pRb and Mcl-1 levels in malignant tissues, besides reducing also the angiogenic marker CD31 expression. Therefore, combination of sorafenib and flavopiridol may provide an additional therapeutic option for the treatment of advanced HER2-positive, EGFR-overexpressing or RAS/RAF mutant breast tumors [3].

Altogether, these findings may help to develop novel more efficient treatment strategies for patients with sorafenib-refractory tumors by applying this multikinase inhibitor in proper combinations with plant-derived flavonoids, acting through targeting different cellular mechanisms for overcoming drug resistance (Figure 4.5). In this regard, a great advantage of flavonoids is their ability to simultaneously affect multiple cellular events involved in decrease in drug efficacy. Therefore, these natural agents definitely merit further preclinical studies to unravel molecular mechanisms under their sensitizing activities, but also investigations at clinical level for applying as potential adjuvant agents in sorafenib-based treatment regimens.

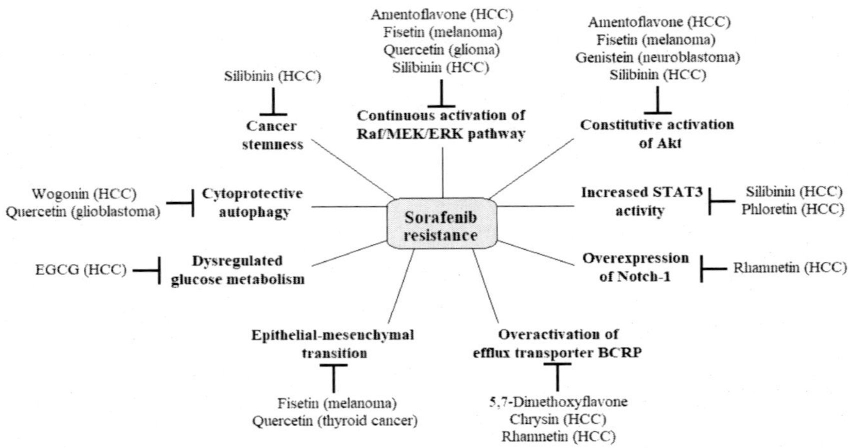


**Figure 4.5.** Overcoming sorafenib resistance and augmenting its antitumor action by flavonoids.

### *4.2.1.7. Sunitinib*

Sunitinib (Sutent) is an orally administered small-molecule multitargeted receptor tyrosine kinase (RTK) inhibitor that induces antiangiogenic and proapoptotic activities through targeting vascular endothelial growth factor receptors (VEGFRs) 1-3, platelet-derived growth factor receptors (PDGFRs) α and β, and stem cell growth factor receptor (KIT) [10, 78-80] (Figure 4.1). Sunitinib is approved by the FDA for treatment of advanced renal cell carcinoma and gastrointestinal stromal tumors, but also for unresectable or metastatic neuroendocrine cancers in the pancreas [10, 79-81]. Renal cell carcinoma is the most common type of adult kidney cancer accounting for 80-85% of all cases, being by far the most lethal urologic malignancy [79, 80]. About 20-30% of renal cell carcinoma patients have metastatic disease already at diagnosis, whereas up to 30% of patients presented with localized tumor at diagnosis develop metastases [80]. In 2020, there were more than 430,000 new kidney cancer cases detected worldwide with almost 180,000 cancer-related deaths [31]. In addition, sunitinib is being investigated for its potential therapeutic use also against other tumors. However, treatment with sunitinib alone may not be sufficient due to the feedback activation of many cellular signaling cascades and compensatory mechanisms, leading to acquired resistance to the drug during treatment course and unsatisfactory response rates of patients [53, 78, 80]. Moreover, sunitinib therapy is often required to be reduced in its dosage or even discontinued because of severe systemic side effects, including fatigue, nausea, diarrhea, anorexia, hypertension, hand-foot syndrome and stomatitis [79, 80]. To overcome these limitations, therapeutic strategies targeting the signaling pathways involved in feedback compensatory mechanisms have been investigated, with the aim to surpass acquired resistance to sunitinib, lower its therapeutic doses and thereby improve clinical outcomes [78, 80]. Plant-derived flavonoids as commonly non-toxic natural agents with a wide range of anticancer bioactivities might be ideal candidates as adjuvants for sunitinib therapy, definitely deserving further attention.

*4.2.1.7.1. Effects of Flavonoids on Pharmacokinetics of Sunitinib*

To date, the only natural flavonoid studied concerning its potential effects on pharmacokinetic profile of sunitinib has been the green tea flavanol EGCG. These results, summarized in Table 4.13, clearly indicate that EGCG can affect the bioavailability of this multikinase inhibitor; however, in an unexpected way. Proceeding from an interesting phenomenon that frequent green tea drinking could intervene in the symptom control of metastatic renal cell carcinoma in a patient under sunitinib treatment, an *in vivo* pharmacokinetic study was designed. As a result, cotreatment of male rats with sunitinib and EGCG led to a significant decrease in the drug bioavailability, reducing the plasma concentrations of sunitinib (both $C_{max}$ and $AUC_{0\text{-}\infty}$). This undesired effect was accompanied by a complex formation between EGCG and sunitinib at concurrent administration, confirmed in the *in vitro* study showing forming of a precipitate after mixing the solutions of sunitinib and EGCG. Sticky semisolid contents were produced also in the stomachs of mice following to co-administration of sunitinib and EGCG. On the other hand, pharmacokinetic parameters of the drug were not affected by EGCG, when a week-long daily administration of this catechin was stopped 12h before sunitinib administration or single EGCG dosage was administered 8h or 4h before the drug, showing that concurrent treatment of both agents is needed for the complex formation [10]. These data unambiguously show that EGCG can reduce the bioavailability of sunitinib and antagonize antitumor effects of the drug when administered simultaneously, for what reason drinking of green tea or

**Table 4.13.** Effects of flavonoids on pharmacokinetic parameters of sunitinib (highlighted rows indicate undesired negative effects on anticancer efficacy)

| Flavonoid and its dosage | Sunitinib and its dosage | Biological system | Effects | Purported mechanism | Ref. |
|---|---|---|---|---|---|
| FLAVANOLS | | | | | |
| EGCG; 100 mg/kg, via direct administration into the stomach | Sunitinib; 30 mg/kg, via direct administration into the stomach, immediately following EGCG | Male Sprague-Dawley rats, 7 w-old | Reduction of sunitinib bioavailability, decrease in $AUC_{0-\infty}$ (51.5%) and $C_{max}$ (47.7%) of plasma sunitinib. (No effect on pharmacokinetics of sunitinib when EGCG was added daily for 7 days until 12h before applying sunitinib or when single dose of EGCG was administered 8h or 4h before sunitinib) | Formation of complex between EGCG and sunitinib (by co-administration) | [10] |

taking EGCG-containing dietary supplements by patients receiving sunitinib therapy should be avoided. Possible pharmacokinetic interactions between sunitinib and additional green tea components as well as other plant-derived flavonoids are needed to be elucidated in future studies.

*4.2.1.7.2. Effects of Flavonoids on Anticancer Potential of Sunitinib*

A few recently reported preclinical studies have been focused on clarifying the possible effects of EGCG on antitumor action of sunitinib, avoiding the direct chemical interaction between these two agents by loading them into nanoparticles or applying sequential administration schedules. The results of these as well as other studies about flavonoids-sunitinib co-effects on preclinical cancer models are presented in Table 4.14 and discussed more closely below.

Specifically, sunitinib-loaded micellar nanocomplex that was formed using PEG-conjugated EGCG as a carrier revealed remarkably enhanced tumor growth inhibitory and proapoptotic effects than sunitinib alone-loaded polymeric micelles in nude mice implanted with ACHN or A498 human renal cell carcinoma (RCC) xenografts. Such improved anticancer efficacy was attributed to the synergy between sunitinib and PEG-EGCG, besides tumor-targeted delivery and greater accumulation of nanocomplex in the xenografts [79]. Also, treatment of human breast cancer cells MCF-7 or human NSCLC lines H460 and H1975 with sunitinib for 24h, followed by replacement of the culture medium and addition of EGCG (20 μM, 50 μM) for additional 12h, led to a synergistic increase in cell growth inhibition, accompanied by augmentation of sunitinib-induced decrease in VEGF secretion. Mechanistically, in H460 cells, this sequential combination suppressed the upregulation of insulin receptor substrate-1 (IRS1) and activation of ERK1/2, induced by exposure to sunitinib as a classical feedback compensatory mechanism regulated by PI3K/AKT/mTOR/S6K cascade inhibition. These superior antitumor effects were further reproduced also in nude mice harboring MCF-7 or H460 xenografts, by adding EGCG at 4h after sunitinib treatment, resulting in a greater tumor shrinkage and antiangiogenic action than with sunitinib alone, via suppression of the drug-induced IRS1/ERK1/2 signaling. Most importantly, this treatment approach was well tolerated by the mice, as no apparent signs of toxicity were detected [78]. Thus, administration of EGCG in a proper sequential regimen with sunitinib therapy, to avoid direct chemical interaction between these two agents, might represent a promising new strategy for overcoming sunitinib resistance and improving therapeutic outcomes in clinical practice.

**Table 4.14.** Effects of flavonoids on anticancer action of sunitinib

| Flavonoid and its dosage | Sunitinib and its dosage | Biological system | Assay method and time | Effect | Mechanisms | Ref. |
|---|---|---|---|---|---|---|
| FLAVANOLS | | | | | | |
| EGCG (sunitinib-loaded micellar nanocomplex formed using PEG-conjugated EGCG); 33 mg/kg (PEG-EGCG), i.v., twice per week | Sunitinib (sunitinib-loaded micellar nanocomplex formed using PEG-conjugated EGCG); 5 mg/kg (equivalent sunitinib), i.v., twice per week | A498 human RCC cells (with Matrigel) inoculated s.c. in the right flank of 5-6 w-old female athymic nude mice | 35 days | Inhibition of tumor growth | Increase in induction of apoptosis and inhibition of proliferation (compared to sunitinib alone-loaded polymeric micelles) | [79] |
| EGCG (sunitinib-loaded micellar nanocomplex formed using PEG-conjugated EGCG); 33 mg/kg (PEG-EGCG), i.v., twice per week | Sunitinib (sunitinib-loaded micellar nanocomplex formed using PEG-conjugated EGCG); 5 mg/kg (equivalent sunitinib), i.v., twice per week | ACHN human RCC cells (with Matrigel) inoculated s.c. in the right flank of 5-6 w-old female athymic nude mice | 35 days | Synergistic inhibition of tumor growth (CI<1, DRI>1) | Increase in induction of apoptosis and inhibition of proliferation (compared to sunitinib alone-loaded polymeric micelles) | [79] |
| EGCG; 20, 50 μM | Sunitinib; 3 μM | MCF-7 human breast cancer cells | MTT; 24h sunitinib followed by 12h EGCG treatment | Synergistic increase in cell growth inhibition (CI<1) | Potentiation of sunitinib-induced decrease in VEGF secretion | [78] |
| EGCG; 50 mg/kg, i.p., once daily, five times per week, 4h after sunitinib | Sunitinib; 40 mg/kg, p.o., daily treatment five times per week | MCF-7 cells injected s.c. in the right flank of female nude mice | 24 days | Increase in antitumor effect of sunitinib; increase in tumor shrinkage, decrease in tumor volume | Potentiation of sunitinib-induced decrease in VEGF secretion and MVD (CD31). Suppression of sunitinib-upregulated IRS1 and p-ERK expression | [78] |

| Flavonoid and its dosage | Sunitinib and its dosage | Biological system | Assay method and time | Effect | Mechanisms | Ref. |
|---|---|---|---|---|---|---|
| EGCG; 10-50 μM | Sunitinib; 3 μM | H460 human NSCLC cells | MTT; 24h sunitinib followed by 12h EGCG treatment | Synergistic increase in cell growth inhibition (CI<1) | Potentiation of sunitinib-induced decrease in VEGF secretion. Inhibition of sunitinib-induced IRS1 upregulation and ERK1/2 activation | [78] |
| EGCG; 20, 50 μM | Sunitinib; 3 μM | H1975 human NSCLC cells | MTT; 24h sunitinib followed by 12h EGCG treatment | Synergistic increase in cell growth inhibition (CI<1) | Potentiation of sunitinib-induced decrease in VEGF secretion | [78] |
| EGCG; 50 mg/kg, i.p., once daily, five times per week, 4h after sunitinib | Sunitinib; 40 mg/kg, p.o., daily treatment five times per week | H460 cells injected s.c. in the right flank of female nude mice | 24 days | Increase in antitumor effect of sunitinib; increase in tumor shrinkage, decrease in tumor volume | Potentiation of sunitinib-induced decrease in VEGF secretion and MVD (CD31) | [78] |
| FLAVONES | | | | | | |
| Hispidulin; 25 μM | Sunitinib; 4 μM | 786-0 human RCC cells | MTT; 48h | Increase in sunitinib-induced decrease in cell viability, sensitization to sunitinib | Increase in G0/G1, decrease in G2 phase cell cycle arrest; increase in apoptosis (activation of caspase-3, cleavage of PARP, decrease in Bcl-2 and survivin). Inhibition of Stat3 signaling | [80] |

**Table 4.14.** (Continued)

| Flavonoid and its dosage | Sunitinib and its dosage | Biological system | Assay method and time | Effect | Mechanisms | Ref. |
|---|---|---|---|---|---|---|
| Hispidulin; 25 μM | Sunitinib; 4 μM | Caki-1 human RCC cells | MTT; 48h | Increase in sunitinib-induced decrease in cell viability, sensitization to sunitinib | Increase in G0/G1, decrease in G2 phase cell cycle arrest; increase in apoptosis (activation of caspase-3, cleavage of PARP, decrease in Bcl-2 and survivin). Inhibition of Stat3 signaling | [80] |
| Hispidulin; 20 mg/kg/day | Sunitinib; 20 mg/kg/day | Caki-1 cells injected s.c. into 8 w-old male athymic BALB/c nu/nu mice | 4 weeks | Potentiation of antitumor effect of sunitinib, decrease in tumor size | Decrease in Ki67 and CD31 labeling | [80] |
| ISOFLAVONES | | | | | | |
| Formononetin; 100 mg/kg/day, i.g. | Sunitinib; 80 mg/kg/day | MDA-MB-231 human breast cancer cells implanted s.c. into female BALB/c nude mice | 24 days | Increase in sunitinib-induced tumor growth inhibition | Blocking of FGFR2 signaling by formononetin | [53] |

Modulation of antitumor efficacy of sunitinib was explored also by inclusion of a natural monomethylated flavone, hispidulin (25 μM), in the treatment protocol of human RCC lines 786-0 and Caki-1. As a result, combination therapy with sunitinib and hispidulin led to a superior decrease in cellular viability, accompanied by enhanced arrest of cell cycle progression in G0/G1 phase and promotion of apoptotic death, achieved through inhibition of Stat3 signaling pathway. Constitutively activated Stat3 has been indeed found to be an independent prognostic indicator for RCC. Moreover, sensitization to sunitinib antitumor efficacy by hispidulin was verified also in Caki-1 xenografts-bearing nude mice, resulting in smaller tumors with reduced expression of proliferative and angiogenic biomarkers, while revealing no obvious toxicities. Combining sunitinib and hispidulin might therefore present a novel therapeutic option for patients with RCC, definitely warranting initiation of clinical trials [80]. Furthermore, sunitinib-induced tumor growth inhibition was enhanced also by isoflavone formononetin in nude mice harboring MDA-MB-231 xenografts, at least in part, by augmenting suppression of tumor angiogenesis via blocking beside sunitinib-dependent VEGFR2 signaling also FGFR2-mediated pathways by formononetin [53].

Much more preclinical studies are required to elucidate the possible role of structurally different natural flavonoids on antitumor action of sunitinib in models of not only renal cell carcinoma, but also gastrointestinal stromal tumor and pancreatic neuroendocrine tumor, for which the sunitinib-based therapy is currently approved. These studies could not only identify potential adjuvant agents for enhancing the antitumor efficacy of sunitinib, but may establish also flavonoid-sunitinib combinations with undesired interactions, thereby helping to avoid impairment of therapeutic outcomes.

- **Inhibitors with an intracellular target**

#### *4.2.1.8. Crizotinib*

Crizotinib (Xalkori) is an orally administered multitargeting tyrosine kinase inhibitor (TKI) with activity against anaplastic lymphoma kinase (ALK), c-MET and ROS1 [82, 83] (Figure 4.1). This drug is approved by the FDA for treatment of locally advanced or metastatic non-small cell lung cancer (NSCLC) patients whose tumors are ALK-positive or ROS1-positive, and for pediatric and young adult patients with relapsed or refractory systemic anaplastic large cell lymphoma that is ALK-positive [82]. About 2-5% of NSCLC tumors present a chromosomal rearrangement that generates a fusion gene between ALK and echinoderm microtubule-associated protein-like 4 (EML4), leading to constitutive kinase activity that contributes to cancer growth and progression [82]. As the kinase activity of the fusion protein is suppressed by crizotinib, patients with ALK-EML4 translocation usually receive clinical benefit from targeted therapy directed to ALK [82]. Crizotinib has been indeed shown to significantly prolong the median progression-free survival and improve response rates in advanced NSCLC patients with ALK rearrangement, as compared to standard chemotherapy [82]. However, despite impressive responses, systemic acquired resistance invariably develops during the treatment course, remaining the major limitation to prolonged clinical efficacy to crizotinib in NSCLC patients [82]. Although the main reason of acquired resistance to crizotinib has been supposed to be formation of tyrosine kinase mutations in ALK, other oncogene kinases might also be additionally activated to circumvent the inhibition of ALK phosphorylation by crizotinib [82]. Therefore, identification of non-toxic adjuvant agents which can contribute to overcoming acquired resistance to crizotinib therapy and thereby prolong the beneficial effects of this ALK-targeted drug is highly needed.

*4.2.1.8.1. Effects of Flavonoids on Anticancer Potential of Crizotinib*

A couple of flavonoids have been tested in respect to their possible effects on antitumor action of crizotinib in some preclinical cancer models. These findings are summarized in Table 4.15 and discussed more closely as follows.

Based on a recent report, the milk thistle-derived flavonolignan silibinin (50 μM) could significantly augment crizotinib-induced suppression of cell viability and thereby reverse acquired resistance in ALK-translocated crizotinib-refractory NSCLC cells that lack mutations in the kinase domain of ALK (H3122/CR), through suppression of the STAT3 signaling. STAT3 activity was indeed shown to be about three-fold higher in crizotinib-resistant H3122/CR cells as compared to the parent crizotinib-sensitive cells (H3122). Moreover, in long-term co-exposure experiments, silibinin promoted both cytostatic and cytotoxic effects of the drug in crizotinib-refractory H3122/CR cells, but abolished also the late proliferative burst of H3122 cells occurring despite the presence of crizotinib, indicating a rapid adaption of ALK-rearranged cells to crizotinib exposure. Silibinin further suppressed also the immune escape in ALK-positive NSCLC cells,

**Table 4.15.** Effects of flavonoids on anticancer action of crizotinib

| Flavonoid and its dosage | Crizotinib and its dosage | Biological system | Assay method and time | Effect | Mechanisms | Ref. |
|---|---|---|---|---|---|---|
| FLAVANOLS | | | | | | |
| EGCG; 80 μg/ml (174.5 μM) | Crizotinib; 50 μM | MG-63 human osteosarcoma cells | Apoptosis assay; 48h | Increase in antitumor effect of crizotinib | Potentiation of crizotinib-induced apoptosis, increase in G1 phase arrest. Inhibition of c-MET expression by EGCG | [83] |
| EGCG; 80 μg/ml (174.5 μM) | Crizotinib; 50 μM | U-2OS human osteosarcoma cells | Apoptosis assay; 48h | Increase in antitumor effect of crizotinib | Potentiation of crizotinib-induced apoptosis. Inhibition of c-MET expression by EGCG | [83] |
| FLAVONOLIGNANS | | | | | | |
| Silibinin; 50 μM | Crizotinib; various | H3122 human NSCLC cells; crizotinib-sensitive, harboring EML4-ALK fusion gene | MTT. Counting; 2, 4, 8 days | Non-significant 1.5-fold decrease in $IC_{50}$ of crizotinib in short-term co-exposure. Full abolishment of late proliferative burst of cells exposed to crizotinib | Inhibition of STAT3 activation. Downregulation of high baseline levels of PD-L1; decrease in EMT markers (Slug, vimentin, CD44) by silibinin | [82] |
| Silibinin; 50 μM | Crizotinib; various | H3122/CR human NSCLC cells; H3122-derived crizotinib-resistant subline with no amplifications or mutations in the kinase domain of ALK | MTT. Counting; 2, 4, 8 days | Synergistic reversal of acquired resistance to crizotinib, more than 5-fold decrease in $IC_{50}$ of crizotinib. Promotion of cytostatic and cytotoxic effects of crizotinib in long-term co-exposure | Inhibition of STAT3 activation. Decrease in upregulation of PD-L1 and EMT markers (Slug, vimentin, CD44) by silibinin | [82] |

by downregulating the high baseline levels of programmed death-ligand 1 (PD-L1) in H3122 cells and reducing the upregulation of PD-L1 expression in H3122/CR cells, accompanied by inhibition of the EMT process and decrease in mesenchymal markers. STAT3 activation seems therefore to be a novel molecular mechanism underlying the resistance to crizotinib, whereas addition of silibinin to crizotinib therapy might reverse this acquired resistance and restore the drug sensitivity in crizotinib-refractory cells. These findings could open new horizons also for the therapeutic use of silibinin as a potential immunogenic enhancer in ALK-positive NSCLC tumors. Further preclinical studies with ALK-targeted drug-resistant cell lines and animal models are definitely needed to fully comprehend the actual therapeutic power of crizotinib-silibinin combination for improving the clinical management of ALK-rearranged lung carcinomas in the future [82]. Another common natural flavonoid, the major green tea flavanol EGCG (174.5 μM), potentiated crizotinib-induced growth inhibitory and apoptotic effects in a couple of human osteosarcoma lines (MG-63 and U-2OS). This sensitization was shown to involve inhibition of c-MET expression by EGCG through upregulation of miR-1 levels [83].

Further *in vitro* studies with structurally different flavonoids are highly needed to select the most promising flavonoid-crizotinib combinations for moving into clinical trials with patients harboring ALK-rearranged tumors.

#### *4.2.1.9. Everolimus*

Everolimus (Afinitor) is an orally administered rapamycin analog, classified as an allosteric inhibitor of mTOR complex 1 (mTORC1) [84] (Figure 4.1). mTORC1 is a highly conserved intracellular serine/threonine kinase that plays a central role in pathways regulating cell growth, proliferation, survival and angiogenesis [84]. Everolimus is approved by the FDA for treatment of several tumors, including advanced renal cell carcinoma, unresectable metastatic pancreatic neuroendocrine tumor, and hormone receptor-positive HER2-negative advanced postmenopausal breast cancer [80, 84]. However, besides its clinical benefits, the use of everolimus has been associated also with several adverse reactions, including stomatitis, rash, fatigue, diarrhea, infections, myelosuppression, anemia, hyperglycemia and hypercholesterolemia, requiring either discontinuation of the treatment or reduction of the drug dosage [84]. Development of resistance to everolimus has also been characterized, initiated by different cellular mechanisms [84]. Therefore, non-toxic adjuvant agents that can sensitize malignant cells to tumoricidal action of everolimus and lower its therapeutically efficient doses, might be of great interest in improving clinical outcomes.

*4.2.1.9.1. Effects of Flavonoids on Anticancer Potential of Everolimus*
To date, the possible modulatory action only of a commonly occurring dietary flavonol quercetin has been investigated on antitumor effects of everolimus in human hormone-dependent breast cancer line MCF-7 (Table 4.16). The results of this study clearly demonstrated that quercetin (loaded into hyaluronic acid nanohydrogel) could synergistically enhance the growth inhibitory and proapoptotic activities of everolimus in breast cancer cells, being of potential importance in improving the therapeutic outcomes of breast cancer management [84].

***4.2.1.10. Vemurafenib***
Vemurafenib (Zelboraf) is an inhibitor of serine/threonine kinase B-Raf. This drug interrupts the B-Raf/MEK step in the B-Raf/MEK/ERK signaling pathway that is constitutively activated by the presence of BRAF V600E mutation [55, 58] (Figure 4.1). Vemurafenib is approved by the FDA for treatment of late-stage or unresectable melanoma with BRAF V600E mutation, leading melanoma cells to apoptosis [85]. About 60% of melanomas harbor this mutation contributing to higher proliferation and enhanced survival of melanoma cells [55, 58]. Melanoma is the most aggressive and lethal form of cutaneous malignancy, being responsible for about 75% of skin cancer deaths and remaining one of the most incurable cancerous neoplasms [55, 58, 85, 86]. This disease presents a high invasive and metastatic potential with a prominent angiogenic ability, forming metastases in many organs like the lungs, bones, liver and brain [55, 58, 85, 86]. In 2020, there were almost 325,000 new melanoma cases diagnosed worldwide, with more than 57,000 cancer-related deaths [31]. Moreover, the incidence rate of melanoma is rising with higher speed than of any other cancer type [55, 58, 85]. Although promising results have been obtained in the treatment of BRAF-mutated metastatic melanoma with Raf/MEK pathway-targeting drugs, the emergence of resistance after long-term use of vemurafenib represents a severe limitation to therapeutic efficacy, ultimately resulting in tumor relapse and progression [55, 85, 86]. Therefore, it is urgent to discover novel non-toxic adjuvant agents that could sensitize advanced melanoma cells to vemurafenib by affecting different cellular mechanisms for improving clinical outcome of antimelanoma therapy. Plant-derived polyphenolic compounds might be attractive candidates to achieve this goal.

**Table 4.16.** Effects of flavonoids on anticancer action of everolimus

| Flavonoid and its dosage | Everolimus and its dosage | Biological system | Assay method and time | Effect | Mechanisms | Ref. |
|---|---|---|---|---|---|---|
| FLAVONOLS | | | | | | |
| Quercetin (hyaluronic acid nanohydrogel of quercetin); 2 mg/ml of total product (equivalent quercetin concentration of 71.4 μM) | Everolimus; 0.05-1000 nM | MCF-7 human breast cancer cells; hormone-dependent | MTT; 24, 48, 72h | Synergistic inhibition of cell growth (CI 0.38); decrease in $IC_{50}$ of everolimus | Increase in apoptosis | [84] |

*4.2.1.10.1. Effects of Flavonoids on Anticancer Potential of Vemurafenib*
Recently, a couple of natural polymethoxylated flavonoids were tested concerning their potential impact on antitumor effects of vemurafenib in human melanoma cells A2058 harboring oncogenic BRAF V600E mutation. Unfortunately, neither centauridin (5,7-dihydroxy-3,4`,6-trimethoxyflavone, 4 μM) nor 3`,5,7-trihydroxy-3,4`,5`,6-tetrahydroxyflavone (2 μM) were able to improve vemurafenib-induced inhibition of proliferation of these highly invasive and metastatic melanoma cells [86]. However, dimeric chalcone, oxyfadichalcone C, synergistically enhanced the cell growth inhibitory and proapoptotic effects of vemurafenib in human melanoma line A375 [85] (Table 4.17). Much more studies with structurally different flavonoids are definitely needed to identify a proper adjuvant agent for improving the therapeutic effects of vemurafenib treatment and overcoming acquired resistance of melanoma cells to this mutated BRAF-targeting drug.

### 4.2.2. Influence of Flavonoids on Therapeutic Action of Pharmacological Inhibitors Prescribed in Hematology

Hematological malignancies are primary cancers occurring in the blood or blood-forming organs, i.e., bone marrow and lymphoid tissues, including leukemia, lymphoma and multiple myeloma. Leukemia or blood cancer is classified into acute lymphocytic leukemia (ALL), acute myelogenous leukemia (AML), chronic lymphocytic leukemia (CLL) and chronic myelogenous leukemia (CML), on the basis of the type of blood cells affected and the nature of malignant progression [87].

#### *4.2.2.1. Imatinib*

Imatinib (Gleevec) is an orally active tyrosine kinase inhibitor, targeting cytoplasmic Bcr-Abl fusion protein through occupation of the ATP-binding pocket in the active site of the enzyme and blocking its autophosphorylation, thereby leading to the inhibition of downstream signaling cascades and inactivation of Bcr-Abl-positive cells [88-91] (Figure 4.6). Bcr-Abl protein is encoded by the Bcr-Abl chimeric oncogene in which the amino terminal sequence of the breakpoint cluster region (Bcr) gene on chromosome 22 is fused with the second exon of the Abelson (Abl) gene on chromosome 9,

**Table 4.17.** Effects of flavonoids on anticancer action of vemurafenib in melanoma models

| Flavonoid and its dosage | Vemurafenib and its dosage | Biological system | Assay method and time | Effect | Mechanisms | Ref. |
|---|---|---|---|---|---|---|
| FLAVONOLS | | | | | | |
| 3`,5,7-Trihydroxy 3,4`,5`,6-tetramethoxyflavone; 4 μM | Vemurafenib; 1-00 μM | A2058 human melanoma cells; metastatic cells from lymph nodes, harboring BRAF V600E mutation, vemurafenib-sensitive | MTT; 72h | No improvement in vemurafenib-induced antiproliferative effect (no significant changes in $IC_{50}$ of vemurafenib) | | [86] |
| 5,7-Dihydroxy-3,4`,6-trimethoxyflavone (santin, centauridin, 3-methylbetuletol); 2 μM | Vemurafenib; 1-100 μM | A2058 human melanoma cells; metastatic cells from lymph nodes, harboring BRAF V600E mutation, vemurafenib-sensitive | MTT; 72h | No improvement in vemurafenib-induced antiproliferative effect (no significant changes in $IC_{50}$ of vemurafenib) | | [86] |
| CHALCONES (dimers) | | | | | | |
| Oxyfadichalcone C; ratio with vemurafenib of $IC_{50}$: $5xIC_{50}$ (μM: μM) | Vemurafenib | A375 human melanoma cells | MTT; 24h | Synergistic inhibition of cell growth (CI<1) | Increase in cell cycle arrest at G1 phase, enhancement of apoptosis | [85] |

constituting a shortened chromosome 22, i.e., the Philadelphia chromosome (Ph) [91-93]. This Philadelphia chromosome is observed in about 90-95% of chronic myelogenous leukemia (CML) cases, where the fusion protein Bcr-Abl constitutively activates tyrosine kinase, contributing to leukemic transformation and malignant progression with a massive influx of immature myeloid lineage cells into the circulation [87, 90, 91, 94]. Therefore, imatinib as the first-generation Bcr-Abl inhibitor is approved by the FDA for treatment of Ph-positive CML in multiple contexts of disease, including chronic phase of disease, accelerated phase of disease as well as blast crisis [95-98]. Moreover, imatinib is approved also for treatment of Ph-positive acute lymphocytic leukemia (ALL) in children [88, 97]. Inhibition of Bcr-Abl tyrosine kinase activity by imatinib results in suppression of uncontrolled cellular proliferation and survival, and facilitates the apoptotic pathways in malignant blood cells [89, 94].

| PHARMACOLOGICAL INHIBITORS PRESCRIBED IN HEMATOLOGY | |
|---|---|
| 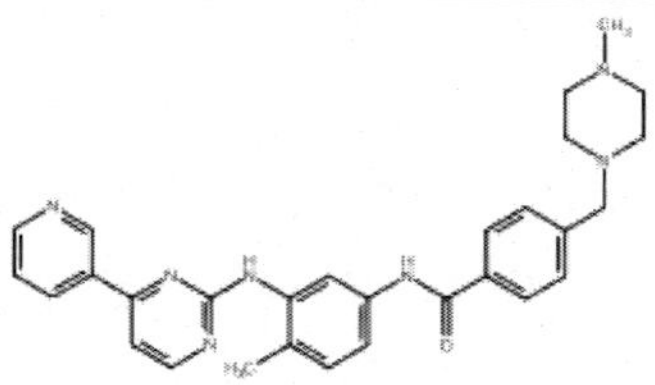 Imatinib (first generation Bcr-Abl inhibitor) | 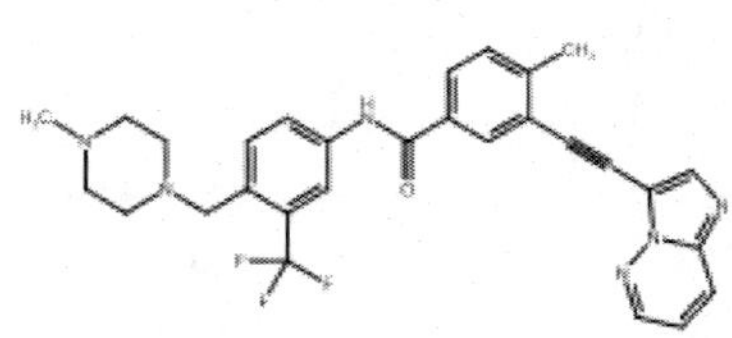 Ponatinib (third generation Bcr-Abl inhibitor) |
| 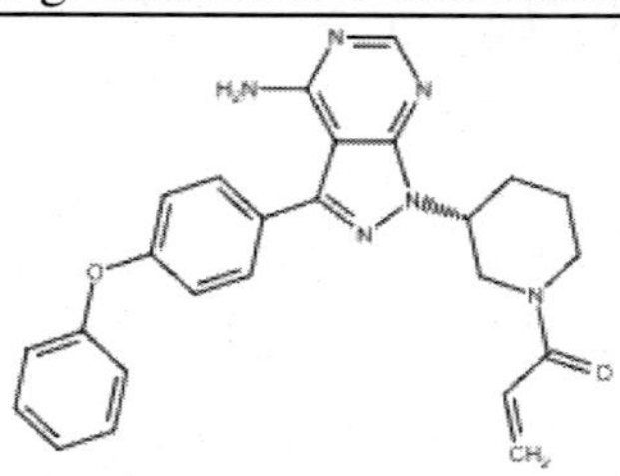 Ibrutinib (BTK inhibitor) | 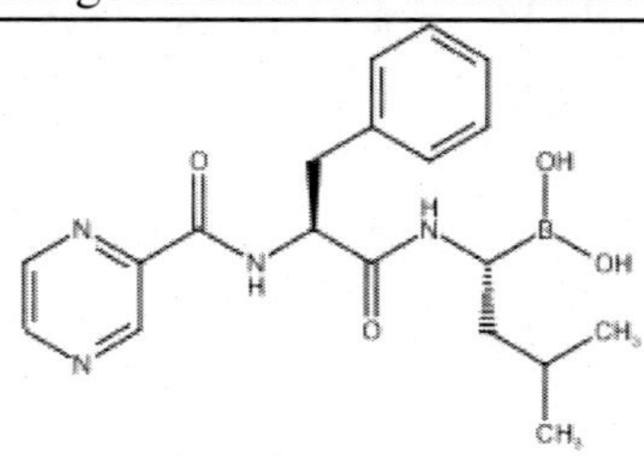 Bortezomib (proteasome inhibitor) |
| 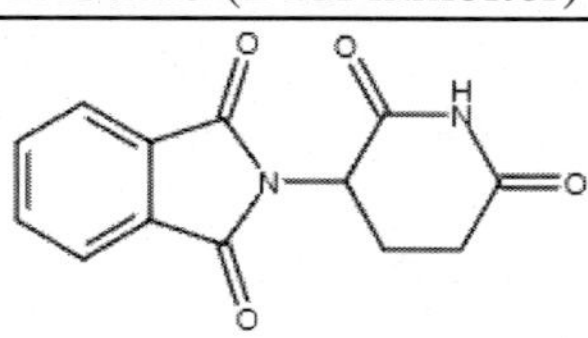 Thalidomide | 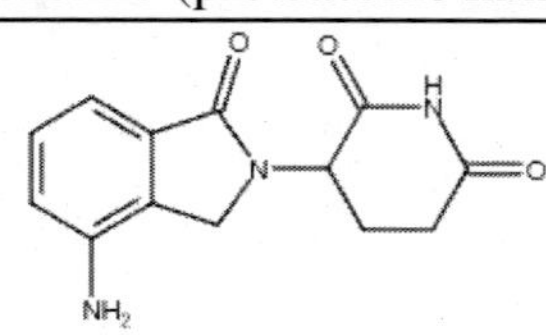 Lenalidomide |

**Figure 4.6**. Structural formulas of pharmacological inhibitors prescribed in hematology, studied in combination with flavonoids.

Although the discovery of imatinib has remarkably improved the clinical management of CML by significantly enhancing the median survival time [89, 94, 99], emergence of drug resistance over time has become a serious problem ultimately leading to disease progression [89, 91, 97, 99]. Development of resistance to imatinib has been shown to be mainly due to point mutations within the ATP-binding site and amplification of the Bcr-Abl gene, but also by overexpression of efflux transporter P-gp and activation of multiple cellular pathways supporting tumor survival, such as Stat5, MAPK and PI3K/Akt signalings [87, 89-91, 93, 94, 100, 101]. Moreover, imatinib has been found to be unable to eradicate leukemia stem cells that drive the disease relapse [90]. Accordingly, the majority of CML patients continue to present with minimal residual disease in the bone marrow microenvironment where malignant cells remain in their protective shelter from the drug attack, while being affected by diverse cytokines and growth factors secreted by surrounding bone marrow stromal cells [93, 99, 101]. In addition, generation of intolerance to this Bcr-Abl tyrosine kinase inhibitor, manifesting as several cardiovascular and metabolic toxicities, also limits the use of imatinib in clinical settings [90]. Furthermore, despite the entry of the second- and third-generation Bcr-Abl inhibitors (dasatinib, nilotinib, bosutinib, ponatinib) into clinical trials to overcome imatinib resistance, emergence of novel mutations counteracting these new drugs will always remain a concern [87, 89, 91, 92]. Therefore, investigation into possibilities to combine imatinib therapy with non-toxic adjuvant agents to circumvent acquired drug resistance would be very important to further improve the clinical outcomes of Bcr-Abl-positive CML.

#### *4.2.2.1.1. Effects of Flavonoids on Pharmacokinetics of Imatinib*

After oral administration, imatinib is predominantly metabolized to N-desmethyl imatinib by cytochrome P450 3A4 (CYP3A4), representing a rate-limiting step in the drug metabolism [88, 95, 96]. N-desmethyl imatinib exerts similar pharmacological activity to imatinib, but has only about 10-15% of area under the plasma concentration-time curve (AUC) as compared to the parent drug [88, 96]. Therefore, modulation of CYP3A4 enzyme by supplementary agents might be of great importance in regulating pharmacokinetics of imatinib, whereas inhibition of the enzymatic activity could contribute to enhanced systemic exposure of the drug [88, 95]. To a lesser extent, imatinib is metabolized also by other CYP enzymes, such as CYP1A2, CYP2C9, CYP2C19 and CYP2D6 [88, 96].

Several common dietary flavonoids have been studied concerning their potential to modulate pharmacokinetic parameters of imatinib in experimental animals. These results are summarized in Table 4.18 and discussed more closely below. As a result, abundant plant-derived flavone apigenin was shown to be able to inhibit imatinib metabolism in the short-term study, with increasing AUC values ($AUC_{0\text{-}t}$, $AUC_{0\text{-}\infty}$) and maximal plasma concentrations ($C_{max}$), and decreasing total body clearance (CL/F) of imatinib in male rats. On the contrary, in long-term study, apigenin accelerated the drug metabolism, reducing AUC values and enhancing both apparent volume of distribution ($V_z$/F) as well as CL/F of imatinib. In neither of these study models did apigenin significantly affect the pharmacokinetic parameters of N-desmethyl imatinib as compared to the control animals. Therefore, dosage schedule of apigenin, i.e., single dose versus long-term oral administration, seems to be critical in determining its effect on imatinib pharmacokinetics, whereas reducing the metabolic rate by short-term treatment with apigenin might lead to enhanced exposure and improved bioavailability of imatinib, potentially accompanying also with stronger adverse reactions. These effects of apigenin are probably regulated through its interactions with CYP enzymes [96]. Another common dietary flavonoid, the soy isoflavone genistein, could similarly increase the metabolism of imatinib in healthy male rats, when genistein was administered as multiple doses in long-term regimen. This was manifested as significantly reduced values of AUC and $C_{max}$ of imatinib, being achieved through induction of CYP3A4 activity by genistein. However, single dose administration of genistein concurrently with imatinib did not affect the metabolism of either the parent drug or its major metabolite, N-desmethyl imatinib [88]. Given the widespread availability of both flavonoids, apigenin and genistein, in food products and dietary supplements, it is important to recognize the modulatory role of these phytochemicals on imatinib pharmacokinetics, when used concurrently with the drug. As short-term exposure to apigenin can lead to higher concentrations of imatinib in the plasma and potentially induce also more adverse reactions, chronic dosing of apigenin or genistein might lead to lower plasma levels of imatinib resulting in reduction of therapeutic efficacy or even treatment failure [88, 96]. On the other hand, milk thistle-derived flavonolignan silibinin inhibited the metabolism of imatinib, increasing AUC values, mean resistance time (MRT) and half-life ($t_{1/2}$) of imatinib in the plasma of healthy male rats, while reducing apparent drug clearance from the body, in both short-term as well as long-term study

**Table 4.18.** Effects of flavonoids on pharmacokinetic parameters of imatinib (highlighted rows indicate undesired negative effects on anticancer efficacy)

| Flavonoid and its dosage | Imatinib and its dosage | Biological system | Effects | Purported mechanism | Ref. |
|---|---|---|---|---|---|
| FLAVONES | | | | | |
| Apigenin; 165 or 252 mg/kg as a single dose, oral administration | Imatinib; 30 mg/kg as a single dose, oral administration after apigenin | Sprague-Dawley male rats | Inhibition of imatinib metabolism in short-term study. Increase in $AUC_{0-t}$, $AUC_{0-\infty}$, and $C_{max}$, decrease in CL/F. No effect on the main pharmacokinetic parameters of N-desmethyl imatinib | Modulation of CYP enzymes | [96] |
| Apigenin; 165 mg/kg for 15 days, oral administration | Imatinib; 30 mg/kg as a single dose, oral administration after the last dose of apigenin | Sprague-Dawley male rats | Acceleration of imatinib metabolism in long-term study. Decrease in $AUC_{0-t}$ and $AUC_{0-\infty}$, increase in CL/F and $V_z/F$. No effect on the main pharmacokinetic parameters of N-desmethyl imatinib | Modulation of CYP enzymes | [96] |
| ISOFLAVONES | | | | | |
| Genistein; 50 or 100 mg/kg as a single dose | Imatinib; 30 mg/kg as a single dose, oral administration after genistein | Male Sprague-Dawley rats | No significant effect on metabolism rate of imatinib. No effect on pharmacokinetic parameters of N-desmethyl imatinib | | [88] |
| Genistein; 50 or 100 mg/kg as multiple doses for 15 consecutive days | Imatinib; 30 mg/kg as a single dose, oral administration after the last dose of genistein | Male Sprague-Dawley rats | Increase in metabolism rate of imatinib. Decrease in $AUC_{0-t}$, $AUC_{0-\infty}$ and $C_{max}$. No effect on pharmacokinetic parameters of N-desmethyl imatinib | Induction of CYP3A4 activity | [88] |
| FLAVONOLIGNANS | | | | | |
| Silibinin; 50 mg/kg as a single dose or as multiple doses for 15 consecutive days | Imatinib; 30 mg/kg, orally, as a single dose after the last administration of silibinin | Male Sprague-Dawley rats | Decrease in metabolism of imatinib. Increase in $AUC_{0-t}$, $AUC_{0-\infty}$, $MRT_{0-t}$, $MRT_{0-\infty}$ and $t_{1/2}$; decrease in apparent clearance (CL/F) (with both multiple-dose and single-dose treatment) | Inhibition of CYP3A4-mediated metabolism | [95] |

| Flavonoid and its dosage | Imatinib and its dosage | Biological system | Effects | Purported mechanism | Ref. |
|---|---|---|---|---|---|
| Silibinin; 0.01-100 μM | Imatinib; 10 μM | Human liver microsomes | Inhibition of imatinib metabolism, decrease in N-desmethyl imatinib generation rate | | [95] |
| Silibinin; 0.01-100 μM | Imatinib; 10 μM | Rat liver microsomes | Inhibition of imatinib metabolism, decrease in N-desmethyl imatinib generation rate | | [95] |

regimens, possibly through inhibition of CYP3A4-mediated drug metabolism by silibinin. Moreover, silibinin suppressed imatinib metabolism also in human and rat liver microsomes *in vitro*, reducing the rate of N-desmethyl imatinib generation. Therefore, much more attention should be paid when imatinib is administered concurrently with silibinin, as the systemic exposure to this Bcr-Abl tyrosine kinase inhibitor might be increased in the presence of silibinin [95]. If further studies will confirm these results, it could be possible further to lower the therapeutically efficient drug doses by combining imatinib with silibinin, thereby allowing also to reduce the intensity of adverse side effects.

#### *4.2.2.1.2. Effects of Flavonoids on Anticancer Potential of Imatinib*

The possible modulatory effects of several flavonoid-type natural agents on anticancer activities of imatinib have also been investigated in preclinical CML models. These results are summarized in Table 4.19 and analyzed by the flavonoid subclasses as follows.

Specifically, the major green tea flavanol EGCG (130 μM) was found to be able to significantly augment imatinib-induced decrease in cellular viability in human CML line K562. While imatinib induced typical apoptosis, EGCG further triggered necrosis via a caspase-independent mechanism, ultimately leading to an additive increase in the dead cell population [89]. However, three commonly occurring flavones, apigenin, luteolin and 5-desmethylsinensetin, could all exert both synergistic as well as antagonistic effects on imatinib cytotoxicity in K562 cells, depending on the selected doses. Such antagonistic responses were related, at least in part, to the increased P-gp activity, promoting drug efflux from the cells. Therefore, treatment of CML cells with imatinib in the presence of apigenin, luteolin or 5-desmethylsinensetin might undesirably facilitate the development of acquired resistance [100]. Cotreatment of K562 cells with imatinib and another flavone, chrysin (40 μM), led to a simple summatory cytotoxicity, without any synergism in apoptotic death [91]. Nevertheless, combination of imatinib with polymethoxylated flavone nobiletin (hexamethoxyflavone, 40 μM or 80 μM) synergistically reduced the viability of K562 cells [90].

**Table 4.19.** Effects of flavonoids on anticancer action of imatinib in chronic myelogenous leukemia (CML) models (highlighted rows indicate undesired negative effects on anticancer efficacy)

| Flavonoid and its dosage | Imatinib and its dosage | Biological system | Assay method and time | Effect | Mechanisms | Ref. |
|---|---|---|---|---|---|---|
| FLAVANOLS | | | | | | |
| EGCG; 130 μM | Imatinib; 50-200 nM | K562 human CML cells | CellTiter-Glo; 48h | Increase in imatinib-induced cell death | Induction of distinct modes of cell death (apoptosis by imatinib, necrosis by EGCG) | [89] |
| FLAVONES | | | | | | |
| 5-Desmethylsinensetin; 50, 100 μM | Imatinib; 1.25, 2.5 μM | K562 human CML cells | MTT; 72h | Antagonism in cytotoxicity (CI>1) (slight synergism at 50 μM 5-desmethylsinensetin + 2.5 μM imatinib) | Increase in necrosis. Increase in P-gp activity | [100] |
| Apigenin; 35, 70 μM | Imatinib; 1.25, 2.5 μM | K562 human CML cells | MTT; 72h | Antagonism in cytotoxicity (CI>1) (slight synergism at 70 μM apigenin + 2.5 μM imatinib) | Increase in necrosis. Increase in P-gp activity | [100] |
| Chrysin; 40 μM | Imatinib; 0.25 μM | K562 human CML cells; Bcr-Abl-positive, imatinib-sensitive | Apoptosis assay; 48h | No synergism in cytotoxicity, simple summatory effect (CI 0.987) | No synergism in apoptosis induction, simple summatory effect | [91] |
| Luteolin; 25, 50 μM | Imatinib; 1.25, 2.5 μM | K562 human CML cells | MTT; 72h | Antagonism in cytotoxicity (CI>1) (synergism at 25 or 50 μM luteolin + 2.5 μM imatinib) | Increase in necrosis. Increase in P-gp activity | [100] |
| Nobiletin; 40, 80 μM | Imatinib; 0.2 μM | K562 human CML cells | MTT; 48h | Synergistic reduction of cell viability (CI 0.6 and 0.7) | | [90] |

**Table 4.19.** (Continued)

| Flavonoid and its dosage | Imatinib and its dosage | Biological system | Assay method and time | Effect | Mechanisms | Ref. |
|---|---|---|---|---|---|---|
| Oroxylin A; 60 μM | Imatinib; 0.25 μM | K562 human CML cells within human stromal cells HS-5-derived conditioned media | Apoptosis assay; 12h with oroxylin A followed by addition of imatinib for 36h | Potentiation of antileukemic activity of imatinib. Reversal of resistance to imatinib | Increase in imatinib-induced apoptosis (activation of caspase-3). Inhibition of Stat3, downregulation of P-gp, Mcl-1, Bcl-xl and survivin | [93] |
| Oroxylin A; 60 μM | Imatinib; 1 μM | K562 human CML cells co-cultured with murine bone marrow stromal cells M2-10B4 | Apoptosis assay; 36h with imatinib | Potentiation of antileukemic action of imatinib, decrease in proliferation. Reversal of resistance to imatinib | Increase in imatinib-induced apoptosis. Inhibition of CXCR7 expression, downregulation of p-ERK, p-BAD and survivin | [99] |
| Oroxylin A; 60 μM | Imatinib; 1 μM | KU812 human CML cells co-cultured with murine bone marrow stromal cells M2-10B4 | Apoptosis assay; 36h with imatinib | Potentiation of antileukemic action of imatinib, decrease in proliferation. Reversal of resistance to imatinib | Increase in imatinib-induced apoptosis. Inhibition of CXCR7 expression, downregulation of p-ERK, p-BAD and survivin | [99] |
| Oroxylin A; 30 mg/kg, i.v., daily | Imatinib; 200 mg/kg, p.o., daily | K562 cells inoculated s.c. into 6-8 w-old NOD/SCID mice | 3 weeks | Potentiation of inhibitory effect of imatinib on tumor growth. Reduction of tumor volume and weight | | [93] |

| Flavonoid and its dosage | Imatinib and its dosage | Biological system | Assay method and time | Effect | Mechanisms | Ref. |
|---|---|---|---|---|---|---|
| Oroxylin A; 80 mg/kg, i.v., once every other day | Imatinib; 200 mg/kg, p.o., daily | K562 cells injected via tail vein into female immunodeficient BALB/c nude mice | 4 weeks | Potentiation of inhibitory effect of imatinib on leukemia development | Decrease in the number of $CD13^+$ (leukemia) cells in bone marrow, peripheral blood and spleen; reverting weight and histology of spleen and liver back to normal. Decrease in p-Stat3, Bcl-xl and Mcl-1 in bone marrow and spleen cells | [93] |
| Oroxylin A; 200 mg/kg | Imatinib; 200 mg/kg | K562 cells co-cultured with murine bone marrow stromal cells M2-10B4 injected via tail vein into 35-40 days-old male BALB/c nude mice | 30 days | Potentiation of antileukemic action of imatinib. Sensitization of cells to imatinib treatment | Reverting weight of spleen and liver back to normal; decrease in $CD13^+$ cells in bone marrow, peripheral blood and spleen. Reduction of CXCR7 and p-ERK expression | [99] |
| Tangeretin; 10-80 µM, ratio with imatinib of 25:1 | Imatinib; 0.4-3.2 µM | K562 human erythroleukemia cells; Bcr-Abl-positive | Apoptosis assay; 48h | Synergistic cytotoxicity (CI<1). Sensitization of cells to imatinib | Synergistic increase in apoptosis (activation of caspases-3 and -9, cleavage of PARP); induction of mitotic arrest | [92] |
| Wogonin; 10-40 µM | Imatinib; 0.5 µM | K562 human CML cells cultured in conditioned medium from HS-5 human stromal cells | Apoptosis assay; 36h. Colony assay; 30 days | Potentiation of inhibitory effect of imatinib on leukemia development, overcoming imatinib resistance | Increase in apoptosis, decrease in $CD34^+$ cell proportion and colony-forming capacity. Downregulation of p-Stat5 and its target genes (Mcl-1, Bcl-2, Bcl-xl) | [101] |

**Table 4.19.** (Continued)

| Flavonoid and its dosage | Imatinib and its dosage | Biological system | Assay method and time | Effect | Mechanisms | Ref. |
|---|---|---|---|---|---|---|
| Wogonin; 40 mg/kg, i.v., once every other day | Imatinib; 200 mg/kg, p.o., daily | K562 cells cultured with conditioned medium from HS-5 stromal cells injected via tail vein into 5-6 w-old NOD/SCID immunodeficient mice | 4 weeks | Potentiation of inhibitory effect of imatinib on leukemia development | Reduction of $CD34^+$ cells in bone marrow and peripheral blood. Decrease in $CD13^+$ cells in bone marrow, peripheral blood and spleen. Restoring the weight and histology of spleen and liver back to normal. Downregulation of p-Stat5, Bcl-xl and Mcl-1 | [101] |
| FLAVONOLS | | | | | | |
| 3-Hydroxyflavone; 5-200 µM | Imatinib; 1 µM | K562-S human CML cells; imatinib-sensitive | MTT; 48h | Increase in cell viability reduction | Increase in apoptosis (cleavage of PARP, activation of caspases-3 and -8). Suppression of p-Bcr-Abl and downstream p-Stat5 expression | [87] |
| 3-Hydroxyflavone; 10-200 µM | Imatinib; 1 µM | K562-R human CML cells; imatinib-resistant | MTT; 48h | Increase in cell viability reduction | Synergistic increase in apoptosis (cleavage of PARP, activation of caspases-3 and -8). Suppression of p-Bcr-Abl and downstream p-Stat5 expression (no effect by imatinib alone) | [87] |

| Flavonoid and its dosage | Imatinib and its dosage | Biological system | Assay method and time | Effect | Mechanisms | Ref. |
|---|---|---|---|---|---|---|
| Fisetin; 40 μM | Imatinib; 0.25 μM | K562 human CML cells; Bcr-Abl-positive, imatinib-sensitive | Apoptosis assay; 48h | No synergism in cytotoxicity, simple summatory effect | No synergism in apoptosis induction, simple summatory effect | [91] |
| Galangin; 40 μM | Imatinib; 0.25 μM | K562 human CML cells; Bcr-Abl-positive, imatinib-sensitive | Apoptosis assay; 48h | Synergistic cytotoxic effect (CI 0.38) | Synergistic increase in apoptotic activity of imatinib | [91] |
| Galangin; 40 μM | Imatinib; 2.5 μM | K562-R human CML cells; Bcr-Abl-positive, imatinib-resistant | Apoptosis assay; 48h | Synergistic cytotoxic effect (CI 0.74) | Synergistic increase in apoptotic activity of imatinib | [91] |
| Galangin; 40 μM | Imatinib; 0.25 μM | KCL22 human CML cells; Bcr-Abl-positive, imatinib-sensitive | Apoptosis assay; 48h | Synergistic cytotoxic effect (CI 0.44) | Synergistic increase in apoptotic activity of imatinib | [91] |
| Galangin; 40 μM | Imatinib; 2.5 μM | KCL22-R human CML cells; Bcr-Abl-positive, imatinib-resistant | Apoptosis assay; 48h | Synergistic cytotoxic effect (CI 0.73) | Synergistic increase in apoptotic activity of imatinib | [91] |
| Quercetin; 40 μM | Imatinib; 0.25 μM | K562 human CML cells; Bcr-Abl-positive, imatinib-sensitive | Apoptosis assay; 48h | Synergistic cytotoxic effect (CI 0.72) | Synergistic increase in apoptotic activity of imatinib | [91] |
| SYNTHETIC FLAVONOIDS | | | | | | |
| Flavopiridol; 150 nM | Imatinib; 50-500 nM | K562 human leukemia cells; Bcr-Abl-positive | Apoptosis assay; 48h | | Synergistic potentiation of imatinib-induced apoptosis (increase in $\Delta\Psi m$ loss; cleavage of procaspases-3, -8, -9, Bid and PARP; cytosolic release of cyt c and Smac/DIABLO; decrease in Bcl-xl and Mcl-1); reduction of cyclin D1 and pRb expression. Upregulation of p-JNK and p-ERK1/2, downregulation of p-CREB | [94] |

**Table 4.19.** (Continued)

| Flavonoid and its dosage | Imatinib and its dosage | Biological system | Assay method and time | Effect | Mechanisms | Ref. |
|---|---|---|---|---|---|---|
| Flavopiridol; 200 nM | Imatinib; 1.5 µM | K562R human leukemia cells; Bcr-Abl-positive, multidrug-resistant | Apoptosis assay; 48h | | About 5-fold increase in imatinib-induced apoptosis (increase in cytosolic release of cyt c) | [94] |
| Flavopiridol; 150 nM | Imatinib; 200 nM | LAMA-84 human leukemia cells; Bcr-Abl-positive | Apoptosis assay; 48h | | Potentiation of imatinib-induced apoptosis | [94] |
| Flavopiridol; 30, 45 or 60 $mg/m^2$, 1h i.v. infusion weekly for 3 weeks every 4 weeks | Imatinib; 400 or 600 mg; p.o., daily | 21 adult patients with CML or Ph-positive ALL (Bcr-Abl-positive) | 1 year (from the end of treatment) | 5 patients responded (4 with CML, 1 with ALL), including 4 sustained responses (one CML patient had a complete response lasting 30 months). 4 patients had stable disease (all CML, imatinib-pretreated) | An average of 21% lowering of imatinib AUC. Tolerable combination: the only frequent toxicities were hematological (anemia, leukopenia, neutropenia, thrombocytopenia); one DLT event (grade 3 cholecystitis) | [97] |

Similarly, tangeretin (pentamethoxyflavone, 10-80 μM) also synergistically sensitized K562 cells to anticancer responses of imatinib, enhancing apoptotic death and inducing mitotic arrest. In doing so, tangeretin did still not exert any significant effects on the expression level of Bcr-Abl fusion gene [92]. One of the most promising results reported so far about the combinatorial action of imatinib and flavonoids in CML models probably include the interactions between imatinib and monomethylated flavone oroxylin A. Specifically, combination of imatinib and oroxylin A (60 μM) resulted in a significant potentiation of antileukemic activity of the drug in K562 cells cultured in human stromal cells HS-5-derived conditioned media. This sensitizing effect was achieved through suppression of stromal cells-secreted soluble factors-induced Stat3 signaling by addition of oroxylin A, leading to downregulation of P-gp efflux pump expression and promoting imatinib-induced apoptosis in CML cells. In addition, oroxylin A potentiated anticancer effects of imatinib also in nude mice inoculated with K562 cells by inhibiting Stat3 signaling pathway, resulting in a substantial decrease in leukemic ($CD13^+$) cells in bone marrow, peripheral blood and spleen, and restoring the normal weight and architecture of the spleen and liver [93]. Moreover, oroxylin A (60 μM) potentiated antileukemic activities of imatinib also in another bone marrow microenvironment-mimicking preclinical model, generated by co-culturing human CML cells K562 or KU812 with murine bone marrow stromal cells M2-10B4. As a result, oroxylin A suppressed stromal cells-secreted chemokine CXCL12-induced CXCR7 pathway in CML cells, inhibiting ERK signaling and ultimately leading to a significant increase in imatinib-induced apoptotic death. While so far, expression of CXCL12-activated CXCR4 chemokine receptors has been associated with the ability of CML cells to home into bone marrow for forming stromal niches that are protected against Bcr-Abl tyrosine kinase inhibitors, CXCL12/CXCR7 axis might also play an important role in emergence of drug resistance. Accordingly, downregulation of CXCR7 expression by oroxylin A can markedly sensitize CML cells to imatinib therapy. Addition of oroxylin A reversed imatinib resistance also in nude mice injected with K562 and M2-10B4 co-cultured cells, manifested as a reduced $CD13^+$ cell population in bone marrow, peripheral blood and spleen, and reverting the weight of spleen and liver back to the normal levels [99]. Therefore, inclusion of oroxylin A in imatinib therapy might enhance the antileukemic action of imatinib by suppressing bone marrow stroma-derived soluble factors-mediated drug resistance, allowing to eradicate minimal residual disease in the bone marrow compartment, avoiding CML relapse and improving patients` prognosis. Another monomethylated flavone from *Scutellaria* radix, wogonin (10-40 μM), also augmented the anticancer effects of imatinib in K562 cells cultured in human stromal cells HS-5-derived conditioned media. Whereas the presence of bone marrow stromal cells-derived conditioned medium was related to enhanced maintenance of CML stem cells during imatinib treatment, addition of wogonin resulted in a significant decrease in the viability of $CD34^+$ cells, representing a subpopulation of leukemic stem cells. These sensitizing activities were achieved through suppression of the Stat5 signaling pathway by combinatorial treatment with imatinib and wogonin, leading to a marked increase in apoptotic death. In addition, combination of imatinib and wogonin augmented drug-induced antileukemic effects also in immunodeficient mice inoculated with K562 cells that were cultured in HS-5-derived conditioned medium. This *in vivo* potentiating action was again accompanied by a substantial decrease in the proportion of $CD34^+$ cells in bone marrow and peripheral blood, as well as reduction of $CD13^+$ leukemic cells in bone marrow, peripheral blood and spleen, mediated by downregulation of Stat5 pathway [101]. Consequently, natural flavones oroxylin A and wogonin may present attractive adjuvant agents for imatinib therapy to overcome bone marrow microenvironment-derived factors-induced resistance to this Bcr-Abl tyrosine kinase inhibitor.

Promising results in suppressing CML development have been reported also by combining imatinib with some commonly occurring natural flavonols. In fact, 3-hydroxyflavone was found to enhance cytotoxic and proapoptotic activities of imatinib in both imatinib-sensitive (K562-S) as well as imatinib-resistant (K562-R) cells, but this potentiating effect was much stronger and even synergistic in drug-refractory CML cells. Mechanistically, combined treatment with imatinib and 3-hydroxyflavone resulted in a significant decrease in activated Bcr-Abl levels with inhibition of the downstream Stat5 pathway, rendering resistant cells susceptible to imatinib therapy. If further studies with experimental animals will verify these results, 3-hydroxyflavone may represent an important adjuvant agent for CML patients with Bcr-Abl-positive imatinib-resistant disease [87]. Another flavonol-type phytochemical, galangin (40 μM), was able to synergistically increase the apoptotic activity of imatinib in both imatinib-sensitive CML lines (K562 and KCL22) as well as imatinib-resistant lines (K562-R and KCL22-R). Although at lower level, quercetin also synergistically increased imatinib-induced mitochondrial apoptosis in K562 cells, while addition of fisetin led only to a simple summatory effect [91].

Besides naturally occurring polyphenolic phytochemicals, a semisynthetic flavonoid-type compound, flavopiridol, has also been tested in combination with imatinib towards the possible co-effects on CML development. As a result, combined treatment with imatinib and flavopiridol (150 nM) synergistically potentiated both death receptor-dependent as well as mitochondrial-mediated apoptotic death in Bcr-Abl-positive CML lines (K562 and LAMA-84), but not in Bcr-Abl-negative leukemic cells (HL-60, U937, Jurkat). This apoptosis-augmenting interaction was associated with activation of ERK1/2 and JNK signaling in K562 cells, with no effects on the expression of Bcr-Abl protein. Moreover, combination of imatinib and flavopiridol enhanced apoptotic death also in drug-resistant K562R cells displaying Bcr-Abl amplification [94]. The translational implications of this novel antileukemic strategy were further investigated in a phase I clinical trial, testing the effect of imatinib-flavopiridol combination in 21 adult patients suffering from Bcr-Abl-positive malignancies (CML or Ph-positive ALL). As a result of this dose-escalation study, encouraging clinical outcomes were observed: five patients met criteria for a response (four with sustained responses) and four patients had stable disease. One CML patient had a complete response that sustained for 30 months. Most importantly, the combination of imatinib and flavopiridol was well tolerated, with only frequent adverse reactions of hematologic toxicities. Despite the promising clinical activities, the study was closed due to introduction of the second-generation Bcr-Abl tyrosine kinase inhibitors dasatinib and nilotinib for treatment of CML patients with imatinib-refractory disease. However, as emergence of novel mutations in the Bcr-Abl kinase domain will always remain a concern in respect to development of therapeutic resistance, combination of these new drugs with flavopiridol presents an attractive future avenue for further improving the clinical outcomes of Bcr-Abl-positive hematological malignancies [97].

Altogether, inclusion of specific naturally occurring plant-derived flavonoids in the treatment of CML with imatinib might be important in overcoming acquired drug resistance and improving therapeutic responses through regulating different cellular mechanisms (Figure 4.7). Further studies are urgently needed to identify the most effective imatinib-flavonoid combinations for circumventing drug resistance, thereby providing valuable input for future clinical trials.

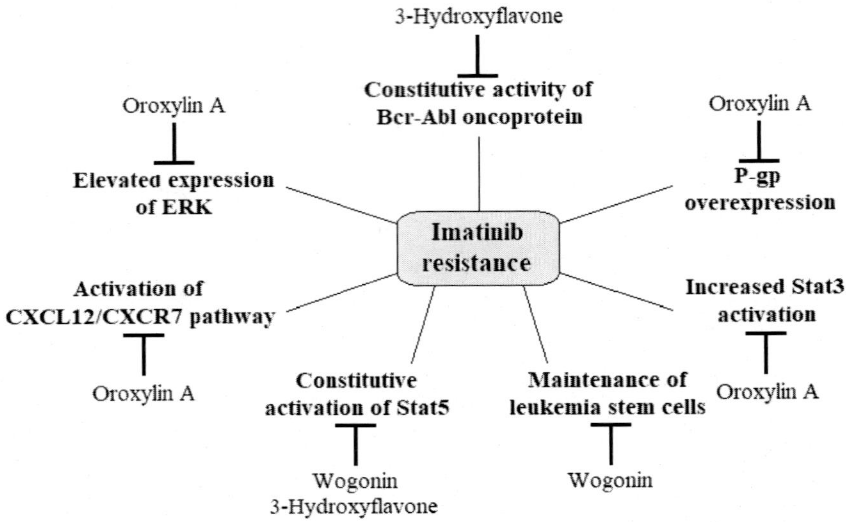


**Figure 4.7.** Overcoming imatinib resistance and augmenting its antitumor action by flavonoids in CML models.

### *4.2.2.2. Ponatinib*

Ponatinib (Iclusig) is an orally active third-generation Bcr-Abl tyrosine kinase inhibitor [102] (Figure 4.6). This drug is approved by the FDA for treatment of chronic myelogenous leukemia (CML) and Philadelphia chromosome (Ph)-positive acute lymphocytic leukemia (ALL), especially for patients with resistance or intolerance to other TKIs [102]. As an abnormal tyrosine kinase activity of Bcr-Abl fusion protein can stimulate diverse cellular signaling pathways associated with malignant transformation and progression, inactivation of Bcr-Abl is currently the major strategy for the treatment of CML patients [102].

#### *4.2.2.2.1. Effects of Flavonoids on Anticancer Potential of Ponatinib*

The only flavonoid that has been investigated to date respecting its possible ability to modulate ponatinib-induced antileukemic activities, is the green tea flavanol EGCG. As a result of this study, EGCG was found to synergistically enhance the antiproliferative and proapoptotic effects of ponatinib in human CML cells K562, accompanied by regulation of the expression profiles of the cell cycle associated genes [102] (Table 4.20). Further studies with structurally different flavonoids are encouraged to elucidate the role of polyphenolic phytochemicals in therapeutic efficacy of ponatinib in Bcr-Abl-positive hematological malignancies, as well as the molecular mechanisms under these co-effects are needed to be unraveled.

**Table 4.20.** Effects of flavonoids on anticancer action of ponatinib in chronic myelogenous leukemia (CML) models

| Flavonoid and its dosage | Ponatinib and its dosage | Biological system | Assay method and time | Effect | Mechanisms | Ref. |
|---|---|---|---|---|---|---|
| FLAVANOLS | | | | | | |
| EGCG; 1-100 μM | Ponatinib; 1-100 nM | K562 human CML cells | WST-1; 24, 48, 72h | Synergistic cytotoxic effect, synergistic inhibition of proliferation (CI 0.658) | Synergistic increase in apoptosis. Downregulation of cyclin D1 and CDC25A, upregulation of TGF-β2 gene | [102] |

### *4.2.2.3. Ibrutinib*

Ibrutinib (Imbruvica) is a small-molecule irreversible inhibitor for Bruton`s tyrosine kinase (BTK) [103] (Figure 4.6). Blocking BTK by ibrutinib impairs the B-cell receptor pathway and suppresses B-cell proliferation and survival. Therefore, this drug is used for the clinical management of B-cell malignancies. To date, ibrutinib is approved by FDA for treatment of chronic lymphocytic leukemia (CLL), mantle cell lymphoma, marginal zone lymphoma, Waldenström`s macroglobulinemia and chronic graft vs host disease.

#### *4.2.2.3.1. Effects of Flavonoids on Pharmacokinetics of Ibrutinib*

Very recently, the findings from an investigation into the effect of dietary flavanone naringenin on pharmacokinetic profile of ibrutinib were reported [103]. In this work, it was shown that the presence of naringenin could inhibit the drug metabolism and increase plasma exposure, by significantly prolonging the half-life, increasing $AUC_{0\text{-}t}$ and reducing clearance time of ibrutinib in male rats. As ibrutinib is mainly metabolized by CYP3A4, it is probable that naringenin can inhibit CYP3A4 activity and thereby intervene in ibrutinib metabolism. Therefore, naringenin or naringenin-containing dietary supplements and herbal medicines can affect pharmacokinetic behavior of ibrutinib, and it should be taken into account by patients receiving ibrutinib therapy [103] (Table 4.21).

So far, no studies have been reported about the possible interactions between ibrutinib and flavonoids on antileukemic activities of this BTK inhibitor in different models of B-cell malignancies. This would be an interesting task for the future, considering a wide application of ibrutinib in the treatment of hematological cancers.

**Table 4.21.** Effects of flavonoids on pharmacokinetic parameters of ibrutinib

| Flavonoid and its dosage | Ibrutinib and its dosage | Biological system | Effects | Purported mechanism | Ref. |
|---|---|---|---|---|---|
| FLAVANONES | | | | | |
| Naringenin; 50 mg/kg, oral administration | Ibrutinib; 10 mg/kg, oral administration | Male Sprague-Dawley rats | Decrease in metabolism and increase in plasma exposure of ibrutinib. Prolongation of $t_{1/2}$, decrease in clearance, increase in $AUC_{0-t}$ (2.99-fold) of ibrutinib | Inhibition of CYP3A-mediated metabolism | [103] |

#### *4.2.2.4. Bortezomib*

Bortezomib (Velcade) is a potent and specific, the first-in-class, proteasome inhibitor [104-106]. This drug is a modified dipeptidyl boronic acid [104, 107] (Figure 4.6). Mechanistically, the boronic acid group reversibly forms an anionic borate adduct with threonine at the chymotrypsin-like active site of the 26S proteasome [105, 108]. Cellular proteasome is a highly conserved multi-subunit key enzymatic complex that is responsible for degradation of ubiquitinated intracellular proteins which are marked for deletion from the cell`s inventory, playing a critical role in cell division, differentiation, proliferation and survival [105, 107, 109, 110]. Inhibition of 26S proteasome by bortezomib blocks inducible IκB degradation and consequently prevents NF-κB activation, restricting the growth of malignant cells and leading them to apoptosis [104, 105, 109, 111, 112]. In addition, accumulation of ubiquitinated unfolded or misfolded proteins triggers the induction of endoplasmic reticulum stress [105, 109]. While endoplasmic reticulum stress can restore homeostasis and thereby support cell survival in the case of low to moderate stress, it initiates apoptosis during severe stress conditions, such as in response to inhibition of proteasome activity by bortezomib [109]. A key player in these stress responses is glucose-regulated protein 78 (GRP78), functioning as a sensor of endoplasmic reticulum stress and subsequent homeostatic control [113].

Bortezomib is approved by the FDA for treatment of relapsed, refractory and newly diagnosed multiple myeloma, and refractory mantle cell lymphoma [105-107, 110]. Although this proteasome inhibitor has been under consideration for the treatment of other cancers as well, so far, it has revealed only poor efficacy in management of chronic lymphocytic leukemia or acute leukemias [104, 109, 114]. Multiple myeloma is a malignant dyscrasia of monoclonal immunoglobulin-producing plasma cells progressing to multiorgan dysfunction, failure and death [115, 116]. This severe disease is the second most common hematological malignancy next to non-Hodgkin's lymphoma, comprising about 10% of all blood cancers [115, 117]. In 2020, there were over 176,000 new multiple myeloma cases diagnosed worldwide, with more than 117,000 cancer-related deaths [31]. Despite an appreciable improvement in the survival rate of multiple myeloma patients after introduction of bortezomib therapy, relapsed and refractory disease has still remained a major challenge to cure, and improvement of the clinical outcome is imperative [106, 115, 117]. The objective response rate of multiple myeloma patients to bortezomib has indeed been shown to be only 43%, with many patients developing resistance to this drug [108, 111, 116]. There are several mechanisms underlying bortezomib resistance, including hyperphosphorylation of NF-κB pathway leading to failure in accumulating proapoptotic proteins and suppressing antiapoptotic proteins, but also induction of autophagy for removing damaged proteins [104, 117]. In addition, the use of bortezomib is associated with several adverse effects, such as thrombocytopenia, neutropenia, fever, neuropathy, asthenia and gastrointestinal toxicity [115, 116, 118]. Therefore, identification of novel non-toxic adjuvant agents that can circumvent resistance to bortezomib and allow to reduce the therapeutically effective doses of this proteasome inhibitor is highly important in improving clinical outcomes of patients suffering from relapsed and refractory multiple myeloma. Flavonoid-type phytochemicals might be especially attractive to achieve this purpose by simultaneously targeting multiple oncogenic signaling cascades activated by malignant cells for compensating bortezomib-inhibited processes.

#### *4.2.2.4.1. Effects of Flavonoids on Anticancer Potential of Bortezomib*

Several structurally different flavonoids have been studied in combination with bortezomib in diverse preclinical cancer models. The results of these works, unexpected and even astonishing in some sense, are summarized in Table 4.22 and discussed more closely as follows.

Somewhat surprisingly, it was recently found that green tea flavanols exert antagonistic interaction with bortezomib, neutralizing its anticancer effects. In detail, green tea constituents with 1,2-benzenediol moiety, i.e., catechol group, especially EGCG but also epicatechin, epigallocatechin (EGC) and epicatechin gallate (ECG), all effectively prevented cytotoxic effects of boronic acid-based proteasome inhibitor bortezomib (Figure 4.8). Indeed, combination of bortezomib and EGCG (2.5 μM and higher) completely prevented bortezomib-induced cell killing and apoptosis in both human multiple myeloma lines (RPMI/8226, U266, MM1) as well as human glioblastoma lines (LN229, U251). Although to a noticeably lower extent, epicatechin, EGC and ECG also neutralized the cytotoxic action of bortezomib in LN229 cells. Mechanistically, combined treatment of RPMI/8226 and LN229 cells with bortezomib and EGCG led to prevention of bortezomib-induced reduction of proteasome activity and accumulation of ubiquitinated proteins, thereby impeding endoplasmic reticulum stress and blocking also bortezomib-triggered apoptosis. Moreover, EGCG could neutralize antitumor effects of bortezomib also in RPMI/8226 xenografts-bearing nude mice, by blocking drug-induced apoptosis and necrosis in malignant tissues. This *in vitro* and *in vivo* antagonistic function was achieved through a direct interaction between the catechol group of flavonoids and boronic acid moiety of bortezomib leading to formation of a covalent cyclic boronate adduct, thereby prohibiting binding of the drug to proteasome and exerting its proteasome inhibitory activities, further preventing initiation of endoplasmic reticulum stress and apoptotic death of malignant cells [109]. Blocking of antiproliferative and proapoptotic effects of bortezomib by EGCG was further demonstrated in human multiple myeloma lines MC/CAR, RPMI8226 and U266, accompanied by prevention of proteasome inhibitory function of the drug. Moreover, antagonistic activity of EGCG on antimyeloma action of bortezomib was observed also in primary myeloma cells obtained from patients. The direct chemical interaction of vicinal diols of EGCG molecule with boronic acid moiety of bortezomib was proven by using the NMR spectroscopy [112]. Similar antagonistic effects were demonstrated also in latter studies, showing a significant decrease in bortezomib-induced cytotoxicity when combined with EGCG in human multiple myeloma lines ARP-1 [108] and RPMI/8226 [105, 107], due to formation of stable cyclic adducts between 1,2-benzenediol moiety of EGCG and boronic acid group of bortezomib, driven and stabilized by electronic and steric effects [105]. Nevertheless, differently from the other studies, EGCG was found to synergistically enhance bortezomib-induced inhibition of cell growth and promotion of apoptosis in human multiple myeloma line KM3, achieved through increase in the inhibition of IκBα degradation and suppression of NF-κB pathway. The reasons behind such contradictory findings might include, at least in part, the use of remarkably higher concentrations of EGCG (25 μM, 50 μM) in the experiments with KM3 cells [111].

Besides multiple myeloma, co-effects of EGCG and bortezomib were studied also in preclinical models of several other cancer types. As a consequence, antagonistic action of EGCG on antitumor activities of bortezomib was observed in human glioblastoma lines (MO59J, U251), neuroblastoma lines (NGP, SH-SY5Y) and melanoma lines (CHL-1, WM266-4) [113]. Additional similar findings for bortezomib inactivation were reported also in human prostate cancer cells PC-3, where addition of EGCG suppressed bortezomib-induced cytotoxicity, apoptosis, proteasome inhibition and endoplasmic reticulum stress. Moreover, the presence of EGCG promoted activation of compensatory autophagy in bortezomib-treated cells, further mitigating endoplasmic reticulum stress by relieving the burden of unfolded proteins and aggregates, and ultimately protecting cells from the apoptotic death [110]. EGCG antagonized bortezomib-induced antitumor action also in CWR22 human prostate tumor fragments-bearing immunocompromised mice, by partially suppressing bortezomib-induced proteasome inhibition in both blood and tumor tissues. However, this antagonistic action appeared only when EGCG levels in the plasma were above 200 μM at the time of bortezomib dosing (attained via intravenous administration of 50 mg/kg EGCG two minutes before bortezomib injection), but not at the lower EGCG concentrations usually achievable via dietary or supplemental intake. Moreover, as bortezomib has a rapid initial distribution phase in its pharmacokinetic profile, with very little amounts present in the plasma at an hour after administration, the time window for potential interaction and complex formation with EGCG can be rather narrow in the real *in vivo* conditions [107].

Besides flavanols, flavonol-type phytochemicals also comprise several catechol moiety-containing compounds and therefore, their co-effects with bortezomib were also investigated (Figure 4.8). As a result, the abundant natural flavonol quercetin (20 μM) was found to be able to completely inhibit bortezomib-induced apoptosis in human malignant B-cell lines (DoHH2, HRC57) as well as primary chronic lymphocytic leukemia (CLL) cells derived from the peripheral blood of CLL patients. Inhibition of bortezomib-induced apoptosis by quercetin (40 μM) was similarly observed also in two human multiple myeloma lines, RPMI-8226 and U266. This antagonism was associated with chemical reactions between catechol moiety of quercetin and boronic acid group of bortezomib, forming cyclic boronate esters, as verified by Raman spectroscopy. In support of this assertion, apoptotic effects induced by bortezomib were blocked also by another catechol-containing dietary flavonol, myricetin (30 μM), in human diffuse large B-cell lymphoma cells DoHH2 [114]. Moreover, decrease in the drug efficacy was further confirmed in a set of human multiple myeloma lines (MC/CAR, RPMI8226, U266), where antiproliferative and proteasome inhibitory functions of bortezomib were blocked by the presence of quercetin and also its sugar conjugate, rutin (quercetin 3-O-rutinoside), leading to reduction of the number of apoptotic cells. In doing so, rutin hydrate revealed essentially lower antagonistic potential than quercetin, with only a marginal inhibitory impact on anticancer activities of bortezomib.

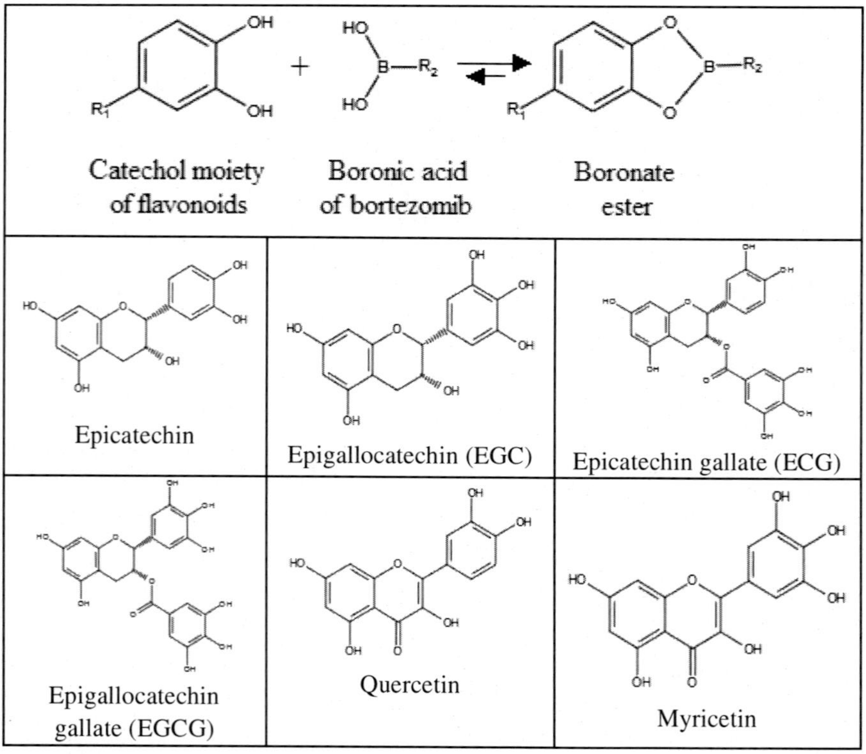


**Figure 4.8.** Complex formation between catechol moiety of flavonoids and boronic acid group of bortezomib. Structural formulas of the most common catechol-containing flavonoids.

**Table 4.22.** Effects of flavonoids on anticancer action of bortezomib (highlighted rows indicate undesired negative effects on anticancer efficacy)

| Flavonoid and its dosage | Bortezomib and its dosage | Biological system | Assay method and time | Effect | Mechanisms | Ref. |
|---|---|---|---|---|---|---|
| FLAVANOLS | | | | | | |
| Epicatechin; 10-40 μM | Bortezomib; 20 nM | RPMI/8226 human multiple myeloma cells | MTT; 48h | Moderate reduction of bortezomib activity | | [105] |
| Epicatechin; 10-40 μM | Bortezomib; 10-50 nM | LN229 human glioblastoma cells | MTT; 48h | Neutralization of cytotoxic effects of bortezomib; weaker cytoprotection than that of EGCG | | [109] |
| ECG; 10-40 μM | Bortezomib; 10-50 nM | LN229 human glioblastoma cells | MTT; 48h | Neutralization of cytotoxic effects of bortezomib; weaker cytoprotection than that of EGCG | | [109] |
| EGC; 10-40 μM | Bortezomib; 10-50 nM | LN229 human glioblastoma cells | MTT; 48h | Neutralization of cytotoxic effects of bortezomib; weaker cytoprotection than that of EGCG | | [109] |
| EGCG; 5-25 μM | Bortezomib; 25 nM | ARP-1 human multiple myeloma cells | MTT; 48h | Inhibition of bortezomib-induced cytotoxicity | Formation of cyclic boronate ester with bortezomib | [108] |

**Table 4.22.** (Continued)

| Flavonoid and its dosage | Bortezomib and its dosage | Biological system | Assay method and time | Effect | Mechanisms | Ref. |
|---|---|---|---|---|---|---|
| EGCG; 25, 50 μM | Bortezomib; 20 nM | KM3 human multiple myeloma cells | Counting; 48h | Synergistic inhibition of cell growth (CI<1) | Synergistic induction of apoptosis (activation of caspases-3, -8, -9, cleavage of PARP). Downregulation of P65, p-P65, p-IκBα; upregulation of IκBα protein | [111] |
| EGCG; 1-100 μM | Bortezomib; 10 nM | MC/CAR human multiple myeloma cells | CellTiter-Glo; 48h | Blocking of antiproliferative (antimyeloma) effect of bortezomib, strong antagonism (CI>1) | Abolishment of proteasome inhibitory function of bortezomib. Blocking of bortezomib-induced apoptosis (decrease in caspases-3, -8, -9 and PARP activities, reduction of bortezomib-induced ΔΨm disruption). Direct chemical interaction between EGCG and bortezomib | [112] |
| EGCG; 5-20 μM | Bortezomib; 10-100 nM | MM1 human multiple myeloma cells | MTT; 48, 72h | Blocking of bortezomib-induced cytotoxic effects, antagonistic function. Increase in $IC_{50}$ of bortezomib | | [109] |
| EGCG; 2.5-20 μM | Bortezomib; 10-100 nM | RPMI/8226 human multiple myeloma cells | MTT; 48h | Blocking of bortezomib-induced cytotoxic effects, antagonistic function. | Prevention of bortezomib-induced proteasome inhibition and ubiquitinated proteins accumulation. | [109] |

| Flavonoid and its dosage | Bortezomib and its dosage | Biological system | Assay method and time | Effect | Mechanisms | Ref. |
|---|---|---|---|---|---|---|
| | | | | Increase in $IC_{50}$ of bortezomib | Prevention of bortezomib-induced apoptosis (blocking of bortezomib-activated caspase-7 and cleaved PARP), maintaining normal cell cycle distribution | |
| EGCG; 1-100 µM | Bortezomib; 10 nM | RPMI8226 human multiple myeloma cells | CellTiter-Glo; 48h | Blocking of antiproliferative (antimyeloma) effect of bortezomib, strong antagonism (CI>1) | Abolishment of proteasome inhibitory function of bortezomib. Blocking of bortezomib-induced apoptosis (decrease in caspases-3, -8, -9 and PARP activities, reduction of bortezomib-induced $\Delta\Psi m$ disruption). Direct chemical interaction between EGCG and bortezomib | [112] |
| EGCG; 10-40 µM | Bortezomib; 20 nM | RPMI/8226 human multiple myeloma cells | MTT; 48h | Reduction of bortezomib-induced cytotoxicity (up to 82%) | Formation of stable cyclic boron adducts between bortezomib and EGCG | [105] |
| EGCG; 0.425-100 µM | Bortezomib; 1-40 nM | RPMI-8226 human multiple myeloma cells | Luminescent ATP-lite assay; 48h | Substantial shift in the potency, increase in $IC_{50}$ of bortezomib | | [107] |
| EGCG; 2.5-20 µM | Bortezomib; 10-100 nM | U266 human multiple myeloma cells | MTT; 48h | Blocking of bortezomib-induced cytotoxic effects, antagonistic function. Increase in $IC_{50}$ of bortezomib | | [109] |

**Table 4.22.** (Continued)

| Flavonoid and its dosage | Bortezomib and its dosage | Biological system | Assay method and time | Effect | Mechanisms | Ref. |
|---|---|---|---|---|---|---|
| EGCG; 1-50 μM | Bortezomib; 10 nM | U266 human multiple myeloma cells | CellTiter-Glo; 48h | Blocking of antiproliferative (antimyeloma) effect of bortezomib, strong antagonism (CI>1) | Abolishment of proteasome inhibitory function of bortezomib. Blocking of bortezomib-induced apoptosis (decrease in caspases-3, -8, -9 and PARP activities, reduction of bortezomib-induced ΔΨm disruption). Direct chemical interaction between EGCG and bortezomib | [112] |
| EGCG; 1-100 μM | Bortezomib; 10 nM | Primary myeloma cells from six patients | CellTiter-Glo; 48h | Blocking of antiproliferative (antimyeloma) activity of bortezomib | | [112] |
| EGCG; 25 or 50 mg/kg, as a single dose via direct administration into the stomach | Bortezomib; 0.5 or 1 mg/kg, as a single dose via i.p. injection | RPMI/8226 cells implanted s.c. into 4-6 w-old male athymic nu/nu mice | 72h | Neutralization of antitumoral effects of bortezomib. Antagonistic effect on bortezomib cytotoxic activity | Blocking of bortezomib-increased apoptosis and necrosis | [109] |
| EGCG; 10-40 μM | Bortezomib; 10-100 nM | LN229 human glioblastoma cells | MTT; 48h. Colony assay; 12-14 days | Blocking of cytotoxic activity, increase in $IC_{50}$ of bortezomib. Antagonistic effect on bortezomib-inhibited colony formation | Prevention of bortezomib-induced proteasome inhibition and ubiquitinated proteins accumulation; prevention of bortezomib-induced GRP78 expression | [109] |

| Flavonoid and its dosage | Bortezomib and its dosage | Biological system | Assay method and time | Effect | Mechanisms | Ref. |
|---|---|---|---|---|---|---|
| EGCG; ratio with bortezomib of 50:1 | Bortezomib; 0.01-0.4 μM | MO59J human glioblastoma cells | SRB; 24h | Inhibition of bortezomib activity (CI>1) | | [113] |
| EGCG; 10, 20 μM | Bortezomib; 10 nM | U251 human glioblastoma cells | Colony assay; 12-14 days | Antagonistic effect on bortezomib-inhibited colony formation | | [109] |
| EGCG; ratio with bortezomib of 50:1 | Bortezomib; 0.01-0.4 μM | U251 human glioblastoma cells | SRB; 24h | Inhibition of bortezomib activity (CI>1) | | [113] |
| EGCG; ratio with bortezomib of 500:1 | Bortezomib; 0.01-0.04 μM | NGP human neuroblastoma cells | SRB; 24h | Inhibition of bortezomib activity (CI>1) | | [113] |
| EGCG; ratio with bortezomib of 500:1 | Bortezomib; 0.01-0.04 μM | SH-SY5Y human neuroblastoma cells | SRB; 24h | Inhibition of bortezomib activity (CI>1) | | [113] |
| EGCG; ratio with bortezomib of 50:1 | Bortezomib; 0.01-0.4 μM | CHL-1 human melanoma cells | SRB; 24h | Inhibition of bortezomib activity (CI>1) | | [113] |
| EGCG; ratio with bortezomib of 50:1 | Bortezomib; 0.01-0.4 μM | WM266-4 human melanoma cells | SRB; 24h | Inhibition of bortezomib activity (CI>1) | | [113] |
| EGCG; 5, 50 μM | Bortezomib; 5-30 nM | PC3 human prostate cancer cells; androgen-independent | WST-1; 48h | Antagonization of bortezomib cytotoxicity; shift of bortezomib dose-response curve to the right | Prevention of bortezomib-induced proteasome inhibition and endoplasmic reticulum stress (decrease in CHOP and p-eIF2α proteins). Promotion of autophagy induction. Inhibition of bortezomib-induced apoptosis (decrease in cleavage of caspase-8 and PARP-1) | [110] |

**Table 4.22.** (Continued)

| Flavonoid and its dosage | Bortezomib and its dosage | Biological system | Assay method and time | Effect | Mechanisms | Ref. |
|---|---|---|---|---|---|---|
| EGCG; 50 mg/kg, i.v. biweekly for 7 doses, about 2 min prior to bortezomib | Bortezomib; 0.8 mg/kg, i.v., biweekly for 7 doses | CWR22 human prostate tumor fragments inoculated into 5-8 w-old male CB-17 SCID mice | 22 days | Antagonistic effect on bortezomib-induced tumor growth inhibition; no antitumor activity | Partial blunting of bortezomib-induced 20S proteasome inhibition in blood and tumor. Prevention of bortezomib-elevated levels of phospho-β-catenin, GADD34 and ATF3 in tumors | [107] |
| EGCG; 50 mg/kg, s.c., biweekly for 7 doses; 30 or 60 min before bortezomib, or 60 min after bortezomib | Bortezomib; 0.8 mg/kg, i.v., biweekly for 7 doses | CWR22 human prostate tumor fragments inoculated into 5-8 w-old male CB-17 SCID mice | 25 days | No antagonistic effect on antitumor activity of bortezomib | Little or no antagonistic effect on bortezomib-induced 20S proteasome inhibition in blood and tumor. No effect on bortezomib-elevated levels of phospho-β-catenin, GADD34 and ATF3 | [107] |
| FLAVONES | | | | | | |
| Dihydroxy-pentamethoxyflavone; 100 μM | Bortezomib; 20 nM | U266 human multiple myeloma cells | Apoptosis assay; 24h | | Potentiation of bortezomib-induced apoptosis. Inhibition of STAT3 activation (by dihydroxy-pentamethoxyflavone) | [122] |
| Scutellarin; 30 mg/kg, co-injected with bortezomib via tail vein, alternate day treatment for 6 times | Bortezomib; 30 mg/kg, i.v., alternate day treatment for 6 times | MM.1S human multiple myeloma cells injected s.c. on the left side of BALB/C nude mice | 12 days | Potentiation of antimyeloma activity of bortezomib, dramatic decrease in tumor weight | Potentiation of bortezomib-induced drop in HDAC1/3, increase in miR-34a expression. Augmentation of bortezomib-induced decline in c-Met, p-Akt, mTOR. Decrease in NF-κB and XIAP levels | [115] |

| Flavonoid and its dosage | Bortezomib and its dosage | Biological system | Assay method and time | Effect | Mechanisms | Ref. |
|---|---|---|---|---|---|---|
| FLAVONOLS | | | | | | |
| Morin; 10, 25 μM | Bortezomib; 20 nM | U-266 human multiple myeloma cells | MTT; 4h with morin followed by 24h with bortezomib | Increase in bortezomib-induced cytotoxicity. Sensitization of cells to bortezomib | Increase in bortezomib-induced apoptosis. Inhibition of STAT3 activation (by morin) | [120] |
| Myricetin; 30 μM | Bortezomib; 20 nM | DoHH2 human diffuse large B-cell lymphoma cells | Apoptosis assay; 1h with myricetin followed by 12h with bortezomib | Blocking of anticancer effects of bortezomib | Inhibition of bortezomib-induced apoptosis | [114] |
| Quercetin dehydrate; 1-100 μM | Bortezomib; 10 nM | MC/CAR human multiple myeloma cells | CellTiter-Glo; 48h | Blocking of antiproliferative (antimyeloma) effect of bortezomib (CI>1) | Abolishment of proteasome inhibitory function of bortezomib. Blocking of bortezomib-induced apoptosis (decrease in caspases-3, -8, -9 and PARP activities, reduction of bortezomib-induced $\Delta\Psi m$ disruption) | [112] |
| Quercetin; 40 μM | Bortezomib; 20 nM | RPMI-8226 human multiple myeloma cells | Apoptosis assay; 1h with quercetin followed by 12h with bortezomib | Blocking of anticancer effects of bortezomib | Complete inhibition of bortezomib-induced apoptosis. Complex formation between quercetin and bortezomib | [114] |

**Table 4.22.** (Continued)

| Flavonoid and its dosage | Bortezomib and its dosage | Biological system | Assay method and time | Effect | Mechanisms | Ref. |
|---|---|---|---|---|---|---|
| Quercetin dehydrate; 1-100 μM | Bortezomib; 10 nM | RPMI8226 human multiple myeloma cells | CellTiter-Glo; 48h | Blocking of antiproliferative (antimyeloma) effect of bortezomib (CI>1) | Abolishment of proteasome inhibitory function of bortezomib. Blocking of bortezomib-induced apoptosis (decrease in caspases-3, -8, -9 and PARP activities, reduction of bortezomib-induced ΔΨm disruption) | [112] |
| Quercetin; 40 μM | Bortezomib; 20 nM | U266 human multiple myeloma cells | Apoptosis assay; 1h with quercetin followed by 12h with bortezomib | Blocking of anticancer effects of bortezomib | Complete inhibition of bortezomib-induced apoptosis. Complex formation between quercetin and bortezomib | [114] |
| Quercetin dehydrate; 1-100 μM | Bortezomib; 10 nM | U266 human multiple myeloma cells | CellTiter-Glo; 48h | Blocking of antiproliferative (antimyeloma) effect of bortezomib (CI>1) | Abolishment of proteasome inhibitory function of bortezomib. Blocking of bortezomib-induced apoptosis (decrease in caspases-3, -8, -9 and PARP activities, reduction of bortezomib-induced ΔΨm disruption) | [112] |

| Flavonoid and its dosage | Bortezomib and its dosage | Biological system | Assay method and time | Effect | Mechanisms | Ref. |
|---|---|---|---|---|---|---|
| Quercetin dehydrate; 1-100 μM | Bortezomib; 10 nM | Primary myeloma cells from six patients | CellTiter-Glo; 48h | Blocking of antiproliferative (antimyeloma) activity of bortezomib | | [112] |
| Quercetin; 50 μM | Bortezomib; 10 nM | BC3 human B-cell line; from primary effusion lymphoma, with latent KSHV | Counting; 24h | Increase in cytotoxicity of bortezomib, decrease in cell survival | | [119] |
| Quercetin; 50 μM | Bortezomib; 10 nM | BCBL1 human B-cell line; from primary effusion lymphoma, with latent KSHV | Counting; 24h | Increase in cytotoxicity of bortezomib, decrease in cell survival | | [119] |
| Quercetin; 20 μM | Bortezomib; 20 nM | DoHH2 human diffuse large B-cell lymphoma cells | Apoptosis assay; 1h with quercetin followed by 12h with bortezomib | Blocking of anticancer effects of bortezomib | Complete inhibition of bortezomib-induced apoptosis (prevention of bortezomib-activated caspases-9 and -3, inhibition of Bax activation and $\Delta\Psi m$ collapse). Complex formation between quercetin and bortezomib | [114] |
| Quercetin; 20 μM | Bortezomib; 20 nM | HRC57 human B cells; EBV-transformed | Apoptosis assay; 1h with quercetin followed by 12h with bortezomib | Blocking of anticancer effects of bortezomib | Complete inhibition of bortezomib-induced apoptosis (inhibition of bortezomib-induced $\Delta\Psi m$ collapse). Complex formation between quercetin and bortezomib | [114] |

**Table 4.22.** (Continued)

| Flavonoid and its dosage | Bortezomib and its dosage | Biological system | Assay method and time | Effect | Mechanisms | Ref. |
|---|---|---|---|---|---|---|
| Quercetin; 20 μM | Bortezomib; 20 nM | Primary CLL cells from patients | Apoptosis assay; 1h with quercetin followed by 12h with bortezomib | Blocking of anticancer effects of bortezomib | Complete inhibition of bortezomib-induced apoptosis (inhibition of bortezomib-induced Bax activation, blocking of cyt c release from mitochondria, inhibition of ROS production and ΔΨm collapse). Complex formation between quercetin and bortezomib | [114] |
| Rutin hydrate; 1-100 μM | Bortezomib; 10 nM | MC/CAR human multiple myeloma cells | CellTiter-Glo; 48h | Marginal inhibitory effect on bortezomib-induced antiproliferative (antimyeloma) activity (CI>1) | Abolishment of proteasome inhibitory function of bortezomib. Blocking of bortezomib-induced apoptosis (decrease in caspases-3, -8, -9 and PARP activities, reduction of bortezomib-induced ΔΨm disruption) | [112] |
| Rutin hydrate; 1-100 μM | Bortezomib; 10 nM | RPMI8226 human multiple myeloma cells | CellTiter-Glo; 48h | Marginal inhibitory effect on bortezomib-induced antiproliferative (antimyeloma) activity | Abolishment of proteasome inhibitory function of bortezomib. Blocking of bortezomib-induced apoptosis (decrease in caspases-3, -8, -9 and PARP activities, reduction of bortezomib-induced ΔΨm disruption) | [112] |

| Flavonoid and its dosage | Bortezomib and its dosage | Biological system | Assay method and time | Effect | Mechanisms | Ref. |
|---|---|---|---|---|---|---|
| Rutin hydrate; 1-100 μM | Bortezomib; 10 nM | U266 human multiple myeloma cells | CellTiter-Glo; 48h | Marginal inhibitory effect on bortezomib-induced antiproliferative (antimyeloma) activity | Abolishment of proteasome inhibitory function of bortezomib. Blocking of bortezomib-induced apoptosis (decrease in caspases-3, -8, -9 and PARP activities, reduction of bortezomib-induced ΔΨm disruption) | [112] |
| Rutin hydrate; 1-100 μM | Bortezomib; 10 nM | Primary myeloma cells from six patients | CellTiter-Glo; 48h | Blocking of antiproliferative (antimyeloma) activity of bortezomib | | [112] |
| Icariside II; 20 μM | Bortezomib; 20, 40 nM | U266 human multiple myeloma cells | MTT; 24h | Increase in bortezomib-induced cytotoxicity | Potentiation of bortezomib-induced apoptosis (increase in caspase-3 activation and PARP cleavage). Inhibition of STAT3 pathway (by icariside II) | [121] |
| ISOFLAVONES | | | | | | |
| Daidzin; 20 μM | Bortezomib; 5 nM | U266 human multiple myeloma cells | MTT; 24h | Synergistic attenuation of cell growth (CI<1) | Augmentation of bortezomib-induced apoptosis (cleavage of caspase-3 and PARP; decrease in Bcl-2, | [116] |
| | | | | | Bcl-xL and survivin). Downregulation of p-JAK1/2, p-Src and p-STAT3. Decrease in cyclin D1 and COX-2 levels | |

**Table 4.22.** (Continued)

| Flavonoid and its dosage | Bortezomib and its dosage | Biological system | Assay method and time | Effect | Mechanisms | Ref. |
|---|---|---|---|---|---|---|
| Formononetin; 50-100 μM | Bortezomib; 10, 20 nM | RPMI 8226 human multiple myeloma cells | MTT; 24h | Augmentation of bortezomib-induced cytotoxicity, synergistic attenuation of cell growth (CI<1) | | [117] |
| Formononetin; 50-100 μM | Bortezomib; 10, 20 nM | U266 human multiple myeloma cells | MTT; 24h | Augmentation of bortezomib-induced cytotoxicity, synergistic attenuation of cell growth (CI<1) | Enhancement of bortezomib-induced apoptosis (activation of caspase-3, cleavage of PARP); mitigation of the levels of tumorigenic proteins (Bcl-2, Bcl-xL, survivin, IAP-1/2, COX-2, VEGF and MMP-9). Augmentation of bortezomib-induced decrease in p-p38 and p-ERK1/2, increase in p-JNK; mitigation of p-IKKα/β, p-IκBα, p-p65, c-Fos and c-Jun proteins | [117] |

| Flavonoid and its dosage | Bortezomib and its dosage | Biological system | Assay method and time | Effect | Mechanisms | Ref. |
|---|---|---|---|---|---|---|
| Formononetin; 20 mg/kg bw, i.p., thrice per week | Bortezomib; 0.25 mg/kg bw, i.p., once per week | U266 cells (with Matrigel) implanted s.c. into the right flank of 5 w-old athymic nu/nu female mice | 21 days | Increase in antitumor action of bortezomib, potentiation of bortezomib-induced decrease in tumor growth and weight | Downregulation of p65, c-Fos, c-Jun levels in tumors; decrease in Ki67 and VEGF expression, increase in apoptosis (cleavage of caspase-3 and PARP). Attenuation of Bcl-2, Bcl-xL, survivin, IAP-1/2, COX-2 and MMP-9 proteins | [117] |
| CHALCONES | | | | | | |
| Butein; 25 μM | Bortezomib; 20 nM | U266 human multiple myeloma cells | Apoptosis assay; 24h | | Potentiation of bortezomib-induced apoptosis. Inhibition of STAT3 activation (by butein) | [123] |
| Flavokawain B; 8.8 μM | Bortezomib; 5 nM | C4-2B human prostate cancer cells | MTT; 24h | Increase in bortezomib-induced growth inhibition | Downregulation of Skp2 protein expression | [4] |
| Flavokawain B; 8.8 μM | Bortezomib; 5 nM | DU145 human prostate cancer cells | MTT; 24h | Increase in bortezomib-induced growth inhibition | Downregulation of Skp2 protein expression | [4] |
| Flavokawain B; 8.8 μM | Bortezomib; 5 nM | PC3 human prostate cancer cells | MTT; 24h | Increase in bortezomib-induced growth inhibition | Downregulation of Skp2 protein expression | [4] |
| SYNTHETIC FLAVONOIDS | | | | | | |
| Flavopiridol; 100 nM | Bortezomib; 5 nM | CCRF-CEM human lymphoid leukemia cells; Bcr-Abl-negative | Apoptosis assay; 24h | | Greater than additive increase in apoptosis | [98] |

**Table 4.22.** (Continued)

| Flavonoid and its dosage | Bortezomib and its dosage | Biological system | Assay method and time | Effect | Mechanisms | Ref. |
|---|---|---|---|---|---|---|
| Flavopiridol; 100 nM | Bortezomib; 3 nM | HL-60 human myeloid leukemia cells; Bcr-Abl-negative | Apoptosis assay; 24h | | Greater than additive increase in apoptosis | [98] |
| Flavopiridol; 100 nM | Bortezomib; 7.5 nM | Jurkat human lymphoid leukemia cells; Bcr-Abl-negative | Apoptosis assay; 24h | | Greater than additive increase in apoptosis | [98] |
| Flavopiridol; 150-200 nM | Bortezomib; 5-8 nM | K562 human leukemia cells; Bcr-Abl-positive | Apoptosis assay; 24, 48h | | Synergistic increase in apoptosis (CI<1) (extensive loss of $\Delta\Psi m$, release of cyt c and Smac/DIABLO, cleavage of PARP). Increase in MKK4, JNK and p38 MAPK phosphorylation; decrease in NF-κB and STAT3/5 activities; downregulation of Bcr-Abl and Bcl-xL | [98] |
| Flavopiridol; 200 nM | Bortezomib; 8 nM | K562-R human leukemia cells; Bcr-Abl-positive, imatinib-resistant (increased Bcr-Abl expression) | Apoptosis assay; 24, 48h | | Increase in apoptosis (cleavage of PARP). Downregulation of Bcr-Abl and Bcl-xL; diminished phosphorylation of Akt, Lyn, Hck and CrkL | [98] |

| Flavonoid and its dosage | Bortezomib and its dosage | Biological system | Assay method and time | Effect | Mechanisms | Ref. |
|---|---|---|---|---|---|---|
| Flavopiridol; 150-200 nM | Bortezomib; 5-8 nM | LAMA84 human leukemia cells; Bcr-Abl-positive | Apoptosis assay; 24, 48h | | Synergistic increase in apoptosis (CI<1) (extensive loss of ΔΨm, release of cyt c and Smac/DIABLO, cleavage of PARP). Increase in MKK4, JNK and p38 MAPK phosphorylation; decrease in NF-κB and STAT3/5 activities; downregulation of Bcr-Abl and Bcl-xL | [98] |
| Flavopiridol; 100 nM | Bortezomib; 5 nM | LAMA84-R human leukemia cells; Bcr-Abl-positive, imatinib-resistant (reduced Bcr-Abl expression) | Apoptosis assay; 24, 48h | | Induction of apoptosis (cleavage of PARP). Downregulation of Bcr-Abl and Bcl-xL; diminished phosphorylation of Akt, Lyn and Hck | [98] |
| Flavopiridol; 100 nM | Bortezomib; 5 nM | Raji human lymphoid leukemia cells; Bcr-Abl-negative | Apoptosis assay; 24h | | Greater than additive increase in apoptosis | [98] |
| Flavopiridol; 100 nM | Bortezomib; 5 nM | U937 human leukemia cells; Bcr-Abl-negative | Apoptosis assay; 24h | | Synergistic enhancement of apoptosis (increase in loss of ΔΨm, cytosolic release of cyt c and Smac/DIABLO, cleavage of PARP). Increase in JNK activation, abrogation of NF-κB activity | [98] |

**Table 4.22.** (Continued)

| Flavonoid and its dosage | Bortezomib and its dosage | Biological system | Assay method and time | Effect | Mechanisms | Ref. |
|---|---|---|---|---|---|---|
| Flavopiridol; 40-80 $mg/m^2$, on days 1 and 8, via i.v. bolus infusion over 30 min, followed by a 4h continuous infusion. Repeated at 3-week cycles | Bortezomib; 1.3 $mg/m^2$, on days 1, 4, 8 and 11; via an i.v. push over 3-5 seconds. Repeated at 3-week cycles | 16 patients, 11 males and 5 females (9 with non-Hodgkin lymphoma, 6 with multiple myeloma, 1 with extramedullary plasmacytoma) | 2-6 courses (median of 4 courses) | 2 complete responses (12%; 1 with NHL, 1 with multiple myeloma) and 5 partial responses (31%; 3 with multiple myeloma, 2 with NHL) with overall response rate of 44% | MTD 1.3 $mg/m^2$ for bortezomib and 30 $mg/m^2$ for flavopiridol (both the 30-min bolus and 4h infusion). Common hematologic toxicities included myelosuppression (leukopenia, lymphopenia, neutropenia, thrombocytopenia). Common non-hematologic toxicities were fatigue, neuropathy, diarrhea | [118] |
| Flavopiridol; 15-90 $mg/m^2$, on days 1, 4, 8 and 11, after bortezomib as i.v. infusion over 1h. Repeated at 3-week cycles | Bortezomib; 1.0-1.3 $mg/m^2$, on days 1, 4, 8 and 11, via an i.v. push over 3-5 seconds. Repeated at 3-week cycles | 44 patients, 12 females and 32 males (24 with multiple myeloma, 18 with non-Hodgkin lymphoma, 2 with Waldenstrom macroglobulinemia) | 1-16 cycles (median of 5 cycles) | 3 complete remissions (8%; 2 with NHL, 1 with multiple myeloma) and 10 partial remissions (26%; 6 with multiple myeloma, 3 with NHL, 1 with Waldenstrom macroglobulinemia) with total response rate of 33% | MTD 1.3 $mg/m^2$ for bortezomib and 40 $mg/m^2$ for flavopiridol. The most common hematologic toxicities included myelosuppression (leukopenia, lymphopenia, neutropenia, thrombocytopenia). The most common non-hematologic toxicities were diarrhea, fatigue, sensory neuropathy | [106] |

Moreover, the inhibitory effect of quercetin and rutin on antiproliferative activities of bortezomib was described also in primary myeloma cells derived from the bone marrow aspirates of patients. Direct chemical interaction of vicinal diol moieties of flavonols with boronic acid group of bortezomib provides a valid explanation to such antagonistic action, converting the active triangular boronic acid of bortezomib to an inactive tetrahedral boronate [112]. Although further works are definitely needed to elucidate the *in vivo* significance of these findings, the total intake of catechol moiety-containing flavonoids is probably determinative in blocking bortezomib antitumor efficacy (Figure 4.8). Nevertheless, in a recent study it was found that quercetin (50 μM) could, conversely, enhance the cytotoxic responses of bortezomib in human aggressive B-cell lines derived from primary effusion lymphoma, BC3 and BCBL1 [119]. Also, a flavonol with no 1,2-benzenediol moiety, morin (10 μM, 25 μM), increased bortezomib-induced cytotoxicity and apoptosis in human multiple myeloma cells U-266, by inhibiting the STAT3 pathway [120]. The presence of a natural prenylated flavonol glycoside, icariside II (20 μM), likewise led to sensitization of U266 cells to bortezomib, by augmenting cytotoxic and apoptotic responses [121]. Although further studies with animal models are needed, addition of morin or icariside II to bortezomib therapy might contribute to overcoming drug resistance in the treatment of relapsed or refractory multiple myeloma.

Two flavone-type compounds were also recently studied in combination with bortezomib in preclinical models of multiple myeloma. The findings of these works revealed that a polymethoxylated flavone, dihydroxy-pentamethoxyflavone (100 μM), could potentiate bortezomib-induced apoptosis in human multiple myeloma cells U266, behaving as a potent blocker of STAT3 pathway [122]. In addition, a flavone glycoside, scutellarin, potentiated antimyeloma activities of bortezomib in human multiple myeloma MM.1S xenografts-bearing nude mice, leading to a dramatic reduction of tumor weight through potentiation of bortezomib-induced decrease in the c-Met/Akt/mTOR pathway, as a downstream signaling of HDAC1/3 and miR-34a expression modulation. Increase in the suppression of NF-κB levels by combined treatment with bortezomib and scutellarin also conferred sensitization of the mice to bortezomib, promoting apoptotic death in malignant cells. Therefore, inclusion of scutellarin in bortezomib therapy might circumvent the drug resistance in the treatment of multiple myeloma, thereby allowing to improve the clinical outcomes and reduce therapeutically effective doses of bortezomib [115].

Recently, an isoflavone glycoside, daidzin (daidzein 7-O-glucoside, 20 μM), was described to synergistically enhance the cell growth inhibitory and proapoptotic effects of bortezomib in human multiple myeloma cells U266, by abrogating activation of STAT3 and its upstream signaling kinases (JAK1/2 and c-Src). These results show that cotreatment with bortezomib and daidzin might provide a novel promising strategy for enhancing therapeutic efficacy in the management of multiple myeloma, while mitigating adverse side effects [116]. Furthermore, another isoflavone, formononetin (50-100 μM), synergistically augmented bortezomib-induced antiproliferative and cytotoxic effects in human multiple myeloma lines RPMI 8226 and U266. In the latter cells, addition of formononetin enhanced drug-induced decrease in ERK1/2 and p38 activation and increase in JNK phosphorylation, further suppressing NF-κB and AP-1 pathways, ultimately leading to mitigation of the levels of a diverse set of tumorigenic gene products involved in cell survival, invasion and angiogenesis. Moreover, treatment with formononetin potentiated growth inhibitory action of bortezomib also in athymic nude mice implanted with U266 cells, resulting in the tumors with remarkably smaller sizes. Combination-treated tumors displayed significantly lower levels of biomarkers of proliferation (Ki67) and angiogenesis (VEGF), while increasing the expression of apoptotic proteins as compared to bortezomib alone-treated mice, in accordance with the downmodulation of NF-κB and AP-1 pathways-related factors. Therefore, formononetin could be employed as an adjuvant agent in bortezomib therapy for treatment of multiple myeloma, regulating the activation of diverse oncogenic proteins that are involved in myeloma development and progression. Further clinical trials are definitely warranted to verify the current preclinical findings in patients with relapsed and refractory multiple myeloma [117].

The potential modulatory action of chalcone-type phytochemicals, butein and flavokawain B, was also tested on bortezomib efficacy in different malignant cell lines, showing that butein (25 μM) could significantly potentiate bortezomib-triggered apoptosis in human multiple myeloma cells U266, despite containing a catechol moiety in its structure. Butein behaved as a potent inhibitor of STAT3 activation, thereby possibly contributing to overcoming of bortezomib resistance [123]. Flavokawain B (8.8 μM) enhanced the growth inhibitory activities of bortezomib in several human prostate cancer lines (C4-2B, DU145, PC3), by downregulating protein levels of S-phase kinase protein 2 (Skp2) via proteasomal degradation, in addition to bortezomib-induced suppression of Skp2 transcription, altogether leading to pronounced upregulation of p21/p27 and activation of caspase cascade [4].

Last but not least, semisynthetic flavonoid flavopiridol has also been studied concerning its potential ability to modulate bortezomib anticancer activity in several leukemia cells. It was found that flavopiridol (150-200 nM) synergistically enhanced bortezomib-induced apoptosis in Bcr-Abl-positive human leukemia cells K562 and LAMA84, through a mechanism involving an increased activation of stress-related kinases (MKK4, JNK and p38 MAPK), decreased NF-κB and STAT3/5 activities, and downregulation of Bcr-Abl expression. The combination of bortezomib and flavopiridol was active in enhancing apoptosis also in drug-resistant K562 (K562-R) and LAMA84 (LAMA84-R) cells, with different resistance mechanisms to imatinib. Moreover, combined treatment with bortezomib and flavopiridol potently induced apoptotic death also in Bcr-Abl-negative human leukemia cells, either from myeloid (U937, HL-60) or lymphoid lineage (Jurkat, Raji, CCRF-CEM) [98]. Driven by these promising preclinical results, two phase I clinical trials were further initiated and conducted to determine the dose-limiting toxicities (DLTs) and maximum tolerated doses (MTDs) for the combination of bortezomib and flavopiridol in patients with various B-cell malignancies. One of them included 16 patients with non-Hodgkin lymphoma (NHL; mantle cell lymphoma, follicular lymphoma), multiple myeloma or extramedullary plasmacytoma, treated with bortezomib (1.3 $mg/m^2$) according to a standard day 1, 4, 8 and 11 schedule, along with flavopiridol (40-80 $mg/m^2$) administered by a hybrid infusional schedule on days 1 and 8 (30 min bolus infusion followed by 4h continuous infusion). Two complete responses and five partial responses were described in this study with the overall response rate of 44% [118]. The other phase I clinical trial included 44 patients with multiple myeloma, NHL (mantle cell lymphoma, follicular lymphoma) or Waldenstrom macroglobulinemia, of whom 39 patients were evaluable for response. All patients received bortezomib (1.0-1.3 $mg/m^2$) by a standard day 1, 4, 8 and 11 schedule, in conjunction with flavopiridol (15-90 $mg/m^2$) given as a 1h intravenous infusion after bortezomib. As a result, three complete responses and ten partial responses were observed, with the total response rate of 33%. In addition, 20 patients had stable disease as their best response [106]. In both studies, the combination of bortezomib and flavopiridol was well tolerable, whereas the most common adverse reactions included hematologic toxicities (neutropenia, leukopenia, thrombocytopenia, lymphopenia) and non-hematologic toxicities (diarrhea, fatigue, neuropathy) [106, 118]. The findings of these phase I studies clearly justify phase II clinical trials for more definite determination of antimyeloma/antilymphoma activities of this novel combinatorial regimen; recommended to apply as a more easily manageable non-hybrid dosing schedule [106].

Collectively, whereas catechol group-containing flavonoids present in the plant-derived food items or herbal supplements exert pronounced antagonistic effects on anticancer potential of bortezomib through direct interaction between two agents and formation of cyclic boronate esters, some other structurally different polyphenolic phytochemicals or their semisynthetic derivatives can significantly augment the antitumor efficacy of bortezomib. There are diverse mechanisms underlying the sensitization of malignant cells to bortezomib by natural flavonoids, summarized in Figure 4.9, providing novel combinatorial strategies for improving therapeutic outcomes of relapsed and refractory multiple myeloma.

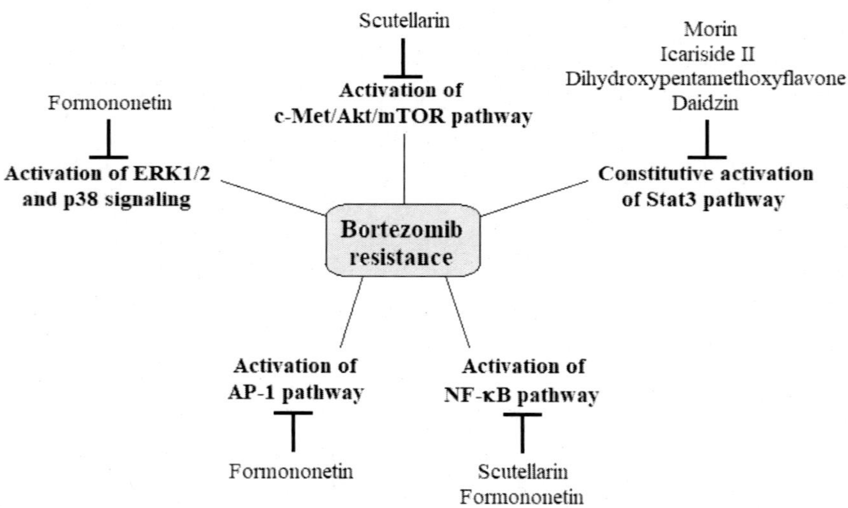


**Figure 4.9.** Overcoming bortezomib resistance and augmenting its antitumor action by flavonoids in multiple myeloma models.

### *4.2.2.4.2. Effects of Flavonoid-Rich Natural Products on Anticancer Efficacy of Bortezomib*

In addition to single flavanols as the constituents of green tea, complete green tea extract has also been tested regarding to its potential impact on anticancer effects of bortezomib. As a result, the presence of green tea extract blocked drug-induced cytotoxicity in both human multiple myeloma lines RPMI/8226 and U266 as well as human glioblastoma line LN229. Therefore, similar to the individual flavanols harboring catechol moiety, complex green tea extract could also provide efficient protection against anticancer activities of bortezomib, showing that drinking lots of green tea or taking supplements of green tea extract should be avoided by multiple myeloma patients undergoing bortezomib therapy [109] (Table 4.23).

**Table 4.23.** Effects of flavonoid-rich natural products on anticancer action of bortezomib (highlighted rows indicate undesired negative effects on anticancer efficacy)

| Flavonoid-rich natural product | Bortezomib and its dosage | Biological system | Assay method and time | Effect | Ref. |
|---|---|---|---|---|---|
| Green tea extract (GTE); 0.1-2.5 μg/ml EGCG in GTE | Bortezomib; 10, 20 nM | RPMI/8226 human multiple myeloma cells | MTT; 48h | Protection from the cytotoxic effects of bortezomib | [109] |
| Green tea extract (GTE); 0.1-2.5 μg/ml EGCG in GTE | Bortezomib; 10-40 nM | U266 human multiple myeloma cells | MTT; 48h | Protection from the cytotoxic effects of bortezomib | [109] |
| Green tea extract (GTE); 0.15-7.5 μg/ml EGCG in GTE | Bortezomib; 10-50 nM | LN229 human glioblastoma cells | MTT; 48h | Protection from the cytotoxic effects of bortezomib | [109] |

#### *4.2.2.5. Thalidomide*

Thalidomide (Thalomid) is an inhibitor of tumor necrosis factor (TNF) expression, modulating intracellular signaling pathways and inducing apoptosis in malignant cells [121-123] (Figure 4.6). This drug is approved for the first-line treatment of multiple myeloma, given in combination with dexamethasone [116]. Although thalidomide has improved the overall prognosis of multiple myeloma patients [120], the use of this drug is associated with substantial non-cancer cell toxicity, leading to a spectrum of adverse effects [115, 116]. Prolonged exposure to thalidomide is associated also with the development of resistance, eventually inducing disease relapses and contributing to short progression-free and overall survival times [120, 122]. Therefore, identification of safe and cost-effective adjuvant agents for sensitizing myeloma cells to thalidomide treatment is highly needed.

##### *4.2.2.5.1. Effects of Flavonoids on Anticancer Potential of Thalidomide*

A few structurally different flavonoids have been studied concerning their potential ability to sensitize human multiple myeloma cells U266 to the treatment with thalidomide. The results of these works are summarized in Table 4.24 and discussed more closely below.

Specifically, combining thalidomide with a polymethoxylated flavone, dihydroxy-pentamethoxyflavone (100 μM) led to a significant increase in the drug-induced apoptotic death in U266 cells [122]. Similarly, addition of flavonol morin (10 μM, 25 μM) [120] and prenylated flavonol glycoside icariside II (20 μM) [121] likewise enhanced the cytotoxic and proapoptotic activities of thalidomide in U266 cells. Thalidomide-evoked apoptotic death of U266 cells was potentiated also by the presence of chalcone butein (25 μM) in cell culture medium [123]. All these natural flavonoids were able to significantly inhibit STAT3 activation, representing a molecular mechanism underlying, at least in part, their sensitizing activities [120-123]. It is indeed well known that expression of constitutively active STAT3 is related to proliferation, survival, invasion, angiogenesis and therapeutic resistance of malignant cells, being characteristic for most tumor types including multiple myeloma [120-123]. Activation of STAT3 pathway has even been correlated with reduced survival in multiple myeloma patients [120]. Therefore, further *in vivo* studies combining thalidomide with these phytochemicals (dihydroxy-pentamethoxyflavone, morin, icariside II, butein) in animal models are warranted, as well as *in vitro* research with other natural small-molecule STAT3 inhibitors is needed to be expanded, to develop the most promising preclinical combination for entering clinical trials for treatment of relapsed and refractory multiple myeloma.

#### *4.2.2.6. Lenalidomide*

Lenalidomide (Revlimid) is a thalidomide analog that downregulates tumor-secreted prosurvival cytokines (TNF, IL-6, IL-8), inhibits tumor proliferation and angiogenesis, and leads malignant cells to apoptotic death [120, 123, 124] (Figure 4.6). This drug is approved by the FDA for treatment of myelodysplastic syndromes, multiple myeloma, relapsed or refractory mantle cell lymphoma, follicular lymphoma and marginal zone lymphoma [123, 124]. Although lenalidomide has improved the overall prognosis of multiple myeloma, it produces several adverse effects [120]. Also, most patients eventually develop resistance to lenalidomide, leading to disease relapses [120]. It is justified to presume that novel adjuvant agents could help to prevent or delay the emergence of lenalidomide resistance and thereby improve the clinical outcomes of multiple myeloma patients.

**Table 4.24.** Effects of flavonoids on anticancer action of thalidomide in multiple myeloma models

| Flavonoid and its dosage | Thalidomide and its dosage | Biological system | Assay method and time | Effect | Mechanisms | Ref. |
|---|---|---|---|---|---|---|
| FLAVONES | | | | | | |
| Dihydroxy-pentamethoxyflavone; 100 μM | Thalidomide; 10 ng/ml | U266 human multiple myeloma cells | Apoptosis assay; 24h | | Potentiation of thalidomide-induced apoptosis. Inhibition of STAT3 activation (by dihydroxy-pentamethoxyflavone) | [122] |
| FLAVONOLS | | | | | | |
| Morin; 10, 25 μM | Thalidomide; 10 μg/ml | U-266 human multiple myeloma cells | MTT; 4h with morin followed by 24h with thalidomide | Increase in thalidomide-induced cytotoxicity. Sensitization of cells to thalidomide | Increase in thalidomide-induced apoptosis. Inhibition of STAT3 activation (by morin) | [120] |
| Icariside II; 20 μM | Thalidomide; 30 μg/ml | U266 human multiple myeloma cells | MTT; 24h | Increase in thalidomide-induced cytotoxicity | Potentiation of thalidomide-induced apoptosis (increase in caspase-3 activation and PARP cleavage). Inhibition of STAT3 pathway (by icariside II) | [121] |
| CHALCONES | | | | | | |
| Butein; 25 μM | Thalidomide; 10 ng/ml | U266 human multiple myeloma cells | Apoptosis assay; 24h | | Potentiation of thalidomide-induced apoptosis. Inhibition of STAT3 activation (by butein) | [123] |

*4.2.2.6.1. Effects of Flavonoids on Anticancer Potential of Lenalidomide*

Despite expectations placed in phytochemicals as potential adjuvant agents for lenalidomide therapy, no preclinical studies have been reported so far about combinatorial treatment of malignant cells with lenalidomide and natural flavonoids. However, a phase I clinical trial was recently conducted studying the role of inclusion of semisynthetic flavonoid flavopiridol in lenalidomide treatment regimen in 39 patients with relapsed and refractory chronic lymphocytic leukemia (CLL) as the most common adult leukemia form. Although the maximum tolerated dose (MTD) remained unreached in this study where flavopiridol was administered as a hybrid infusional schedule (bolus infusion followed by continuous infusion), dose-limiting toxicities (DLTs) included grade 3-4 transaminitis and grade 3 absolute neutrophil count. The most common adverse reactions were reported to be hematologic toxicities (neutropenia, thrombocytopenia, anemia, lymphopenia), gastrointestinal toxicities (diarrhea), metabolic toxicities (transaminitis, hyperglycemia, hypophosphatemia, hypokalemia, hypocalcemia, hyperkalemia) and tumor lysis syndrome. Moreover, significant clinical activity was demonstrated among 31 evaluable patients, with an overall response rate of 51% (all partial responses). Therefore, combination of lenalidomide and flavopiridol might represent a promising novel therapy for patients requiring disease debulking before undergoing allogeneic transplantation [124] (Table 4.25).

### 4.2.3. Conclusions from Preclinical Knowledge with Dietary Recommendations to Patients under Pharmacological Inhibitors

Several pharmacological inhibitors targeting either membrane receptors or specific intracellular molecules have been developed and also approved for the treatment of certain cancer types, both solid tumors as well as hematological malignancies. However, the great breakthrough initially expected with the discovery of targeted biological drugs has not been realized yet, being impeded by several obstacles. Actually, although EGFR TKIs have revealed significant antitumor responses in diverse tumor models, their clinical application is still limited due to development of resistance through different cellular mechanisms, mainly by emerging of secondary mutations in EGFR gene and activation of alternative receptor tyrosine kinases that bypass the need for EGFR signaling. Acquired resistance has

**Table 4.25.** Effects of flavonoids on anticancer action of lenalidomide

| Flavonoid and its dosage | Lenalidomide and its dosage | Biological system | Assay method and time | Effect | Mechanisms | Ref. |
|---|---|---|---|---|---|---|
| SYNTHETIC FLAVONOIDS | | | | | | |
| Flavopiridol; 30 mg/$m^2$ i.v. bolus + 30 mg/$m^2$ continuous i.v. infusion in cycle 1 day 1 and 30 mg/$m^2$ i.v. bolus + 50 mg/$m^2$ continuous i.v. infusion in cycle 1 days 8, 15 and cycles 2-8 days 3, 10, 17 | Lenalidomide; 15 mg, orally, daily, cycles 2-8, days 1-21 | 39 patients with relapsed and refractory CLL | 1-8 cycles (median of 4 cycles) | Significant clinical activity with 51% overall response rate (31 patients evaluable for response completing at least 2 cycles). No effect on lenalidomide pharmacokinetic parameters | MTD not reached. DLTs in 3 patients (grade 3-4 transaminitis, grade 3 absolute neutrophil count). The most common grade 3-4 adverse events were hematologic (neutropenia, thrombocytopenia, anemia, lymphopenia), gastrointestinal (diarrhea), metabolic (transaminitis, hyperglycemia, hypophosphatemia, hypokalemia) and TLS | [124] |

remained an important obstacle also in administering small-molecule multikinase inhibitors, directed to either membrane receptors or specific intracellular targets (like ALK, mTOR, BRAF, Bcr-Abl, proteasome). The molecular mechanisms under losing sensitivity to these drugs over time are likewise diverse and complex, including development of novel mutations in the active site of the targeted tyrosine kinases and activation of multiple intracellular pathways for compensating the inhibited signaling. In addition, an enhanced efflux of the drugs by ATP-binding cassette transporters, such as P-gp and BCRP, precludes their accumulation in cancer cells at doses sufficient for antitumor activities. Moreover, in hematological malignancies, formation of sanctuary stromal niches in the bone marrow compartment which are protected against antileukemic action of targeted drugs further contributes to maintenance of minimal residual disease, inducing cancer recurrence. Further to the above, toxicity manifesting at higher doses of pharmacological inhibitors is another critical factor that often limits their therapeutic use in clinical settings. Therefore, the need for natural and safe adjuvant agents that could circumvent acquired resistance and resensitize malignant cells to targeted pharmacological inhibitors, lowering also the efficient drug doses, is urgently important. Specific plant-derived flavonoids have been shown to reveal a great promise in performing all these tasks.

- Based on the current *in vitro* and *in vivo* results, several plant-derived flavonoids could augment the antitumor action of EGFR-directed pharmacological inhibitor ERLOTINIB in diverse preclinical cancer models, targeting different cellular mechanisms related to erlotinib resistance. Briefly, remarkable beneficial effects have been described when erlotinib was combined with EGCG (NSCLC, HNSCC), kaempferol (pancreatic cancer), fisetin (NSCLC), ampelopsin (NSCLC) or silibinin (NSCLC). Further preclinical studies are definitely required to unravel the precise molecular mechanisms behind these sensitizing effects, and clinical trials are imperative to verify these results and elaborate optimal dosing, before giving any advice to patients concerning the use of these phytochemicals under treatment with erlotinib. However, we must acknowledge that the percentage of NSCLC patients benefiting from erlotinib therapy might be significantly increased when the drug is properly combined with specific plant-derived flavonoids. In addition, the spectrum of cancer types profiting from erlotinib therapy might also be remarkably wider (besides NSCLC and pancreatic cancer) when erlotinib is combined with certain flavonoids in the future.

- Several natural flavonoids can work synergistically to enhance the sensitivity and overcome resistance of malignant cells to EGFR-targeted drug GEFITINIB. Current preclinical studies have shown some promise in combining gefitinib with EGCG (NSCLC, HNSCC), apigenin (NSCLC), genistein (NSCLC) or silibinin (NSCLC, HCC). If further clinical trials will confirm these results, it could be possible to improve not only the progression-free survival but also the overall survival rate of NSCLC patients receiving the treatment with gefitinib, by preventing or retarding the development of acquired resistance and lowering efficient doses of the drug by applying adjuvant flavonoids. Therefore, clinical studies with combined regimens are urgently needed to be designed and conducted for developing novel treatment strategies and improving the therapeutic outcomes of patients with EGFR-overactivated tumors.
- Specific natural flavonoids can behave as SORAFENIB sensitizers, leading to reversal of sorafenib resistance through affecting different cellular mechanisms and reducing the severity of adverse effects via lowering therapeutically efficient doses of the drug. Current *in vitro* and *in vivo* preclinical studies have provided evidence and revealed some promise as potent adjuvant agents of sorafenib therapy for EGCG (HCC), chrysin (HCC), wogonin (HCC), amentoflavone (HCC), fisetin (melanoma), quercetin (thyroid cancer, glioma), rhamnetin (HCC), genistein (neuroblastoma), silibinin (HCC) and phloretin (HCC). Moreover, the presence of Thai-black ginger-derived 5,7-dimethoxyflavone could increase the plasma and tissue exposure to sorafenib and decrease the systemic drug clearance (in murine experiments) indicating that reduced doses of the drug might be needed to achieve therapeutic responses. Therefore, it is possible that inclusion of these phytochemicals in sorafenib treatment regimens might benefit patients with advanced hepatocellular carcinoma, further improving their prognosis, pointing to the urgent need to design and conduct clinical trials with the respective combinations of sorafenib and flavonoids. If successful, such combined multitargeted therapies might make the clinical management of patients with sorafenib-resistant tumors even more personalized in the future.

- Based on the current best knowledge obtained from preclinical studies driven by a patient case report, the major green tea flavanol EGCG can directly interact with multikinase inhibitor SUNITINIB, reducing the drug bioavailability and potentially impeding its antitumor efficacy, accompanying with a complex formation between sunitinib and EGCG. Therefore, drinking of green tea or consuming of EGCG-containing dietary supplements concurrently with taking sunitinib should be avoided by patients treated with this small-molecule targeted drug. However, when direct chemical interaction between EGCG and sunitinib can be prevented (by applying sequential administration schedules or delivered on specific nanoparticles), these two agents might reveal synergistic antitumor activities, shown in preclinical settings for renal cell carcinoma, but also breast and lung cancer models. Antitumor responses of renal cell carcinomas to sunitinib might be augmented also by hispidulin supplements, if further clinical trials will confirm the current promising preclinical findings.
- Milk thistle-derived flavonolignan silibinin might be an attractive adjuvant agent for overcoming acquired resistance to ALK-targeted drug CRIZOTINIB. If further preclinical studies and clinical trials will confirm the current promising *in vitro* findings, non-small cell lung cancer patients with tumors harboring ALK rearrangement might get benefit from silibinin supplements in prolonging and improving therapeutic responses to crizotinib.
- On the basis of the experimental studies with healthy rats, common dietary flavonoids apigenin and genistein can significantly modulate the pharmacokinetic profile of Bcr-Abl fusion protein-targeted drug IMATINIB, dependent on the dosing time of these natural agents. CML patients receiving imatinib therapy should be aware that concurrent long-term administration of food products or dietary supplements containing apigenin or genistein might accelerate the drug metabolism in the body, resulting in lower plasma levels and potential impairment of antileukemic efficacy of imatinib. On the contrary, intake of milk thistle-derived flavonolignan silibinin containing supplements might decrease the metabolism of imatinib, elevating systemic exposure to the drug and augmenting therapeutic responses (and also adverse reactions). Moreover, the presence of several naturally occurring flavonoids like oroxylin A, wogonin and 3-hydroxyflavone can augment also anticancer activities of imatinib

in preclinical models of CML, contributing to overcoming the drug resistance through regulating different cellular mechanisms. If these findings will be verified in future clinical trials, therapeutic regimens combining imatinib with specific flavonoids might remarkably postpone the emergence of imatinib resistance and improve the outcomes in clinical management of CML patients.

- Current preclinical studies have evidently proven that natural flavonoids containing catechol group can form direct chemical complexes with boronic acid moiety of proteasome inhibitor BORTEZOMIB, thereby antagonizing anticancer effects and impairing therapeutic efficacy of this drug. Such phytochemicals harboring catechol group include some common dietary flavonoids like epicatechin, epigallocatechin, epicatechin gallate, EGCG, myricetin and quercetin. Although more information about the doses of flavonoids at which such inhibitory effects appear *in vivo* as well as the possibilities to reach these levels in the plasma is clearly needed, it would be still justified to recommend that multiple myeloma patients receiving bortezomib therapy avoid an excessive exposure to the food items and dietary supplements containing these phytochemicals, in order to not deteriorate bortezomib-induced therapeutic responses. In particular, abundant consumption of green tea products might be contraindicated for patients treated with bortezomib. On the other hand, some structurally distinct flavonoids without catechol group in their molecular composition, especially scutellarin and isoflavones daidzin and formononetin, can contrary augment anticancer potential of bortezomib, definitely requiring further *in vivo* studies and clinical trials. If verified in the future, therapeutic regimens combining bortezomib with specific plant-derived phytochemicals might be an important strategy for overcoming drug resistance and lowering effective drug doses, thereby improving clinical outcomes of multiple myeloma management and reducing also severe toxicities associated with bortezomib therapy.

It is highly possible that combination of targeted pharmacological inhibitors, like HER family-directed TKIs or small-molecule multikinase inhibitors designed for specific membranous or intracellular proteins, with specific plant-derived flavonoids might represent a new and even more personalized coming of targeted anticancer drugs, ultimately leading to the success that was initially expected from the discovery of targeted biological therapies.

## References

[1] Park SJ, Kim MJ, Kim YK, Kim SM, Park JY, Myoung H. Combined cetuximab and genistein treatment shows additive anti-cancer effect on oral squamous cell carcinoma. *Cancer Lett* 2010; 292: 54-63.

[2] Liskova A, Samec M, Koklesova L, Brockmueller A, Zhai K, Abdellatif B, Siddiqui M, Biringer K, Kudela E, Pec M, Gadanec LK, Sudomova M, Hassan STS, Zulli A, Shakibaei M, Giordano FA, Büsselberg D, Golubnitschaja O, Kubatka P. Flavonoids as an effective sensitizer for anti-cancer therapy: insights into multi-faceted mechanisms and applicability towards individualized patient profiles. *EPMA J* 2021; 12: 155-76.

[3] Nagaria TS, Williams JL, Leduc C, Squire JA, Greer PA, Sangrar W. Flavopiridol synergizes with sorafenib to induce cytotoxicity and potentiate antitumorigenic activity in EGFR/HER-2 and mutant RAS/RAF breast cancer models systems. *Neoplasia* 2013; 15: 939-51.

[4] Li X, Pham V, Tippin M, Fu D, Rendon R, Song L, Uchio E, Hoang BH, Zi X. Flavokawain B targets protein neddylation for enhancing the anti-prostate cancer effect of Bortezomib via Skp2 degradation. *Cell Commun Signal* 2019; 17: 25.

[5] Bae S, D`Cunha R, Shao J, An G. Effect of 5,7-dimethoxyflavone on Bcrp1-mediated transport of sorafenib in vitro and in vivo in mice. *Eur J Pharm Sci* 2018; 117: 27-34.

[6] Guney Eskiler G, Deveci AO, Bilir C, Kaleli S. Synergistic effects of nobiletin and sorafenib combination on metastatic prostate cancer cells. *Nutr Cancer* 2019; 71: 1299-1312.

[7] Haque A, Rahman MA, Chen ZG, Saba NF, Khuri FR, Shin DM, Ruhul Amin AR. Combination of erlotinib and EGCG induces apoptosis of head and neck cancers through posttranscriptional regulation of Bim and Bcl-2. *Apoptosis* 2015; 20: 986-95.

[8] Daveri E, Adamo AM, Alfine E, Zhu W, Oteiza PI. Hexameric procyanidins inhibit colorectal cancer cell growth through both redox and non-redox regulation of the epidermal growth factor signaling pathway. *Redox Biol* 2021; 38: 101830.

[9] Huang WC, Hsieh YL, Hung CM, Chien PH, Chien YF, Chen LC, Tu CY, Chen CH, Hsu SC, Lin YM, Chen YJ. BCRP/ABCG2 inhibition

sensitizes hepatocellular carcinoma cells to sorafenib. *PLoS One* 2013; 8: e83627.

[10] Ge J, Tan BX, Chen Y, Yang L, Peng XC, Li HZ, Lin HJ, Zhao Y, Wei M, Cheng K, Li LH, Dong H, Gao F, He JP, Wu Y, Qiu M, Zhao YL, Su JM, Hou JM, Liu JY. Interaction of green tea polyphenol epigallocatechin-3-gallate with sunitinib: potential risk of diminished sunitinib bioavailability. *J Mol Med* 2011; 89: 595-602.

[11] Hu WJ, Liu J, Zhong LK, Wang J. Apigenin enhances the antitumor effects of cetuximab in nasopharyngeal carcinoma by inhibiting EGFR signaling. *Biomed Pharmacother* 2018; 102: 681-8.

[12] Park MH, Hong JE, Hwang CJ, Choi M, Choi JS, An YJ, Son DJ, Hong JT. Synergistic inhibitory effect of cetuximab and tectochrysin on human colon cancer cell growth via inhibition of EGFR signal. *Arch Pharm Res* 2016; 39: 721-9.

[13] Honndorf VS, Wiehr S, Rolle AM, Schmitt J, Kreft L, Quintanilla-Martinez L, Kohlhofer U, Reischl G, Maurer A, Boldt K, Schwarz M, Schmidt H, Pichler BJ. Preclinical evaluation of the anti-tumor effects of the natural isoflavone genistein in two xenograft mouse models monitored by [18F]FDG, [18F]FLT, and [64Cu]NODAGA-cetuximab small animal PET. *Oncotarget* 2016; 7: 28247-61.

[14] Lattrich C, Lubig J, Springwald A, Goerse R, Ortmann O, Treeck O. Additive effects of trastuzumab and genistein on human breast cancer cells. *Anticancer Drugs* 2011; 22: 253-61.

[15] Nahta R, Trent S, Yang C, Schmidt EV. Epidermal growth factor receptor expression is a candidate target of the synergistic combination of trastuzumab and flavopiridol in breast cancer. *Cancer Res* 2003; 63: 3626-31.

[16] Liu W, Xu J, Liu Y, Yu X, Tang X, Wang Z, Li X. Anthocyanins potentiate the activity of trastuzumab in human epidermal growth factor receptor 2-positive breast cancer cells in vitro and in vivo. *Mol Med Rep* 2014; 10: 1921-6.

[17] Wu K, Wang C, D`Amico M, Lee RJ, Albanese C, Pestell RG, Mani S. Flavopiridol and trastuzumab synergistically inhibit proliferation of breast cancer cells: association with selective cooperative inhibition of cyclin D1-dependent kinase and Akt signaling pathways. *Mol Cancer Ther* 2002; 1: 695-706.

[18] Jandial DD, Krill LS, Chen L, Wu C, Ke Y, Xie J, Hoang BH, Zi X. Induction of G2M arrest by flavokawain A, a kava chalcone, increases the responsiveness of HER2-overexpressing breast cancer cells to herceptin. *Molecules* 2017; 22: 462.

[19] Nahta R, Iglehart JD, Kempkes B, Schmidt EV. Rate-limiting effects of Cyclin D1 in transformation by ErbB2 predicts synergy between herceptin and flavopiridol. *Cancer Res* 2002; 62: 2267-71.
[20] Li X, Wang X, Zhang M, Li A, Sun Z, Yu Q. Quercetin potentiates the antitumor activity of rituximab in diffuse large B-cell lymphoma by inhibiting STAT3 pathway. *Cell Biochem Biophys* 2014; 70: 1357-62.
[21] Kay C, Martinez-Perez C, Meehan J, Gray M, Webber V, Dixon JM, Turnbull AK. Current trends in the treatment of HR+/HER2+ breast cancer. *Future Oncol* 2021; 17: 1665-81.
[22] Liu J, Zhong T, Yi P, Fan C, Zhang Z, Liang G, Xu Y, Fan Y. A new epigallocatechin gallate derivative isolated from Anhua dark tea sensitizes the chemosensitivity of gefitinib via the suppressing of PI3K/mTOR and epithelial-mesenchymal transition. *Fitoterapia* 2020; 143: 104590.
[23] Aichinger G, Pahlke G, Nagel LJ, Berger W, Marko D. Bilberry extract, its major polyphenolic compounds, and the soy isoflavone genistein antagonize the cytostatic drug erlotinib in human epithelial cells. *Food Funct* 2016; 7: 3628-36.
[24] Chang CM, Chang PY, Tu MG, Lu CC, Kuo SC, Amagaya S, Lee CY, Jao HY, Chen MY, Yang JS. Epigallocatechin gallate sensitizes CAL-27 human oral squamous cell carcinoma cells to the anti-metastatic effects of gefitinib (Iressa) via synergistic suppression of epidermal growth factor receptor and matrix metalloproteinase-2. *Oncol Rep* 2012; 28: 1799-807.
[25] Meng J, Chang C, Chen Y, Bi F, Ji C, Liu W. EGCG overcomes gefitinib resistance by inhibiting autophagy and augmenting cell death through targeting ERK phosphorylation in NSCLC. *Onco Targets Ther* 2019; 12: 6033-43.
[26] Cufi S, Bonavia R, Vazquez-Martin A, Oliveras-Ferraros C, Corominas-Faja B, Cuyas E, Martin-Castillo B, Barrajon-Catalan E, Visa J, Segura-Carretero A, Joven J, Bosch-Barrera J, Micol V, Menendez JA. Silibinin suppresses EMT-driven erlotinib resistance by reversing the high miR-21/low miR-200c signature in vivo. *Sci Rep* 2013; 3: 2459.
[27] Chen Z, Tian D, Liao X, Zhang Y, Xiao J, Chen W, Liu Q, Chen Y, Li D, Zhu L, Cai S. Apigenin combined with gefitinib blocks autophagy flux and induces apoptotic cell death through inhibition of HIF-1α, c-Myc, p-EGFR, and glucose metabolism in EGFR L858R+T790M-mutated H1975 cells. *Front Pharmacol* 2019; 10: 260.
[28] Zhu H, Cheng H, Ren Y, Liu ZG, Zhang YF, De Luo B. Synergistic inhibitory effects by the combination of gefitinib and genistein on NSCLC with acquired drug-resistance in vitro and in vivo. *Mol Biol Rep* 2012; 39: 4971-9.

[29] Milligan SA, Burke P, Coleman DT, Bigelow RL, Steffan JJ, Carroll JL, Williams BJ, Cardelli JA. The green tea polyphenol EGCG potentiates the antiproliferative activity of c-Met and epidermal growth factor receptor inhibitors in non-small cell lung cancer cells. *Clin Cancer Res* 2009; 15: 4885-94.

[30] Cromie MM, Liu Z, Gao W. Epigallocatechin-3-gallate augments the therapeutic effects of benzo[a]pyrene-mediated lung carcinogenesis. *Biofactors* 2017; 43: 529-39.

[31] Sung H, Ferlay J, Siegel RL, Laversanne M, Soerjomataram I, Jemal A, Bray F. Global cancer statistics 2020: GLOBOCAN estimates of incidence and mortality worldwide for 36 cancers in 185 countries. *CA Cancer J Clin* 2021; 71: 209-49.

[32] Zhang L, Huang Y, Zhuo W, Zhu Y, Zhu B, Chen Z. Fisetin, a dietary phytochemical, overcomes Erlotinib-resistance of lung adenocarcinoma cells through inhibition of MAPK and AKT pathways. *Am J Transl Res* 2016; 8: 4857-68.

[33] Wu Z, Xu B, Yu Z, He Q, Hu Z, Zhou S, Chen M, Zhu L. Trifolium flavonoids overcome gefitinib resistance of non-small-cell lung cancer cell by suppressing ERK and STAT3 signaling pathways. *Biomed Res Int* 2020; 2020: 2491304.

[34] Ambrosio R, Ombra MN, Gridelli C, Picariello G, DI Stasio M, Volpe MG. Isoflavone extracts enhance the effect of epidermal growth factor receptor inhibitors in NSCLC cell lines. *Anticancer Res* 2016; 36: 5827-33.

[35] Corominas-Faja B, Oliveras-Ferraros C, Cuyas E, Segura-Carretero A, Joven J, Martin-Castillo B, Barrajon-Catalan E, Micol V, Bosch-Barrera J, Menendez JA. Stem cell-like ALDH(bright) cellular states in EGFR-mutant non-small cell lung cancer: a novel mechanism of acquired resistance to erlotinib targetable with the natural polyphenol silibinin. *Cell Cycle* 2013; 12: 3390-404.

[36] Rho JK, Choi YJ, Jeon BS, Choi SJ, Cheon GJ, Woo SK, Kim HR, Kim CH, Choi CM, Lee JC. Combined treatment with silibinin and epidermal growth factor receptor tyrosine kinase inhibitors overcomes drug resistance caused by T790M mutation. *Mol Cancer Ther* 2010; 9: 3233-43.

[37] Cufi S, Bonavia R, Vazquez-Martin A, Corominas-Faja B, Oliveras-Ferraros C, Cuyas E, Martin-Castillo B, Barrajon-Catalan E, Visa J, Segura-Carretero A, Bosch-Barrera J, Joven J, Micol V, Menendez JA. Silibinin meglumine, a water-soluble form of milk thistle silymarin, is an orally active anti-cancer agent that impedes the epithelial-to-

mesenchymal transition (EMT) in EGFR-mutant non-small-cell lung carcinoma cells. *Food Chem Toxicol* 2013; 60: 360-8.

[38] Zhang X, Zhang H, Tighiouart M, Lee JE, Shin HJ, Khuri FR, Yang CS, Chen Z, Shin DM. Synergistic inhibition of head and neck tumor growth by green tea (-)-epigallocatechin-3-gallate and EGFR tyrosine kinase inhibitor. *Int J Cancer* 2008; 123: 1005-14.

[39] Ruhul Amin AR, Khuri FR, Chen ZG, Shin DM. Synergistic growth inhibition of squamous cell carcinoma of the head and neck by erlotinib and epigallocatechin-3-gallate: the role of p53-dependent inhibition of nuclear factor-kappaB. *Cancer Prev Res* 2009; 2: 538-45.

[40] Hong SW, Park NS, Noh MH, Shim JA, Ahn BN, Kim YS, Kim D, Lee HK, Hur DY. Combination treatment with erlotinib and ampelopsin overcomes erlotinib resistance in NSCLC cells via the Nox2-ROS-Bim pathway. *Lung Cancer* 2017; 106: 115-24.

[41] Zhang Z, Guo Y, Chen M, Chen F, Liu B, Shen C. Kaempferol potentiates the sensitivity of pancreatic cancer cells to erlotinib via inhibition of the PI3K/AKT signaling pathway and epidermal growth factor receptor. *Inflammopharmacology* 2021; 29: 1587-601.

[42] Haque A, Rahman MA, Chen ZG, Shin DM, Ruhul Amin AR. Abstract 2269: Combination of erlotinib and epigallocatechin-3-gallate induces apoptosis of squamous cell carcinoma of the head and neck through posttranslational regulation of Bim and Bcl-2. *Cancer Res* 2014; 74Suppl: 2269.

[43] Sakurai MA, Ozaki Y, Okuzaki D, Naito Y, Sasakura T, Okamoto A, Tabara H, Inoue T, Hagiyama M, Ito A, Yabuta N, Nojima H. Gefitinib and luteolin cause growth arrest of human prostate cancer PC-3 cells via inhibition of cyclin G-associated kinase and induction of miR-630. *PLoS One* 2014; 9: e100124.

[44] Tiwari H, Karki N, Pal M, Basak S, Verma RK, Bal R, Kandpal ND, Bisht G, Sahoo NG. Functionalized graphene oxide as a nanocarrier for dual drug delivery applications: The synergistic effect of quercetin and gefitinib against ovarian cancer cells. *Colloids Surf B Biointerfaces* 2019; 178: 452-9.

[45] Parashar P, Tripathi CB, Arya M, Kanoujia J, Singh M, Yadav A, Kumar A, Guleria A, Saraf SA. Biotinylated naringenin intensified anticancer effect of gefitinib in urethane-induced lung cancer in rats: favourable modulation of apoptotic regulators and serum metabolomics. *Artif Cells Nanomed Biotechnol* 2018; 46Suppl3: S598-610.

[46] Castillo-Pichardo L, Dharmawardhane SF. Grape polyphenols inhibit Akt/mammalian target of rapamycin signaling and potentiate the effects of gefitinib in breast cancer. *Nutr Cancer* 2012; 64: 1058-69.

[47] Shen Y, TanTai J. Co-delivery anticancer drug nanoparticles for synergistic therapy against lung cancer cells. *Drug Des Devel Ther* 2020; 14: 4503-10.

[48] Markaverich BM, Vijjeswarapu M, Shoulars K, Rodriguez M. Luteolin and gefitinib regulation of EGF signaling pathway and cell cycle pathway genes in PC-3 human prostate cancer cells. *J Steroid Biochem Mol Biol* 2010; 122: 219-31.

[49] Gu HR, Park SC, Choi SJ, Lee JC, Kim YC, Han CJ, Kim J, Yang KY, Kim YJ, Noh GY, No SH, Jeong JH. Combined treatment with silibinin and either sorafenib or gefitinib enhances their growth-inhibiting effects in hepatocellular carcinoma cells. *Clin Mol Hepatol* 2015; 21: 49-59.

[50] Zhang L, Liu Q, Huang L, Yang F, Liu A, Zhang J. Combination of lapatinib and luteolin enhances the therapeutic efficacy of lapatinib on human breast cancer through the FOXO3a/NQO1 pathway. *Biochem Biophys Res Commun* 2020; 531: 364-71.

[51] Mitchell C, Yacoub A, Hossein H, Martin AP, Bareford MD, Eulitt P, Yang C, Nephew KP, Dent P. Inhibition of MCL-1 in breast cancer cells promotes cell death in vitro and in vivo. *Cancer Biol Ther* 2010; 10: 903-17.

[52] Sirin N, Elmas L, Secme M, Dodurga Y. Investigation of possible effects of apigenin, sorafenib and combined applications on apoptosis and cell cycle in hepatocellular cancer cells. *Gene* 2020; 737: 144428.

[53] Wu XY, Xu H, Wu ZF, Chen C, Liu JY, Wu GN, Yao XQ, Liu FK, Li G, Shen L. Formononetin, a novel FGFR2 inhibitor, potently inhibits angiogenesis and tumor growth in preclinical models. *Oncotarget* 2015; 6: 44563-78.

[54] Jia H, Yang Q, Wang T, Cao Y, Jiang QY, Ma HD, Sun HW, Hou MX, Yang YP, Feng F. Rhamnetin induces sensitization of hepatocellular carcinoma cells to a small molecular kinase inhibitor or chemotherapeutic agents. *Biochim Biophys Acta* 2016; 1860: 1417-30.

[55] Pal HC, Diamond AC, Strickland LR, Kappes JC, Katiyar SK, Elmets CA, Athar M, Afaq F. Fisetin, a dietary flavonoid, augments the anti-invasive and anti-metastatic potential of sorafenib in melanoma. *Oncotarget* 2016; 7: 1227-41.

[56] Jakubowicz-Gil J, Langner E, Badziul D, Wertel I, Rzeski W. Quercetin and sorafenib as a novel and effective couple in programmed cell death induction in human gliomas. *Neurotox Res* 2014; 26: 64-77.

[57] Wei CT, Chen LC, Hsiang YP, Hung YJ, Chien PH, Pan HL, Chen YJ. Chrysin-induced ERK1/2 phosphorylation enhances the sensitivity of human hepatocellular carcinoma cells to sorafenib. *Anticancer Res* 2019; 39: 695-701.

[58] Pal HC, Baxter RD, Hunt KM, Agarwal J, Elmets CA, Athar M, Afaq F. Fisetin, a phytochemical, potentiates sorafenib-induced apoptosis and abrogates tumor growth in athymic nude mice implanted with BRAF-mutated melanoma cells. *Oncotarget* 2015; 6: 28296-311.

[59] Rong LW, Wang RX, Zheng XL, Feng XQ, Zhang L, Zhang L, Lin Y, Li ZP, Wang X. Combination of wogonin and sorafenib effectively kills human hepatocellular carcinoma cells through apoptosis potentiation and autophagy inhibition. *Oncol Lett* 2017; 13: 5028-34.

[60] Lin MT, Lin CL, Lin TY, Cheng CW, Yang SF, Lin CL, Wu CC, Hsieh YH, Tsai JP. Synergistic effect of fisetin combined with sorafenib in human cervical cancer HeLa cells through activation of death receptor-5 mediated caspase-8/caspase-3 and the mitochondria-dependent apoptotic pathway. *Tumour Biol* 2016; 37: 6987-96.

[61] Mao J, Yang H, Cui T, Pan P, Kabir N, Chen D, Ma J, Chen X, Chen Y, Yang Y. Combined treatment with sorafenib and silibinin synergistically targets both HCC cells and cancer stem cells by enhanced inhibition of the phosphorylation of STAT3/ERK/AKT. *Eur J Pharmacol* 2018; 832: 39-49.

[62] Celano M, Maggisano V, Bulotta S, Allegri L, Pecce V, Abballe L, Damante G, Russo D. Quercetin improves the effects of sorafenib on growth and migration of thyroid cancer cells. *Endocrine* 2020; 67: 496-8.

[63] Izkhakov E, Sharon O, Knoll E, Aizic A, Fliss DM, Kohen F, Stern N, Somjen D. A sorafenib-sparing effect in the treatment of thyroid carcinoma cells attained by co-treatment with a novel isoflavone derivative and 1,25 dihydroxyvitamin D3. *J Steroid Biochem Mol Biol* 2018; 182: 81-6.

[64] Li S, Wu L, Feng J, Li J, Liu T, Zhang R, Xu S, Cheng K, Zhou Y, Zhou S, Kong R, Chen K, Wang F, Xia Y, Lu J, Zhou Y, Dai W, Guo C. In vitro and in vivo study of epigallocatechin-3-gallate-induced apoptosis in aerobic glycolytic hepatocellular carcinoma cells involving inhibition of phosphofructokinase activity. *Sci Rep* 2016; 6: 28479.

[65] Wang C, Su L, Wu C, Wu J, Zhu C, Yuan G. RGD peptide targeted lipid-coated nanoparticles for combinatorial delivery of sorafenib and quercetin against hepatocellular carcinoma. *Drug Dev Ind Pharm* 2016; 42: 1938-44.

[66] Lee JH, Mohan CD, Shanmugam MK, Rangappa S, Sethi G, Siveen KS, Chinnathambi A, Alahmadi TA, Alharbi SA, Basappa S, Rangappa KS, Ahn KS. Vitexin abrogates invasion and survival of hepatocellular carcinoma cells through targeting STAT3 signaling pathway. *Biochimie* 2020; 175: 58-68.

[67] Nair B, Anto RJ, Sabitha M, Nath LR. Kaempferol-mediated sensitization enhances chemotherapeutic efficacy of sorafenib against hepatocellular carcinoma: An in silico and in vitro approach. *Adv Pharm Bull* 2020; 10: 472-6.

[68] Wu MH, Chiu YF, Wu WJ, Wu PL, Lin CY, Lin CL, Hsieh YH, Liu CJ. Synergistic antimetastatic effect of cotreatment with licochalcone A and sorafenib on human hepatocellular carcinoma cells through the inactivation of MKK4/JNK and uPA expression. *Environ Toxicol* 2018; 33: 1237-44.

[69] Saraswati S, Alhaider A, Abdelgadir AM, Tanwer P, Korashy HM. Phloretin attenuates STAT-3 activity and overcomes sorafenib resistance targeting SHP-1-mediated inhibition of STAT3 and Akt/VEGFR2 pathway in hepatocellular carcinoma. *Cell Commun Signal* 2019; 17: 127.

[70] Chen WL, Hsieh CL, Chen JH, Huang CS, Chen WT, Kuo YC, Chen CY, Hsu FT. Amentoflavone enhances sorafenib-induced apoptosis through extrinsic and intrinsic pathways in sorafenib-resistant hepatocellular carcinoma SK-Hep1 cells in vitro. *Oncol Lett* 2017; 14: 3229-34.

[71] Rigalli JP, Ciriaci N, Arias A, Ceballos MP, Villanueva SS, Luquita MG, Mottino AD, Ghanem CI, Catania VA, Ruiz ML. Regulation of multidrug resistance proteins by genistein in a hepatocarcinoma cell line: impact on sorafenib cytotoxicity. *PLoS One* 2015; 10: e0119502.

[72] Zou H, Cao X, Xiao Q, Sheng X, Ren K, Quan M, Song Z, Li D, Zheng Y, Zeng W, Cao J, Peng Y. Synergistic inhibition of characteristics of liver cancer stem-like cells with a combination of sorafenib and 8-bromo-7-methoxychrysin in SMMC-7721 cell line. *Oncol Rep* 2016; 36: 1731-8.

[73] Li B, Feng F, Jia H, Jiang Q, Cao S, Wei L, Zhang Y, Lu J. Rhamnetin decelerates the elimination and enhances the antitumor effect of the molecular-targeting agent sorafenib in hepatocellular carcinoma cells via the miR-148a/PXR axis. *Food Funct* 2021; 12: 2404-17.

[74] Youssef MM, Tolba MF, Badawy NN, Liu AW, El-Ahwany E, Khalifa AE, Zada S, Abdel-Naim AB. Novel combination of sorafenib and biochanin-A synergistically enhances the anti-proliferative and pro-apoptotic effects on hepatocellular carcinoma cells. *Sci Rep* 2016; 6: 30717.

[75] Tsai JJ, Hsu FT, Pan PJ, Chen CW, Kuo YC. Amentoflavone enhances the therapeutic efficacy of sorafenib by inhibiting anti-apoptotic potential and potentiating apoptosis in hepatocellular carcinoma in vivo. *Anticancer Res* 2018; 38: 2119-25.

[76] Ferrari SM, Antonelli A, Guidi P, Bernardeschi M, Scarcelli V, Fallahi P, Frenzilli G. Genotoxicity evaluation of the soybean isoflavone genistein

in human papillary thyroid cancer cells. Study of its potential use in thyroid cancer therapy. *Nutr Cancer* 2019; 71:1335-44.

[77] Roy Choudhury S, Karmakar S, Banik NL, Ray SK. Synergistic efficacy of sorafenib and genistein in growth inhibition by down regulating angiogenic and survival factors and increasing apoptosis through upregulation of p53 and p21 in malignant neuroblastoma cells having N-Myc amplification or non-amplification. *Invest New Drugs* 2010; 28: 812-24.

[78] Zhou Y, Tang J, Du Y, Ding J, Liu JY. The green tea polyphenol EGCG potentiates the antiproliferative activity of sunitinib in human cancer cells. *Tumour Biol* 2016; 37: 8555-66.

[79] Yongvongsoontorn N, Chung JE, Gao SJ, Bae KH, Yamashita A, Tan MH, Ying JY, Kurisawa M. Carrier-enhanced anticancer efficacy of sunitinib-loaded green tea-based micellar nanocomplex beyond tumor-targeted delivery. *ACS Nano* 2019; 13: 7591-602.

[80] Gao H, Jiang Q, Han Y, Peng J, Wang C. Hispidulin potentiates the antitumor effect of sunitinib against human renal cell carcinoma in laboratory models. *Cell Biochem Biophys* 2015; 71: 757-64.

[81] Albassam AA, Markowitz JS. An appraisal of drug-drug interactions with green tea (Camellia sinensis). *Planta Med* 2017; 83: 496-508.

[82] Cuyas E, Perez-Sanchez A, Micol V, Menendez JA, Bosch-Barrera J. STAT3-targeted treatment with silibinin overcomes the acquired resistance to crizotinib in ALK-rearranged lung cancer. *Cell Cycle* 2016; 15: 3413-8.

[83] Zhu K, Wang W. Green tea polyphenol EGCG suppresses osteosarcoma cell growth through upregulating miR-1. *Tumour Biol* 2016; 37: 4373-82.

[84] Quagliariello V, Iaffaioli RV, Armenia E, Clemente O, Barbarisi M, Nasti G, Berretta M, Ottaiano A, Barbarisi A. Hyaluronic acid nanohydrogel loaded with quercetin alone or in combination to a macrolide derivative of rapamycin RAD001 (everolimus) as a new treatment for hormone-responsive human breast cancer. *J Cell Physiol* 2017; 232: 2063-74.

[85] Peng X, Wang Z, Liu Y, Peng X, Liu Y, Zhu S, Zhang Z, Qiu Y, Jin M, Wang R, Zhang Q, Kong D. Oxyfadichalcone C inhibits melanoma A375 cell proliferation and metastasis via suppressing PI3K/Akt and MAPK/ERK pathways. *Life Sci* 2018; 206: 35-44.

[86] Goncalves de Oliveira-Junior R, Marcoult-Freville N, Prunier G, Beaugeard L, Beserra de Alencar Filho E, Simoes Mourao ED, Michel S, Quintans-Junior LJ, Guedes da Silva Almeida JR, Grougnet R, Picot L. Polymethoxyflavones from Gardenia oudiepe (Rubiaceae) induce

cytoskeleton disruption-mediated apoptosis and sensitize BRAF-mutated melanoma cells to chemotherapy. *Chem Biol Interact* 2020; 325: 109109.

[87] Kim JH, Song M, Kang GH, Lee ER, Choi HY, Lee C, Kim JH, Kim Y, Koo BN, Cho SG. Combined treatment of 3-hydroxyflavone and imatinib mesylate increases apoptotic cell death of imatinib mesylate-resistant leukemia cells. *Leuk Res* 2012; 36: 1157-64.

[88] Wang Z, Wang L, Xia MM, Sun W, Huang CK, Cui X, Hu GX, Lian QQ, Wang ZS. Pharmacokinetics interaction between imatinib and genistein in rats. *Biomed Res Int* 2015; 2015: 368976.

[89] Iwasaki R, Ito K, Ishida T, Hamanoue M, Adachi S, Watanabe T, Sato Y. Catechin, green tea component, causes caspase-independent necrosis-like cell death in chronic myelogenous leukemia. *Cancer Sci* 2009; 100: 349-56.

[90] Yen JH, Lin CY, Chuang CH, Chin HK, Wu MJ, Chen PY. Nobiletin promotes megakaryocytic differentiation through the MAPK/ERK-dependent EGR1 expression and exerts anti-leukemic effects in human chronic myeloid leukemia (CML) K562 cells. *Cells* 2020; 9: 877.

[91] Tolomeo M, Grimaudo S, Di Cristina A, Pipitone RM, Dusonchet L, Meli M, Crosta L, Gebbia N, Invidiata FP, Titone L, Simoni D. Galangin increases the cytotoxic activity of imatinib mesylate in imatinib-sensitive and imatinib-resistant Bcr-Abl expressing leukemia cells. *Cancer Lett* 2008; 265: 289-97.

[92] Lust S, Vanhoecke B, Van Gele M, Philippe J, Bracke M, Offner F. The flavonoid tangeretin activates the unfolded protein response and synergizes with imatinib in the erythroleukemia cell line K562. *Mol Nutr Food Res* 2010; 54: 823-32.

[93] Li X, Miao H, Zhang Y, Li W, Li Z, Zhou Y, Zhao L, Guo Q. Bone marrow microenvironment confers imatinib resistance to chronic myelogenous leukemia and oroxylin A reverses the resistance by suppressing Stat3 pathway. *Arch Toxicol* 2015; 89: 121-36.

[94] Yu C, Krystal G, Dent P, Grant S. Flavopiridol potentiates STI571-induced mitochondrial damage and apoptosis in BCR-ABL-positive human leukemia cells. *Clin Cancer Res* 2002; 8: 2976-84.

[95] Wang L, Wang Z, Xia MM, Wang YY, Wang HY, Hu GX. Inhibitory effect of silybin on pharmacokinetics of imatinib in vivo and in vitro. *Can J Physiol Pharmacol* 2014; 92: 961-4.

[96] Liu XY, Xu T, Li WS, Luo J, Geng PW, Wang L, Xia MM, Chen MC, Yu L, Hu GX. The effect of apigenin on pharmacokinetics of imatinib and its metabolite N-desmethyl imatinib in rats. *Biomed Res Int* 2013; 2013: 789184.

[97] Bose P, Perkins EB, Honeycut C, Wellons MD, Stefan T, Jacobberger JW, Kontopodis E, Beumer JH, Egorin MJ, Imamura CK, Douglas Figg W Sr, Karp JE, Koc ON, Cooper BW, Luger SM, Colevas AD, Roberts JD, Grant S. Phase I trial of the combination of flavopiridol and imatinib mesylate in patients with Bcr-Abl+ hematological malignancies. *Cancer Chemother Pharmacol* 2012; 69: 1657-67.

[98] Dai Y, Rahmani M, Pei XY, Dent P, Grant S. Bortezomib and flavopiridol interact synergistically to induce apoptosis in chronic myeloid leukemia cells resistant to imatinib mesylate through both Bcr/Abl-dependent and -independent mechanisms. *Blood* 2004; 104: 509-18.

[99] Li W, Ding Q, Ding Y, Lu L, Wang X, Zhang Y, Zhang X, Guo Q, Zhao L. Oroxylin A reverses the drug resistance of chronic myelogenous leukemia cells to imatinib through CXCL12/CXCR7 axis in bone marrow microenvironment. *Mol Carcinog* 2017; 56: 863-76.

[100] Danisman Kalindemirtas F, Birman H, Candöken E, Bilgis Gazioglu S, Melikoglu G, Kuruca S. Cytotoxic effects of some flavonoids and imatinib on the K562 chronic myeloid leukemia cell line: Data analysis using the combination index method. *Balkan Med J* 2019; 36: 96-105.

[101] Xu X, Zhang X, Liu Y, Yang L, Huang S, Lu L, Wang S, Guo Q, Zhao L. BM microenvironmental protection of CML cells from imatinib through Stat5/NF-κB signaling and reversal by Wogonin. *Oncotarget* 2016; 7: 24436-54.

[102] Goker B, Caliskan C, Onur Caglar H, Kayabasi C, Balci T, Erbaykent Tepedelen B, Aygunes D, Yilmaz Susluer S, Mutlu Z, Selvi Gunel N, Korkmaz M, Saydam G, Gunduz C, Biray Avci C. Synergistic effect of ponatinib and epigallocatechin-3-gallate induces apoptosis in chronic myeloid leukemia cells through altering expressions of cell cycle regulatory genes. *J BUON* 2014; 19: 992-8.

[103] Liu J, Liu H, Zeng Q. The effect of naringenin on the pharmacokinetics of ibrutinib in rat: A drug-drug interaction study. *Biomed Chromatogr* 2019; 33: e4507.

[104] Jia L, Liu FT. Why bortezomib cannot go with 'green'? *Cancer Biol Med* 2013; 10: 206-13.

[105] Glynn SJ, Gaffney KJ, Sainz MA, Louie SG, Petasis NA. Molecular characterization of the boron adducts of the proteasome inhibitor bortezomib with epigallocatechin-3-gallate and related polyphenols. *Org Biomol Chem* 2015; 13: 3887-99.

[106] Holkova B, Kmieciak M, Perkins EB, Bose P, Baz RC, Roodman GD, Stuart RK, Ramakrishnan V, Wan W, Peer CJ, Dawson J, Kang L, Honeycutt C, Tombes MB, Shrader E, Weir-Wiggins C, Wellons M,

Sankala H, Hogan KT, Colevas AD, Doyle LA, Figg WD, Coppola D, Roberts JD, Sullivan D, Grant S. Phase I trial of bortezomib (PS-341; NSC 681239) and "nonhybrid" (bolus) infusion schedule of alvocidib (flavopiridol; NSC 649890) in patients with recurrent or refractory indolent B-cell neoplasms. *Clin Cancer Res* 2014; 20: 5652-62.

[107] Bannerman B, Xu L, Jones M, Tsu C, Yu J, Hales P, Monbaliu J, Fleming P, Dick L, Manfredi M, Claiborne C, Bolen J, Kupperman E, Berger A. Preclinical evaluation of the antitumor activity of bortezomib in combination with vitamin C or with epigallocatechin gallate, a component of green tea. *Cancer Chemother Pharmacol* 2011; 68: 1145-54.

[108] Pamu S, Chen D, Morin F, Huo C, Cui Q, Dou QP, Chan TH. Inhibitory effect of bortezomib on human multiple myeloma cells when combined with epigallocatechin-gallate (EGCG) analogs. *Med Chem Commun* 2012: 3: 229-32.

[109] Golden EB, Lam PY, Kardosh A, Gaffney KJ, Cadenas E, Louie SG, Petasis NA, Chen TC, Schönthal AH. Green tea polyphenols block the anticancer effects of bortezomib and other boronic acid-based proteasome inhibitors. *Blood* 2009; 113: 5927-37.

[110] Modernelli A, Naponelli V, Giovanna Troglio M, Bonacini M, Ramazzina I, Bettuzzi S, Rizzi F. EGCG antagonizes Bortezomib cytotoxicity in prostate cancer cells by an autophagic mechanism. *Sci Rep* 2015; 5: 15270.

[111] Wang Q, Li J, Gu J, Huang B, Zhao Y, Zheng D, Ding Y, Zeng L. Potentiation of (-)-epigallocatechin-3-gallate-induced apoptosis by bortezomib in multiple myeloma cells. *Acta Biochim Biophys Sin* 2009; 41: 1018-26.

[112] Kim TY, Park J, Oh B, Min HJ, Jeong TS, Lee JH, Suh C, Cheong JW, Kim HJ, Yoon SS, Park SB, Lee DS, Korean Multiple Myeloma Working Party (KMMWP). Natural polyphenols antagonize the antimyeloma activity of proteasome inhibitor bortezomib by direct chemical interaction. *Br J Haematol* 2009; 146: 270-81.

[113] Martin S, Lamb HK, Brady C, Lefkove B, Bonner MY, Thompson P, Lovat PE, Arbiser JL, Hawkins AR, Redfern CP. Inducing apoptosis of cancer cells using small-molecule plant compounds that bind to GRP78. *Br J Cancer* 2013; 109: 433-43.

[114] Liu FT, Agrawal SG, Movasaghi Z, Wyatt PB, Rehman IU, Gribben JG, Newland AC, Jia L. Dietary flavonoids inhibit the anticancer effects of the proteasome inhibitor bortezomib. *Blood* 2008; 112: 3835-46.

[115] Li L, Zheng Y, Zhang W, Hou L, Gao Y. Scutellarin circumvents chemoresistance, promotes apoptosis, and represses tumor growth by

HDAC/miR-34a-mediated down-modulation of Akt/mTOR and NF-κB-orchestrated signaling pathways in multiple myeloma. *Int J Clin Exp Pathol* 2020; 13: 212-9.

[116] Yang MH, Jung SH, Chinnathambi A, Alahmadi TA, Alharbi SA, Sethi G, Ahn KS. Attenuation of STAT3 signaling cascade by daidzin can enhance the apoptotic potential of bortezomib against multiple myeloma. *Biomolecules* 2020; 10: 23.

[117] Kim C, Lee JH, Ko JH, Chinnathambi A, Alharbi SA, Shair OHM, Sethi G, Ahn KS. Formononetin regulates multiple oncogenic signaling cascades and enhances sensitivity to bortezomib in a multiple myeloma mouse model. *Biomolecules* 2019; 9: 262.

[118] Holkova B, Perkins EB, Ramakrishnan V, Tombes MB, Shrader E, Talreja N, Wellons MD, Hogan KT, Roodman GD, Coppola D, Kang L, Dawson J, Stuart RK, Peer C, Figg WD Sr, Kolla S, Doyle A, Wright J, Sullivan DM, Roberts JD, Grant S. Phase I trial of bortezomib (PS-341; NSC 681239) and alvocidib (flavopiridol; NSC 649890) in patients with recurrent or refractory B-cell neoplasms. *Clin Cancer Res* 2011; 17: 3388-97.

[119] Granato M, Rizzello C, Gilardini Montani MS, Cuomo L, Vitillo M, Santarelli R, Gonnella R, D`Orazi G, Faggioni A, Cirone M. Quercetin induces apoptosis and autophagy in primary effusion lymphoma cells by inhibiting PI3K/AKT/mTOR and STAT3 signaling pathways. *J Nutr Biochem* 2017; 41: 124-36.

[120] Gupta SC, Phromnoi K, Aggarwal BB. Morin inhibits STAT3 tyrosine 705 phosphorylation in tumor cells through activation of protein tyrosine phosphatase SHP1. *Biochem Pharmacol* 2013; 85: 898-912.

[121] Kim SH, Ahn KS, Jeong SJ, Kwon TR, Jung JH, Yun SM, Han I, Lee SG, Kim DK, Kang M, Chen CY, Lee JW, Kim SH. Janus activated kinase 2/signal transducer and activator of transcription 3 pathway mediates icariside II-induced apoptosis in U266 multiple myeloma cells. *Eur J Pharmacol* 2011; 654: 10-6.

[122] Phromnoi K, Prasad S, Gupta SC, Kannappan R, Reuter S, Limtrakul P, Aggarwal BB. Dihydroxypentamethoxyflavone down-regulates constitutive and inducible signal transducers and activators of transcription-3 through the induction of tyrosine phosphatase SHP-1. *Mol Pharmacol* 2011; 80: 889-99.

[123] Pandey MK, Sung B, Ahn KS, Aggarwal BB. Butein suppresses constitutive and inducible signal transducer and activator of transcription (STAT) 3 activation and STAT3-regulated gene products through the induction of a protein tyrosine phosphatase SHP-1. *Mol Pharmacol* 2009; 75: 525-33.

[124] Maddocks K, Wei L, Rozewski D, Jiang Y, Zhao Y, Adusumilli M, Pierceall WF, Doykin C, Cardone MH, Jones JA, Flynn J, Andritsos LA, Grever MR, Byrd JC, Johnson AJ, Phelps MA, Blum KA. Reduced occurrence of tumor flare with flavopiridol followed by combined flavopiridol and lenalidomide in patients with relapsed chronic lymphocytic leukemia (CLL). *Am J Hematol* 2015; 90: 327-33.

# Index

## W



## X